Renal Cell Cancer

Editors

BRADLEY A. MCGREGOR
TONI K. CHOUEIRI

HEMATOLOGY/ONCOLOGY CLINICS OF NORTH AMERICA

www.hemonc.theclinics.com

Consulting Editors
GEORGE P. CANELLOS
EDWARD J. BENZ JR.

October 2023 • Volume 37 • Number 5

ELSEVIER

1600 John F. Kennedy Boulevard • Suite 1800 • Philadelphia, Pennsylvania, 19103-2899

http://www.theclinics.com

HEMATOLOGY/ONCOLOGY CLINICS OF NORTH AMERICA Volume 37, Number 5
October 2023 ISSN 0889-8588, ISBN 13: 978-0-323-93899-0

Editor: Stacy Eastman
Developmental Editor: Shivank Joshi

Hematology/Oncology Clinics (ISSN 0889-8588) is published bimonthly by Elsevier Inc., 360 Park Avenue South, New York, NY 10010-1710. Months of issue are February, April, June, August, October, and December. Business and Editorial Offices: 1600 John F. Kennedy Blvd., Ste. 1800, Philadelphia, PA 19103–2899. Customer Service Office: 3251 Riverport Lane, Maryland Heights, MO 63043. Periodicals postage paid at New York, NY and at additional mailing offices. Subscription prices are $470.00 per year (domestic individuals), $1190.00 per year (domestic institutions), $100.00 per year (domestic students/residents), $495.00 per year (Canadian individuals), $100.00 per year (Canadian students/residents), $1232.00 per year (Canadian institutions) $563.00 per year (international individuals), $1232.00 per year (international institutions), and $255.00 per year (international students/residents). International air speed delivery is included in all *Clinics* subscription prices. All prices are subject to change without notice. **POSTMASTER:** Send address changes to *Hematology/Oncology Clinics of North America*, Elsevier Health Sciences Division, Subscription Customer Service, 3251 Riverport Lane, Maryland Heights, MO 63043. Customer Service (orders, claims, online, change of address): Elsevier Health Sciences Division, Subscription **Customer Service, 3251 Riverport Lane, Maryland Heights, MO 63043. Tel: 1-800-654-2452 (U.S. and Canada); 314-447-8871 (outside U.S. and Canada). Fax: 314-447-8029. E-mail: journalscustomerservice-usa@elsevier.com (for print support); journalsonlinesupport-usa@elsevier.com (for online support).**

Reprints. For copies of 100 or more, of articles in this publication, please contact the Commercial Reprints Department, Elsevier Inc., 360 Park Avenue South, New York, New York 10010-1710; Tel.: 212-633-3874, Fax: 212-633-3820, E-mail: reprints@elsevier.com.

Hematology/Oncology Clinics of North America is covered in *MEDLINE/PubMed (Index Medicus), EMBASE/Excerpta Medica, and BIOSIS.*

Contributors

CONSULTING EDITORS

GEORGE P. CANELLOS, MD
William Rosenberg Professor of Medicine, Department of Medical Oncology, Dana-Farber Cancer Institute, Boston, Massachusetts, USA

EDWARD J. BENZ Jr, MD
President and CEO Emeritus, Dana-Farber Cancer Institute, Director Emeritus, Dana-Farber/Harvard Cancer Center, Richard and Susan Smith Distinguished Professor of Medicine, Professor of Pediatrics, Professor of Genetics, Harvard Medical School, Boston, Massachusetts, USA

EDITORS

BRADLEY A. McGREGOR, MD
Director of Clinical Research, Lank Center for Genitourinary Oncology, Assistant Professor of Medicine, Harvard Medical School, Dana-Farber Cancer Institute, Boston, Massachusetts, USA

TONI K. CHOUEIRI, MD
Director, Lank Center for Genitourinary Oncology, Medical Director, International Strategic Initiatives, Department of Medical Oncology, Dana-Farber Cancer Institute, Co-Leader, Kidney Cancer Program, Dana-Farber/Harvard Cancer Center, Jerome and Nancy Kohlberg Professor of Medicine, Harvard Medical School, Boston, Massachusetts, USA

AUTHORS

ZIAD BAKOUNY, MD, MSc
Department of Medical Oncology, Dana-Farber Cancer Institute, Harvard Medical School, Department of Medicine, Brigham and Women's Hospital, Boston, Massachusetts, USA

REGINA BARRAGAN-CARRILLO, MD
Department of Medical Oncology and Therapeutics Research, City of Hope Comprehensive Cancer Center, Duarte, California, USA; Department of Hematology and Oncology, Instituto Nacional de Ciencias Médicas y Nutrición "Salvador Zubiran," Mexico City, Mexico

STEPHANIE A. BERG, DO
Instructor of Medicine, Department of Medical Oncology, Dana-Farber Cancer Institute, Boston, Massachusetts, USA

AXEL BEX, MD, PhD
Specialist Centre for Kidney Cancer, Royal Free London NHS Foundation Trust, Professor of Urology, Division of Surgery and Interventional Science, University College London,

London, United Kingdom; Department of Urology, The Netherlands Cancer Institute, Amsterdam, the Netherlands

DAVID A. BRAUN, MD, PhD
Center of Molecular and Cellular Oncology, Yale Cancer Center, Yale School of Medicine, New Haven, Connecticut, USA

MARIA I. CARLO, MD
Assistant Professor of Medicine, Weill Cornell Medical College, Assistant Attending, Genitourinary Oncology Service, Clinical Genetics Service, Memorial Sloan Kettering Cancer Center, New York, New York, USA

DANIEL S. CARSON, MD
Department of Urology, University of Washington, Seattle, Washington, USA

ABHISHEK A. CHAKRABORTY, PhD
Department of Cancer Biology, Lerner Research Institute, Cleveland Clinical, Case Comprehensive Cancer Center, Case Western Reserve University, Cleveland, Ohio, USA

STEVEN LEE CHANG, MD, MS
Division of Urological Surgery, Brigham and Women's Hospital, Harvard Medical School, Boston, Massachusetts, USA

TONI K. CHOUEIRI, MD
Director, Lank Center for Genitourinary Oncology, Medical Director, International Strategic Initiatives, Department of Medical Oncology, Dana-Farber Cancer Institute, Co-Leader, Kidney Cancer Program, Dana-Farber/Harvard Cancer Center, Jerome and Nancy Kohlberg Professor of Medicine, Harvard Medical School, Boston, Massachusetts, USA

MARC EID, MD, MSc
Department of Medical Oncology, Dana-Farber Cancer Institute, Boston, Massachusetts, USA

NOURHAN EL AHMAR, MD
Postdoctoral Research Fellow, Department of Pathology, Brigham and Women's Hospital, Harvard Medical School, Boston, Massachusetts, USA

MATTHEW S. ERNST, MD, FRCPC
Department of Oncology, Tom Baker Cancer Centre, University of Calgary, Calgary, Alberta, Canada

ANDREA FLATEN
Division of Hematology and Oncology, Department of Internal Medicine, UT Southwestern Medical Center, Harold C. Simmons Comprehensive Cancer Center, Dallas, Texas, USA

GIANNICOLA GENOVESE, MD, PhD
Department of Genitourinary Medical Oncology, David H. Koch Center for Applied Research of Genitourinary Cancers, Department of Genomic Medicine, TRACTION Platform, Division of Therapeutic Discoveries, The University of Texas MD Anderson Cancer Center, Houston, Texas, USA

FATME GHANDOUR, MD
Postdoctoral Research Fellow, Department of Pathology, Brigham and Women's Hospital, Harvard Medical School, Boston, Massachusetts, USA

AMEISH GOVINDARAJAN, MD
Department of Medical Oncology and Therapeutics Research, City of Hope
Comprehensive Cancer Center, Duarte, California, USA

ELSHAD HASANOV, MD, PhD
Medical Oncology Fellow, Division of Cancer Medicine, The University of Texas MD
Anderson Cancer Center, Houston, Texas, USA

DANIEL Y.C. HENG, MD, MPH, FRCPC
Department of Oncology, Tom Baker Cancer Centre, University of Calgary, Calgary,
Alberta, Canada

ERIC JONASCH, MD
Professor, Department of Genitourinary Medical Oncology, Division of Cancer Medicine,
The University of Texas MD Anderson Cancer Center, Houston, Texas, USA

WILLIAM G. KAELIN Jr, MD
Dana-Farber Cancer Institute, Brigham and Women's Hospital, Harvard Medical School,
Boston, Massachusetts, USA; Howard Hughes Medical Institute

KATHERINE M. KRAJEWSKI, MD
Staff Radiologist, Brigham and Women's Hospital, Assistant Professor of Radiology,
Harvard Medical School, Dana-Farber Cancer Institute, Boston, Massachusetts, USA

TEELE KUUSK, MD, PhD
Homerton University Hospital, Specialist Centre for Kidney Cancer, Royal Free London
NHS Foundation Trust, London, United Kingdom; Department of Urology, The
Netherlands Cancer Institute, Amsterdam, the Netherlands

CHRIS LABAKI, MD
Department of Medical Oncology, Dana-Farber Cancer Institute, Department of
Medicine, Beth Israel Deaconess Medical Center, Boston, Massachusetts, USA

YASMIN NABIL LAIMON, MD
Postdoctoral Research Fellow, Department of Pathology, Brigham and Women's
Hospital, Harvard Medical School, Boston, Massachusetts, USA

ALY-KHAN LALANI, MD, FRCPC
Juravinski Cancer Centre, McMaster University, Hamilton, Ontario, Canada

JONATHAN E. LEEMAN, MD
Department of Radiation Oncology, Dana-Farber Cancer Institute/Brigham and Women's
Hospital, Boston, Massachusetts, USA

AUDREYLIE LEMELIN, MD
Department of Oncology, Tom Baker Cancer Centre, University of Calgary, Calgary,
Alberta, Canada

CARMEL MALVAR, BS
University of California, San Diego, Moores Cancer Center, La Jolla, California, USA

SAYED MATAR, MD
Postdoctoral Research Fellow, Department of Pathology, Brigham and Women's
Hospital, Harvard Medical School, Boston, Massachusetts, USA

RANA R. McKAY, MD
University of California, San Diego, Moores Cancer Center, La Jolla, California, USA

PAVLOS MSAOUEL, MD, PhD
Department of Genitourinary Medical Oncology, Department of Translational Molecular Pathology, David H. Koch Center for Applied Research of Genitourinary Cancers, The University of Texas MD Anderson Cancer Center, Houston, Texas, USA

ELLEN NEIN, MD
Division of Hematology and Oncology, Department of Internal Medicine, UT Southwestern Medical Center, Dallas, Texas, USA

JOSÉ IGNACIO NOLAZCO, MD, MMSc
Servicio de Urología, Hospital Universitario Austral, Universidad Austral, Pilar, Argentina; Division of Urological Surgery, Brigham and Women's Hospital, Harvard Medical School, Boston, Massachusetts, USA

SUMANTA K. PAL, MD
Department of Medical Oncology and Therapeutics Research, City of Hope Comprehensive Cancer Center, Duarte, California, USA

ELIZABETH PAN, MD
University of California, San Diego, Moores Cancer Center, La Jolla, California, USA

SARAH P. PSUTKA, MD, MSc
Associate Professor, Department of Urology, University of Washington, Seattle Cancer Care Alliance, Harborview Medical Center, Seattle, Washington, USA

QIAN QIN, MD
Assistant Professor, Division of Hematology and Oncology, Department of Internal Medicine, UT Southwestern Medical Center, Dallas, Texas, USA; Harold C. Simmons Comprehensive Cancer Center

ADAM ROCK, MD
Department of Medical Oncology and Therapeutics Research, City of Hope Comprehensive Cancer Center, Duarte, California, USA

EDDY SAAD, MD, MSc
Department of Medical Oncology, Dana-Farber Cancer Institute, Boston, Massachusetts, USA

RENÉE MARIA SALIBY, MD, MSc
Department of Medical Oncology, Dana-Farber Cancer Institute, Boston, Massachusetts, USA; Center of Molecular and Cellular Oncology, Yale Cancer Center, Yale School of Medicine, New Haven, Connecticut, USA

KHOSCHY SCHAWKAT, MD, PhD
Fellow in Abdominal Imaging and Intervention, Brigham and Women's Hospital, Harvard Medical School, Boston, Massachusetts, USA

KARL SEMAAN, MD, MSc
Department of Medical Oncology, Dana-Farber Cancer Institute, Boston, Massachusetts, USA

MICHAEL T. SERZAN, MD
Instructor of Medicine, Department of Medical Oncology, Dana-Farber Cancer Institute, Boston, Massachusetts, USA

NITIN H. SHIROLE, PhD
Dana-Farber Cancer Institute, Boston, Massachusetts, USA

SABINA SIGNORETTI, MD
Professor, Department of Pathology, Brigham and Women's Hospital, Harvard Medical School, Department of Oncologic Pathology, Dana-Farber Cancer Institute, Boston, Massachusetts, USA; Broad Institute of MIT and Harvard, Cambridge, Massachusetts, USA

RUBENS C. SPERANDIO, MD
Centro de Oncologia e Hematologia Einstein Família Dayan-Daycoval, Hospital Israelita Albert Einstein, São Paulo, Brazil

KOSUKE TAKEMURA, MD, MPH, PhD
Department of Oncology, Tom Baker Cancer Centre, University of Calgary, Calgary, Alberta, Canada

NIZAR M. TANNIR, MD
Department of Genitourinary Medical Oncology, The University of Texas MD Anderson Cancer Center, Houston, Texas, USA

DANIELLE URMAN, BA
University of California, San Diego, Moores Cancer Center, La Jolla, California, USA

SRINIVAS R. VISWANATHAN, MD, PhD
Harvard Medical School, Department of Medical Oncology, Dana-Farber Cancer Institute, Boston, Massachusetts, USA

TOVA WEISS, MD
Department of Urology, University of Washington, Seattle, Washington, USA

WENXIN XU, MD
Instructor of Medicine, Department of Medical Oncology, Dana-Farber Cancer Institute, Harvard Medical School, Boston, Massachusetts, USA

LISA XINYUAN ZHANG, MD
Department of Urology, University of Washington, Seattle, Washington, USA

TIAN ZHANG, MD, MHS
Associate Professor, Division of Hematology and Oncology, Department of Internal Medicine, UT Southwestern Medical Center, Dallas, Texas, USA; Harold C. Simmons Comprehensive Cancer Center

Contents

The most common form of kidney cancer is clear cell renal cell carcinoma
(ccRCC). Biallelic VHL tumor suppressor gene inactivation is the usual initiating event in both hereditary (VHL Disease) and sporadic ccRCCs. The
VHL protein, pVHL, earmarks the alpha subunits of the HIF transcription
factor for destruction in an oxygen-dependent manner. Deregulation of
HIF2 drives ccRCC pathogenesis. Drugs inhibiting the HIF2-responsive
growth factor VEGF are now mainstays of ccRCC treatment. A first-in-
class allosteric HIF2 inhibitor was recently approved for treating VHL Disease-associated neoplasms and appears active against sporadic ccRCC
in early clinical trials.

The treatment of advanced renal cell carcinoma (RCC) has changed dramatically with immune checkpoint inhibitors, yet most patients do not
have durable responses. There is consequently a tremendous need for
novel therapeutic development. RCC, and particularly the most common
histology clear cell RCC, is an immunobiologically and metabolically distinct tumor. An improved understanding of RCC-specific biology will be
necessary for the successful identification of new treatment targets for
this disease. In this review, we discuss the current understanding of
RCC immune pathways and metabolic dysregulation, with a focus on
topics important for future clinical development.

Up to 5% of renal cell carcinomas (RCCs) can be associated with a known
hereditary RCC syndrome. In addition to the well-characterized RCC syndromes, there are also emerging syndromes associated with increased
RCC risk. In the last few years, consensus guidelines have outlined recommendations for who should be referred for genetic evaluation, and what
screening should be done for early detection of RCC. Although much progress has been made, work is still needed—guidelines are still mostly
based on expert opinion and the role of emerging genetic associations
will need to be clarified.

therapy and surgery should be made through a multidisciplinary approach tailored to each individual patient.

In locally advanced renal cell carcinoma (RCC), 6 phase 3 randomized controlled trials (RCTs) were designed in the perioperative setting with immune checkpoint inhibitor (ICI) monotherapy or combinations. Adjuvant trials with atezolizumab, pembrolizumab, and nivolumab with ipilimumab reported results, as did the only perioperative trial with nivolumab. Of these, only 1 year of adjuvant pembrolizumab improved disease-free survival (DFS) versus placebo, with the other trials showing no improvement in DFS. In the purely neoadjuvant setting, phase 1 b/2 ICI trials have demonstrated safety, efficacy, and dynamic changes of immune infiltrates, and provide a rationale for randomized trial concepts.

Initial studies of radiotherapy in renal cell carcinoma (RCC) failed to demonstrate significant clinical impact. With the advent of stereotactic body radiotherapy (SBRT) that allows for delivery of more effective radiation doses in a precise fashion, radiotherapy has become an essential component in the multidisciplinary management of patients with RCC both in the setting of localized and metastatic disease beyond the traditional role of palliative treatment. Recent evidence has demonstrated high rates of long-term local control ($\sim$95%) when SBRT is delivered to kidney tumors with limited toxicity risks and only minor impact on renal function.

As many new systemic therapy options have recently emerged, the standard of care for patients with metastatic renal cell carcinoma (mRCC) is gradually changing. The increasing complexity of treatment options requires more personalized treatment strategies. This evolution in the systemic therapy landscape comes with a need for validated stratification models that facilitate decision making and patient counseling for clinicians through a risk-adapted approach. This article summarizes the available evidence on risk stratification and prognostic models for mRCC, including the International mRCC Database Consortium and Memorial Sloan Kettering Cancer Center models, as well as their association with clinical outcomes.

Patients with metastatic clear cell renal cell carcinoma (mccRCC) experience highly heterogeneous outcomes when treated with standard-of-care systemic regimens. Therefore, valid biomarkers are needed to predict the clinical response to these therapies and help guide management. In this review, the authors outline relevant and promising biomarkers for patients with mccRCC receiving systemic therapies, with a focus on immunotherapy-based regimens.

Defining metastatic renal-cell carcinoma as a favorable risk depends on clinical risk-stratification tools such as the International Metastatic Renal Cell Carcinoma Database Consortium or the Memorial Sloan-Kettering Cancer Center scores. The favorable-risk disease tends to have better prognosis and survival compared with disease stratified as either intermediate or poor risk and can be attributed in part to an indolent tumor biology. Several phase 3 clinical trials have demonstrated an improvement in progression-free survival and objective response rate, but not overall survival benefit with combinations of immunotherapy and vascular endothelial growth factor tyrosine kinase inhibitors compared with sunitinib in favorable-risk disease.

Combination therapies with immune checkpoint blockers have shown improvements in overall response rate, progression free survival, and overall survival over monotherapy with sunitinib in intermediate and poor risk subgroups. Identification of best upfront therapy may be guided by future clinical trials utilizing adaptive strategies, triplet therapy, or novel biomarkers.

Treatment of metastatic renal cell carcinoma (mRCC) after first-line immune checkpoint inhibitors (ICIs) lacks standardization, with limited evidence from small trials and retrospective data. Vascular endothelial growth factor receptor (VEGFR) inhibition through tyrosine kinase inhibitors (TKIs) is the most widely adopted second-line treatment. Encouraging results have been seen with VEGFR-TKIs in the second-line after exposure to an ICI-based combination, achieving a response rate of 30%, and 75% of patients achieving disease control. Rechallenge with ICI alone seems safe but has limited clinical benefit. Promising regimens with combination therapies and novel drugs are being evaluated in phase 3 trials.

The term variant histology renal cell carcinomas (vhRCCs), also known as non-clear cell RCCs, refers to a diverse group of malignancies with distinct biologic and therapeutic considerations. The management of vhRCC subtypes is often based on extrapolating results from the more common clear cell RCC studies or basket trials that are not specific to each histology. The unique management of each vhRCC subtype necessitates accurate pathologic diagnosis and dedicated research efforts. Herein, we discuss tailored recommendations for each vhRCC histology informed by ongoing research and clinical experience.

Systemic treatments for metastatic renal cell carcinoma have expanded to include antiangiogenic agents targeting either vascular endothelial growth factor receptor, immune checkpoint inhibitors against cytotoxic T-lymphocyte antigen 4, or programmed cell death 1 pathways, and combinations of these treatments. The hypoxia inducible factor-2 inhibitors are emerging, whereas mammalian target of rapamycin (inhibitors) role is fading. To sustain optimal efficacy of these agents, potential toxicities must be recognized early and clinically managed. Here, the authors discuss the adverse events attributable to these treatments and management strategies.

The development of brain metastases is a poor prognostic indicator in renal cell carcinoma. Regular imaging and clinical examinations are necessary to monitor the brain before or during systemic therapy. Central nervous system-targeted radiation therapy, including stereotactic radiosurgery, whole-brain radiation therapy, and surgical resection, is a standard treatment option. Clinical trials are currently investigating the role of targeted therapy and immune checkpoint inhibitor combinations in treating brain metastases and decreasing intracranial disease progression.

Targeted therapies have revolutionized the treatment of renal cell carcinoma (RCC). The VHL/HIF pathway is responsible for the regulation of oxygen homeostasis and is frequently altered in RCC. Targeting this pathway as well as the mTOR pathway have yielded remarkable advances in the treatment of RCC. Here, we review the most promising novel targeted therapies for the treatment of RCC, including HIF2α, MET, metabolic targeting, and epigenomic reprogramming.

Immunotherapy has revolutionized treatment for patients with advanced and metastatic renal cell carcinoma. Nevertheless, many patients do not benefit or eventually relapse, highlighting the need for novel immune targets to overcome primary and acquired resistance. This review discusses 2 strategies currently being investigated: disabling inhibitory stimuli that maintain immunosuppression ("brakes") and priming the immune system to target tumoral cells ("gas pedals"). We explore each class of novel immunotherapy, including the rationale behind it, supporting preclinical and clinical evidence, and limitations.

HEMATOLOGY/ONCOLOGY CLINICS OF NORTH AMERICA

THE CLINICS ARE AVAILABLE ONLINE!
Access your subscription at:
www.theclinics.com

Preface

Renal Cell Cancer

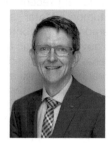 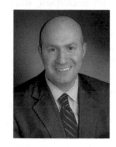

Bradley A. McGregor, MD   Toni K. Choueiri, MD

Editors

Since the last renal cell carcinoma (RCC) issue of *Hematology/Oncology Clinics of North America* in 2011, the management of this disease has changed dramatically with more than 10 different approvals by the Food and Drug Administration for this indication across treatment settings. New options now exist for some hereditary syndromes; adjuvant therapy, and most importantly, combination therapies are now the standard for front line, with new options available for patients with metastatic disease. At the time of this writing, several other new therapies are on the horizon. In this new issue, we worked with internationally recognized thought leaders in the field to provide a comprehensive and up-to-date review of current management of RCC and future directions.

The approach to molecular therapy in RCC continues to evolve, moving beyond targeting vascular endothelial growth factor (VEGF) and mammalian target of rapamycin to direct inhibition of the transcription factor hypoxia-inducible factor 2 alpha (Kaelin and Shirole [Kaelin was the 2019 Nobel Prize Laureate in Physiology or Medicine]). With better understanding of the tumor/immune microenvironment and metabolism of RCC (Braun and Chakraborty), the use of dual immune checkpoint inhibitors (ICI) and ICI combinations with VEGF inhibitors has transformed therapy in the metastatic setting. In fact, median survival with combination therapies has surpassed 4 years across risk groups. Choosing the most suitable therapy remains critical: clinical prognostic classification systems (Lemelin and colleagues) are currently used for choosing the right treatment for a patient presenting with metastatic disease, with degree of benefit for different combinations varying between those with favorable risk (Pan and colleagues) or intermediate-/poor-risk (Serzan and colleagues) disease. Work is ongoing to develop molecular biomarkers (Saliby and colleagues) in both the metastatic and the localized settings to better predict what therapy (if any) should be used by each patient.

Hematol Oncol Clin N Am 37 (2023) xvii–xix
https://doi.org/10.1016/j.hoc.2023.05.019
0889-8588/23/© 2023 Published by Elsevier Inc.

hemonc.theclinics.com

Beyond the role of a medical oncologist, involvement of a multidisciplinary team is critical to optimally manage RCC outside of the traditional tandem of the urologic and medical oncologists. Early recognition of genetic syndromes and consultation with a genetic counselor when appropriate can help minimize long-term treatment-related morbidities (Carlo). To that end, close collaboration with pathology colleagues is critical to properly diagnose RCC histologic subtypes, especially following recent updates to World Health Organization classification of renal tumors (Matar and colleagues), which may provide additional insight into certain hereditary syndromes. Small renal masses are no longer managed by urology alone, as novel radiologic assessments and PET tracers can help characterize indeterminate renal masses to aid in assessing the benefit-to-risk ratio of an active surveillance approach (Krajewski and Schawkat, Psutka and colleagues). When imaging or pathology is consistent with RCC, surgical management of localized disease can preserve renal function without compromising long-term outcomes (Psutka and colleagues). Most importantly, high-risk patients now have an option to reduce risk of recurrence with the first approved adjuvant ICI (Bex and Kuusk) as the role of perioperative systemic therapy continues to evolve. Even in the metastatic setting, while cytoreductive nephrectomy is no longer the de facto standard of care, surgery continues to play a pivotal role (Chang and Nolazco). At the same time, modern radiation techniques have refuted the long-held belief that RCC is a radioresistant tumor (Leeman).

Ultimately, many challenges must still be addressed in the ever-changing management of RCC. One such challenge is the management of RCC with variant histologies (Msaouel and colleagues). More basic questions include how to best sequence therapies in the treatment-refractory setting (Pal and colleagues) and how to select therapy for those patients with central nervous system metastases (Jonasch and Hasanov). As combination therapies intensify, managing the toxicities associated with VEGF and ICI as well as their overlapping toxicities is critical to maximizing therapeutic benefit (Zhang and colleagues). Despite improvements in the standard of care, many patients will progress through all available treatment options, and novel therapies will therefore be critical to build upon advances made in the past 12 years. Efforts in advancing both targeted therapy and immunotherapy are ongoing (Saliby and colleagues).

Thank you for your interest in this topic. I hope you enjoy these expert summaries and perspectives, and are, like us, proud of what the field has accomplished in improving the outlook for this disease and achieving more cures. These are our priorities for our patients and their caregivers. The best is yet to come—Onward!

ACKNOWLEDGMENTS

We would like to thank Kevin Pels, PhD from the Lank Center for Genitourinary Oncology at Dana Farber Cancer Institute for editorial assistance. This book is dedicated to our families, our patients and our colleagues at the Lank Center who make every day possible!

Bradley A. McGregor, MD
Lank Center for Genitourinary Oncology
Dana Farber Cancer Institute
Boston, MA 02215, USA

Toni K. Choueiri, MD
Lank Center for Genitourinary Oncology
Dana Farber Cancer Institute
Boston, MA 02215, USA

E-mail addresses:
bradley_mcgregor@dfci.harvard.edu (B.A. McGregor)
Toni_Choueiri@dfci.harvard.edu (T.K. Choueiri)

von-Hippel Lindau and Hypoxia-Inducible Factor at the Center of Renal Cell Carcinoma Biology

Nitin H. Shirole, PhD[a], William G. Kaelin Jr, MD[a,b,c],*

KEYWORDS

- Hypoxia-inducible factor • Kidney cancer • Renal cell carcinoma
- von Hippel-Lindau disease • Belzutifan

KIDNEY CANCER

Kidney cancer is one of the 10 most common cancers in the developed world and is increasing in incidence. In 2020 there were more than 400,000 new cases of kidney cancer and almost 179,368 deaths from this disease worldwide.[1] In the United States it is estimated that there will be 81,800 new cases of kidney cancer and 14,890 deaths in 2023.[2] Risk factors for kidney cancer include older age, tobacco use, obesity, hypertension, certain chronic kidney diseases, certain industrial exposures, and a positive family history of kidney cancer.[3]

Several subtypes of kidney cancer are well recognized based on their histological appearances and characteristic molecular changes, including clear cell renal cell carcinoma (ccRCC), papillary renal cell carcinoma, chromophobe renal cell carcinoma, collecting duct tumors, and oncocytoma.[4–7] ccRCC is by far the most common form of kidney cancer, followed by papillary renal cell carcinoma.[8,9] Our understanding of the molecular pathogenesis of these kidney cancers has been aided immeasurably by the study of rare families that are at high risk of kidney cancer by virtue of germline genetic variants.[10–13] ccRCC is a prominent feature of von Hippel-Lindau (VHL) disease, described later. Families with germline loss-of-function fumarate hydratase mutations are at increased risk of papillary RCC and smooth muscle tumors (leiomyomas) of the uterus and skin.[14–16] Familial papillary RCC has also been linked to germline gain-of-function *MET* mutations.[17] Individuals with Birt-Hogg-Dube disease, which is caused by germline loss-of-function *FLCN* mutations,[18] are at increased risk primarily of oncocytomas and chromophobe tumors but can also develop ccRCC and papillary RCC.[19] Patients with Birt-Hogg-Dube disease are also

[a] Dana-Farber Cancer Institute, 450 Brookline Avenue, Boston, MA 02215, USA; [b] Brigham and Women's Hospital, Harvard Medical School; [c] Howard Hughes Medical Institute
* Corresponding author. Dana-Farber Cancer Institute, M457, 450 Brookline Avenue, Boston, MA 02215.
E-mail address: William_Kaelin@dfci.harvard.edu

Hematol Oncol Clin N Am 37 (2023) 809–825
https://doi.org/10.1016/j.hoc.2023.04.011
0889-8588/23/© 2023 Elsevier Inc. All rights reserved.

at increased risk for a variety of benign skin tumors including fibrofolliculomas, trichodiscomas, perifollicular fibromas, and acrochordons[20,21] (**Table 1**). *BAP1* is mutated in the germline of some individuals with familial mesothelioma.[22] *BAP1* mutation carriers are also at increased risk of several other tumors, including ccRCC.[23,24] Lastly, a frameshift mutation in *PBRM1* was reported in a family with unexplained history of ccRCC.[25]

VON HIPPEL-LINDAU DISEASE

Individuals with germline (or, less commonly, mosaic) loss-of-function mutations of the *VHL* tumor suppressor gene are at increased risk of developing a variety of tumors including ccRCC, blood vessel tumors called hemangioblastomas of the eye, brain, and spinal cord; paragangliomas; pancreatic neuroendocrine tumors; endolymphatic sac tumors; and epididymal and broad ligament cystadenomas.[26–28] Intraadrenal paragangliomas are referred to as pheochromocytomas. Tumor development in this setting is due to mutational inactivation, loss, or silencing of the remaining wild-type *VHL* allele in a susceptible cell.[29–32]

There are reproducible genotype-phenotype correlations in VHL Disease. Some *VHL* alleles result in a low risk of paraganglioma (type 1 VHL disease) and others high risk of paraganglioma (type 2 VHL disease).[33,34] Type 2 VHL disease alleles are subdivided into those associated with the usual stigmata of VHL disease, but with a low risk of ccRCC (type 2A disease); those associated with the classical stigmata of VHL disease, including a high risk of ccRCC (type 2B disease); and those causing familial paraganglioma without the usual stigmata of VHL disease (type 2C disease). In particular, ccRCC is observed in type 1 VHL disease and type 2B VHL disease but is not a feature of type 2A and 2C disease[28] (**Table 2**). Patients with VHL disease can develop hundreds of renal cysts, which are believed to be precancerous, in addition

Table 1				
Hereditary renal cancer syndromes				
Hereditary Renal Cancer Syndromes	**Altered Gene**	**Affected Protein**	**Renal Cancers**	**Other Tumors and Clinical Features**
Birt-Hogg-Dube syndrome	*FLCN*	Folliculin	Oncocytic, chromophobe, ccRCC, pRCC	Fibrofolliculomas with trichodiscomas and acrochordons, perifollicular fibromas, lung cysts with or without pneumothorax
Hereditary leiomyomatosis and renal cell cancer (HLRCC)	*FH*	Fumarate hydratase	pRCC	Cutaneous and uterine leiomyomas
Hereditary papillary renal cell carcinoma (HPRCC)	*MET*	c-Met	pRCC	NA
von Hippel-Lindau (VHL) disease	*VHL*	pVHL	ccRCC	Hemangioblastomas, paragangliomas, pancreatic neuroendocrine tumors, renal and pancreatic cysts

Table 2
Types of von Hippel-Lindau disease, effect on hypoxia-inducible factor stability, and the associated tumors

Types of VHL Disease	VHL Mutations	Amount of HIF	ccRCC	Hemangioblastoma	Paraganglioma
Type 1	Deletion, missense, nonsense	High	+	+	−
Type 2A	Missense	Modest	−	+	+
Type 2B	Missense	Intermediate	+	+	+
Type 2C	Missense	Minimal	−	−	+

to ccRCCs.[35] ccRCC in VHL disease can be multifocal and bilateral, consistent with germline *VHL* mutations causing a field defect.

VON HIPPEL-LINDAU AND SPORADIC CLEAR CELL RENAL CELL CARCINOMA

As expected from the knowledge that germline *VHL* mutations predispose to ccRCC, biallelic *VHL* inactivation is the initiating or "truncal" event in most sporadic ccRCCs.[36–39] The prevalence of *VHL* mutations in sporadic ccRCC varies from 40% to greater than 80%.[8,32,40–42] These differences likely reflect differences in the histological criteria used to diagnose ccRCC, with a higher percentage of *VHL* mutations found in ccRCCs with pure, rather than mixed, ccRCC histology, and differences in the DNA sequencing technologies used and sample preparation methods. For example, the percentage of *VHL* mutation in ccRCC seems higher when using modern sequencing technologies that are less likely to be confounded by wild-type DNA contributed by contaminating host cells. Biallelic *VHL* inactivation in ccRCC is usually the result of an intragenic *VHL* mutation followed by loss of a large segment of chromosome 3p that includes the *VHL* gene at chromosome 3p25. Some ccRCC without *VHL* mutations have transcriptionally silenced both *VHL* alleles by hypermethylation.[32,43] Importantly, almost all classic ccRCCs have a molecular signature consistent with *VHL* inactivation (see later discussion).[44]

COOPERATING MUTATIONS

Inactivation of the *VHL* tumor suppressor gene, although the usual initiating event in ccRCC, is not sufficient to cause ccRCC.[45–47] In that sense *VHL* seems to be a "gatekeeper" in ccRCC, analogous to other cancer gatekeepers such as *APC* in colorectal cancer. Stereotypical cooperating mutations in both VHL disease–associated and sporadic ccRCCs include chromosomal arm level copy number changes and intragenic mutations. The former typically consists of low-level amplification of chromosome 5q and loss of chromosome 3p and 14q.[44] Intragenic mutation in ccRCC include loss-of-function mutations of *PBRM1* or *BAP1*, loss-of-function *SETD2* mutations, intragenic mutations that activate mammalian target of rapamycin (mTOR) signaling (such as *PTEN* or *TSC1* mutations), and intragenic mutations that alter the response to DNA damage such as *ATM1* mutations.[8,48–52] *PBRM1* encodes BAF180, which is a component of the PBAF chromatin remodeling complex, *BAP1* encodes a ubiquitin hydrolase, and *SETD2* encodes a histone methyltransferase, all of which are implicated in regulation of the epigenome. Importantly, all 3 of these genes are located on chromosome 3p. Therefore, loss of chromosome 3p can serve as the second hit for multiple ccRCC suppressor genes in addition to VHL.[43]

THE VON HIPPEL-LINDAU TUMOR SUPPRESSOR PROTEIN

The *VHL* gene is expressed in all human cells examined to date and is highly conserved throughout evolution. The *VHL* messenger RNA encodes at least 2 protein isoforms by virtue of 2 alternative in-frame translational initiation codons.[28] For simplicity we refer to both here as "pVHL," as they behave similarly in most biochemical and biologically assays performed to date. pVHL is primarily a cytosolic protein but can also dynamically shuttle to and from the nucleus.[28] Some pVHL can also be found associated with the endoplasmic reticulum and mitochondria.[28]

pVHL forms a stable complex with several other proteins including Elongin B, Elongin C, Cullin-2, and Rbx1.[53–57] This complex functions as an E3 ubiquitin ligase that covalently attaches a polypeptide called polyubiquitin to substrate proteins.[58–62] The polyubiquitylated protein is then destroyed by the proteasome. Missense mutations identified in VHL disease families cluster in 1 of 2 areas of the pVHL protein. One cluster defines the alpha domain, which is necessary and sufficient for recruitment of the Elongins, Cullin-2, and Rbx1.[53,57,63] The other cluster defines the beta domain, which has served as the substrate docking site for the best documented pVHL substrate—the alpha subunits of the heterodimeric transcription factor called hypoxia-inducible factor (HIF).[62,63]

THE HYPOXIA-INDUCIBLE FACTOR TRANSCRIPTION FACTOR

HIF is a master regulator of genes that promote adaptation to low oxygen (hypoxia). It consists of a normally unstable alpha subunit and a constitutively stable beta subunit. HIF is actually a generic term because humans have 3 *HIFα* genes (*HIF1α, HIF2α, HIF3α*) and 2 *HIFβ* genes.[64] The latter are usually referred to by the alternative names of aryl hydrocarbon receptor nuclear translocator genes (ARNT and ARNT2). As their names suggest, ARNT and ARNT2 can form dimers with other nuclear proteins in addition to HIFα. The canonical, best studied, "HIF" consists of HIF1α and ARNT.

Both the HIFαs and ARNTs are basic helix–loop–helix *Per*-aryl hydrocarbon receptor nuclear translocator (*ARNT*)-Sim (bHLH-*PAS*) domain proteins.[64,65] Their bHLH and PAS domains mediate DNA-binding and heterodimerization, respectively. Both HIF1α and HIF2α contain 2 transactivation domains, called the N-terminal transactivation domain and C-terminal transactivation domain, that enable them to drive transcription once bound to DNA elements called hypoxia response elements (HREs)[66,67] (**Fig. 1**). HIF1α is ubiquitously expressed, whereas HIF2α expression is

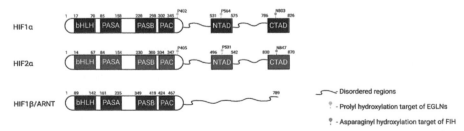

Fig. 1. HIF1α, HIF2α, and HIF1β/ARNT. bHLH, basic helix loop helix domain; C-TAD, C terminal transactivation domain; N-TAD, N terminal transactivation domain; PAC, PAS associated C-terminal motif; PAS, per-arnt-sim domain. (Created with BioRender.com.)

much more restricted to specific cell types. HIF3α undergoes extensive splicing such that many of its protein products lack a transactivation domain and hence cannot activate transcription.

When oxygen is plentiful HIF1α and HIF2α are recognized by the pVHL ubiquitin ligase complex, which earmarks them for proteasomal degradation. When oxygen levels are low, or when pVHL is defective, HIF1α and HIF2α accumulate and dimerize with an ARNT, which allows them to bind to HREs and activate transcription[68] (**Fig. 2**). The binding of pVHL to HIFα is oxygen-dependent because it requires that HIFα is first hydroxylated on 1 of 2 conserved prolyl residues by members of the EgIN prolyl hydroxylase families.[69–71] These enzymes use molecular oxygen to hydroxylate HIFα and have low oxygen affinities, rendering them sensitive to changes in oxygen availability over a physiologically relevant range of oxygen concentrations.[64]

HIF1α and HIF2α have both shared and paralog-specific transcriptional targets.[72,73] For example, many genes devoted to glycolysis, such as *PGK* and *LDHA*, are exclusively regulated by HIF1α,[74] whereas genes such as *PAI-1*, *Cited-2*, and *EPO* are exclusively regulated by HIF2α.[75–77] A caveat when discussing HIF target genes is the knowledge that the precise repertoire of HIF-responsive genes varies in different cells and tissues as does, in some cases, the relative contribution of HIF1α versus HIF2α to the control of those genes. This context-dependence likely stems from differences in the availability of other transcription factors, including cis-acting DNA-binding transcription factors, that cooperate with HIF as well as context-dependent epigenomic differences that govern HRE accessibility. It is also clear that different HIF target genes have different dose-response characteristics with respect to HIF levels and their transcriptional induction.[78,79] As a result, not all HIF target genes are simultaneously induced as HIF levels increase, with some requiring higher levels of HIF for their transcriptional induction than others. Finally, some HIF target genes are primarily

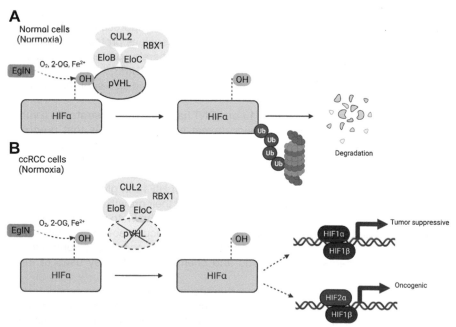

Fig. 2. Role of VHL in the regulation of HIFα abundance in normal and ccRCC cells under normoxia. (Created with BioRender.com.)

driven by the HIFα NTADs and others by the HIFα CTADs; this is important because the HIF1α CTAD, and to a lesser extent the HIF2α CTAD, is subject to oxygen-dependent asparaginyl hydroxylation by FIH1, which prevents the CTADs from recruiting the coactivators p300 and CBP. As a result, the HIF1α that accumulates in cells lacking pVHL (or the EgINs) is enfeebled as a transcriptional activator for HIF1α CTAD–dependent genes. EgINs are more sensitive to oxygen deprivation than FIH1. It is therefore thought that intermediate levels of hypoxia inhibit EgIN more so than FIH1, leading to a stabilized, but partially inactive, HIF1α, while worsening hypoxia would progressively inhibit FIH1 and fully activate HIF1α.[80,81]

Kidney cancer is notoriously rich in blood vessels and, on occasion, stimulates excess red blood cell production (paraneoplastic erythrocytosis). The former is linked to the HIF target *VEGF* and the latter to the HIF target *EPO*. Indeed, these clinical features were important clues that tied pVHL to HIF and oxygen sensing.

HIF1α AND CANCER

HIF1α has been highly touted as a potential cancer target based on epidemiologic data and plausibility arguments. With respect to the former, upregulation of HIF1α is almost universally associated with a poor prognosis in cancer.[72] A caveat, however, is that it is impossible from this association to infer causality. In particular, this correlation could arise because HIF1α promotes aggressive tumor growth but could also reflect the fact that aggressive tumors outgrow their blood supplies, become hypoxic, and upregulate HIF1α.[82]

The plausibility arguments rest on the knowledge that (1) solid tumors, in contrast to most normal tissues, are typically hypoxic, (2) HIF1α promotes adaptation to acute and chronic hypoxia, and (3) many HIF1α target genes, such as *VEGF*, are known or highly suspected of promoting tumor growth. A caveat to this line of reasoning is that HIF1α also activates many genes that one would predict would suppress tumor growth. Thematically, HIF1α activates many genes that suppress ATP utilization, in part by suppressing the synthesis of macromolecules such as proteins. For example, HIF1α activates *REDD1*, which inhibits mTOR and thereby protein synthesis.[83–85] HIF1α also promotes autophagy through proteins such as BNIP3,[86] which can be pro-tumorigenic or antitumorigenic in different contexts, and can also suppress proliferation by antagonizing c-Myc.[87]

Nonetheless, a requirement for HIF1α or ARNT has been demonstrated in a variety of preclinical mouse models.[72] A major caveat here, however, is that preclinical models based on subcutaneous implantation of tumor cells seem to consistently reveal a requirement for HIF1α (or vascular endothelial growth factor [VEGF]), perhaps reflecting the need of ectopic tumor cells in this anatomical space to rapidly induce new blood vessels. In one study, deletion of HIF1α in glioma cells inhibited their ability to grow subcutaneously but accelerated their growth when grown ortho-topically in the brain.[88] Deletion of *HIF1α* has also been shown to promote the growth of teratomas[89] and acute leukemias.[90] Many of the subcutaneous xenograft studies that explored HIF1α as a therapeutic target also failed to completely control for potential off-target effects of the genetic and chemical agents they used to inhibit HIF1α.

The probability of success for any new therapeutic target, including cancer targets, increases when there is strong genetic validation linking that target to the pathophysiology of the disease of interest. Cancer-associated gain-of-function *HIF1A* mutations have not been described, which argues against the idea that increasing HIF1α activity would provide a fitness advantage to tumor cells. In fact, deletion of HIF1α confers a slight fitness advantage to most cancer cell lines, at least when grown under standard cell culture conditions.[91] In contrast, *VHL* loss confers a fitness disadvantage to most cancer cell lines under these conditions (https://depmap.org/portal/gene/VHL?tab=overview).

HIF2α AND CLEAR CELL RENAL CELL CARCINOMA

Given these considerations, it was important to determine whether HIF1α, HIF2α, both, or neither drives the development of pVHL-defective ccRCC. Reintroduction of wild-type pVHL into some pVHL-defective human ccRCC lines suppresses their ability to form subcutaneous or orthotopic tumors in immunocompromised mice.[92] Notably, the effect of pVHL on these cells ex vivo is often subtle, although it can be magnified under certain media conditions or in 3-dimensional growth models. These assays provided a platform for interrogating HIFα-dependence in ccRCC.

In such pVHL-defective ccRCC lines, downregulating HIF2α with siRNAs, shRNAs,[87,93,94] or CRISPR/Cas9-based gene editing suppresses their growth in xenograft assays. Conversely, reactivation of HIF2α using HIF2α variants that escape recognition by pVHL overrides ccRCC suppression by pVHL.[95,96] Unexpectedly, HIF1α has the opposite effect in such assays.[87,97,98] In short, these preclinical studies strongly suggested that HIF2α drives the formation of pVHL-defective ccRCC, whereas HIF1α constrains pVHL-defective ccRCC.[43] With respect to the latter, loss-of-function *HIF1A* mutations have been described in pVHL-defective ccRCC lines and *HIF1A* resides on chromosome 14q, which is frequently lost in ccRCC.[52,98,99] It remains possible that HIF1α is protumorigenic during the early initiation of pVHL-defective ccRCCs but constrains ccRCC during and after the later stages of tumor progression.

Importantly, not all pVHL-defective ccRCC lines are HIF2α-dependent[100–102]; this could suggest that HIF2α plays no role in the pathogenesis of a subset of ccRCC or, alternatively, that all pVHL-defective ccRCCs are initially HIF2α-dependent but become HIF2α-independent during the course of tumor progression or during cell line initiation and propagation. Clinical data suggest the latter (see later discussion).

A number of correlative observations also support a role of HIF2α in ccRCC. Careful examination of early kidney lesions arising in patients with VHL disease revealed that the appearance of HIF2α in such lesions coincides with worsening cellular atypia.[103,104] HIF2α levels are higher in renal cells engineered to express type 1 and type 2B *VHL* mutations, which are associated with a high risk of ccRCC, than in cells engineered to express type 2A or type 2C *VHL* mutations, which have a low risk of ccRCC.[27] *PBRM1* mutations, which are the second most common intragenic mutations in ccRCC after *VHL* mutations, amplify the HIF2α response in pVHL-defective cells.[105–107] Finally, an *EPAS1* (gene encoding HIF2α) genetic variant in the human population has been linked to the risk of ccRCC.[108]

CLEAR CELL RENAL CELL CARCINOMA THERAPEUTICS BASED ON HIF2α BIOLOGY

ccRCC is a highly angiogenic tumor. In fact, in the preCT era renal angiograms were often used to diagnose this disease. In ccRCC HIF2α drives the expression of the angiogenic growth factor VEGF, which supports endothelial cell growth, and platelet-derived growth factor subunit B, which promotes the growth and maturation of pericytes (**Table 3**). Among common solid tumors ccRCCs have the highest VEGF levels.[109] These considerations provided a conceptual foundation for testing VEGF inhibitors in ccRCC and for recognizing that the response of ccRCC in an early trial of the Raf inhibitor sorafenib was likely due to its ability to inhibit the kinase insert domain

Table 3
Representative HIF2α target genes that are implicated in clear cell renal cell carcinoma tumorigenesis

HIF2a Target Genes	Function	Effect on ccRCC Xenografts
VEGF	Promotes angiogenesis	Required for ccRCC growth
PDGF	Supports expansion of pericytes and survival of endothelial cells	Required for ccRCC growth
CCND1	Cell-cycle progression by inhibiting the Rb tumor suppressor	Required for ccRCC growth
TGF-alpha	Acts as EGFR ligand	Promotes EGFR-mediated ccRCC growth
CXCR4 and CXCL 12	Promotes angiogenesis and metastasis	Promotes invasive ability of ccRCC
GLUT1	Glucose transporter	Tumor suppressive effect on ccRCC
SLC7A5	Amino acid transporter activates mTORC1	Required for ccRCC growth
IGFBP3	Binds to IGF1 and IGF2	Tumor suppressive effect on ccRCC

receptor (KDR) for VEGF as an off-target effect. Eight drugs that inhibit VEGF or KDR are now approved for ccRCC treatment in the United States.[110]

In most cell types HIF downregulates *CCND1*, which encodes cyclin D1, but in the cells that give rise to ccRCC HIF2α transcriptionally upregulates *CCND1*[96,111–114] (**Table 3**). Cyclin D1, together with Cdk4 or Cdk6, drives cell-cycle progression by phosphorylating the retinoblastoma tumor suppressor protein.[115,116] In preclinical models inhibiting cyclin D1 or Cdk4/6 inhibits pVHL-defective ccRCC.[117–119] Moreover, *VHL*−/− cells seem to have an increased requirement for Cdk4/6 activity irrespective of HIF2α.[119] Three Cdk4/6 inhibitors have been approved for the treatment of breast cancer and are now being tested in ccRCC.

In ccRCC HIF2α also drives the expression of TGFα, which is a ligand for the epidermal growth factor receptor[120] (**Table 3**). Loss of pVHL also leads to enhanced EGFR stability and signaling.[121,122] Consistent with these observations, EGFR is abundantly expressed in human ccRCCs. In preclinical models inhibiting the EGFR inhibits pVHL-defective ccRCC.[123,124] Surprisingly, however, EGFR inhibitors have not proved active against ccRCC in human clinical trials. The reason for this is unclear but could reflect compensation by other receptor tyrosine kinases such as MET. The importance of MET in mouse experiments is often underestimated because of species differences between mice and men with respect to MET and its ligand HGF.[125] The dual KDR/MET inhibitor cabozantinib is highly active against ccRCC and approved by Food and Drug Administration for its treatment,[126,127] but it is impossible from the existing clinical data to determine whether MET inhibition actually contributes to its efficacy.

Inhibiting HIF2α itself would theoretically be more efficacious than inhibiting any one HIF2α transcriptional target. Despite the conventional wisdom that HIF2α was undruggable, Rick Bruick and Kevin Gardner, who were then at UTSW, identified a potentially druggable hydrophobic pocket in the second of HIF2α's 2 PAS B domains (the HIF2α PAS B domain). Moreover, they discovered, using high-throughput screening technologies, small organic molecules that could bind to this pocket and alter the folding of HIF2α such that it could no longer dimerize to ARNT.[128–131] These initial chemicals were outlicensed to Peloton Therapeutics, which was later acquired by Merck. The medicinal chemists at Peloton further optimized these chemicals with respect to their potency and bioavailability while retaining their specificity. These efforts beget the first-in-class compound PT-2385[132,133] and the later compound PT-2977 (also called MK-6482 or belzutifan [Welireg]).[134] Notably, the corresponding pocket in HIF1α is considerably smaller and thus far has proved undruggable.

HIF2α INHIBITORS AND CANCER

PT-2385 was tested in a single-arm phase 1 trial of 51 patients with heavily pretreated ccRCC in dose-escalation (26) or expansion (25) phases. Complete response, partial response, and stable disease as best response were achieved by 2%, 12%, and 52% of patients, respectively.[135] It became apparent that PT-2385 had a metabolic liability that led to highly variable drug exposure. A post hoc analysis showed that the clinical outcomes were significantly better in the patients with higher drug exposures.[110,135]

PT-2977, which lacks the metabolic liability of PT-2385, was then likewise tested in heavily pretreated ccRCC in a dose-escalation/expansion clinical trial. The initial report described a response rate of 25%, and median progression-free survival of 14.5 months, in the 55 patients who received the projected phase 2 dose.[136] The median duration of response had still not been reached with more than 3 years of follow-up. On-mechanism toxicities included anemia and hypoxia. Curiously, the clinical responses that were observed in this patient population developed slowly, often requiring many months of therapy. The reason for these slow kinetics is not clear.[110]

A truism in medical oncology is that most cancer drugs are more active when used in early lines of therapy compared with later lines of therapy. Peloton, and then Merck, supported a phase 2 trial of 61 patients with VHL disease with measurable kidney tumors that were being monitored in careful surveillance programs in an attempt to delay or prevent the need for surgery. With more than 3 years of follow-up the objective response rate was 64%, with virtually all the kidney tumors exhibiting at least some tumor shrinkage, and the median duration of response had not been reached.[137] Gratifyingly, responses were also seen for some of the incidental nonrenal tumors in these patients, including hemangioblastomas and pancreatic neuroendocrine tumors.[137,138] Based on these findings, Belzutifan was approved by the FDA for the treatment of VHL Disease-associated neoplasms in August 2021.

Belzutifan is also currently being explored in combination with other agents that are active in ccRCC. Combination partners being explored include cabozantinib, nivolumab, pembrolizumab and lenvatinib, palbociclib, and abemaciclib. Other HIF2α inhibitors that have entered the clinic include NKT-2152 (NiKang Therapeutics) and DFF332 (Novartis),[139] which bind to the same pocket as Belzutifan, and ARO-HIF2,[140] which is siRNA-based (**Table 4**). MBM-02 (Tempol) has also been touted as a HIF2α (and HIF1α) inhibitor but its mechanism of action is less clear.[141] A caveat when considering

Table 4
Summary of HIF2α inhibitors that are in clinical trials for clear cell renal cell carcinoma

HIF2a-Inhibitor	Mode of Action	Class	Company
MK-6482	Inhibits dimerization of HIF2a-ARNT	Small molecule	Merck
DFF-32	Inhibits dimerization of HIF2a-ARNT	Small molecule	Novartis
NKT-2152	Inhibits dimerization of HIF2a-ARNT	Small molecule	Nikang Therapeutics
ARO-HIF2	Decrease HIF2a expression by RNAi	dsRNA RNAi trigger	Arrowhead Pharmaceuticals

HIF1α and HIF2α antagonists is that HIF1α and HIF2α have short half-lives and therefore are among the first proteins to be downregulated when cells are confronted with toxins that directly or indirectly suppress transcription or translation.

There are currently no robust biomarkers to predict which pVHL-defective ccRCCs are most likely to respond to HIF2α inhibitors. An early suggestion that responsiveness to HIF2α inhibitors required an intact p53 response pathway based on correlative data from a limited number of cell lines proved incorrect.[101,102] *EPAS1* or *ARNT* mutations have been described in small number of cases of acquired resistance to belzutifan. The former compromise the binding of belzutifan to HIF2α and the latter increase the affinity of ARNT for belzutifan-bound HIF2α.[100,131] Such mutations provide formal genetic proof that belzutifan's activity against pVHL-defective ccRCC is on-target. It remains to be seen how frequently such mutations will arise with increased used of this new class of drugs.

CLINICS CARE POINTS

- Genetic data from patients with VHL disease and preclinical laboratory experiments have established that HIF2α is a key driver of ccRCC linked to *VHL* gene inactivation.

- A first-in-class allosteric HIF2α inhibitor has been approved for VHL disease–associated tumors, and HIF2α inhibitors seem promising for the treatment of sporadic ccRCC based on emerging clinical trial data.

- Multiple clinical trials exploring combinations of a HIF2α inhibitor with other agents are ongoing as is the search for predictive biomarkers to identify which patients with ccRCC are most likely to benefit from this new class of drugs.

ACKNOWLEDGMENTS

The authors thank the members of the Kaelin Laboratory for their helpful comments. Supported by an NIH R35 (W.G. Kaelin), HHMI, United States (W.G. Kaelin), and Hope Funds for Cancer Research Sakonnet Family Fellowship (N.H. Shirole). The authors apologize to our colleagues for any omissions that might have arisen due to our ignorance or oversight. Please bring errors and egregious omissions to our attention.

W.G. Kaelin declares the following commercial or financial conflicts: Lilly Pharmaceuticals, Tango Therapeutics, Circle Pharmaceuticals, IconOVir Bio, Fibrogen, LifeMine Therapeutics, Casdin Capital, and Nextech Invest. He also has a royalty interest in Belzutifan (Welireg). N.H. Shirole has no commercial or financial conflicts.

REFERENCES

1. Sung H, et al. Global Cancer Statistics 2020: GLOBOCAN Estimates of Incidence and Mortality Worldwide for 36 Cancers in 185 Countries. CA Cancer J Clin 2021;71(3):209–49.
2. Siegel RL, et al. Cancer statistics, 2022. CA Cancer J Clin 2022;72(1):7–33.
3. Scelo G, Larose TL. Epidemiology and Risk Factors for Kidney Cancer. J Clin Oncol 2018;36(36). JCO2018791905.
4. Kovacs G, et al. The Heidelberg classification of renal cell tumours. J Pathol 1997;183(2):131–3.
5. Lopez-Beltran A, et al. 2004 WHO classification of the renal tumors of the adults. Eur Urol 2006;49(5):798–805.

6. Srigley JR, et al. The International Society of Urological Pathology (ISUP) Vancouver Classification of Renal Neoplasia. Am J Surg Pathol 2013;37(10): 1469–89.
7. Moch H, et al. The 2016 WHO Classification of Tumours of the Urinary System and Male Genital Organs-Part A: Renal, Penile, and Testicular Tumours. Eur Urol 2016;70(1):93–105.
8. Cancer Genome Atlas Research N. Comprehensive molecular characterization of clear cell renal cell carcinoma. Nature 2013;499(7456):43–9.
9. Cancer Genome Atlas Research N, et al. Comprehensive Molecular Characterization of Papillary Renal-Cell Carcinoma. N Engl J Med 2016;374(2):135–45.
10. Coleman JA. Familial and hereditary renal cancer syndromes. Urol Clin North Am 2008;35(4):563–72.
11. Verine J, et al. Hereditary renal cancer syndromes: an update of a systematic review. Eur Urol 2010;58(5):701–10.
12. Haas NB, Nathanson KL. Hereditary kidney cancer syndromes. Adv Chronic Kidney Dis 2014;21(1):81–90.
13. Linehan WM, Zbar B. Focus on kidney cancer. Cancer Cell 2004;6(3):223–8.
14. Wei MH, et al. Novel mutations in FH and expansion of the spectrum of phenotypes expressed in families with hereditary leiomyomatosis and renal cell cancer. J Med Genet 2006;43(1):18–27.
15. Smit DL, et al. Hereditary leiomyomatosis and renal cell cancer in families referred for fumarate hydratase germline mutation analysis. Clin Genet 2011; 79(1):49–59.
16. Stewart L, et al. Association of germline mutations in the fumarate hydratase gene and uterine fibroids in women with hereditary leiomyomatosis and renal cell cancer. Arch Dermatol 2008;144(12):1584–92.
17. Schmidt L, et al. Germline and somatic mutations in the tyrosine kinase domain of the MET proto-oncogene in papillary renal carcinomas. Nat Genet 1997;16(1): 68–73.
18. Nickerson ML, et al. Mutations in a novel gene lead to kidney tumors, lung wall defects, and benign tumors of the hair follicle in patients with the Birt-Hogg-Dube syndrome. Cancer Cell 2002;2(2):157–64.
19. Pavlovich CP, et al. Evaluation and management of renal tumors in the Birt-Hogg-Dube syndrome. J Urol 2005;173(5):1482–6.
20. Birt AR, Hogg GR, Dube WJ. Hereditary multiple fibrofolliculomas with trichodiscomas and acrochordons. Arch Dermatol 1977;113(12):1674–7.
21. Scalvenzi M, et al. Hereditary multiple fibrofolliculomas, trichodiscomas and acrochordons: syndrome of Birt-Hogg-Dube. J Eur Acad Dermatol Venereol 1998;11(1):45–7.
22. Testa JR, et al. Germline BAP1 mutations predispose to malignant mesothelioma. Nat Genet 2011;43(10):1022–5.
23. Farley MN, et al. A novel germline mutation in BAP1 predisposes to familial clear-cell renal cell carcinoma. Mol Cancer Res 2013;11(9):1061–71.
24. Popova T, et al. Germline BAP1 mutations predispose to renal cell carcinomas. Am J Hum Genet 2013;92(6):974–80.
25. Benusiglio PR, et al. A germline mutation in PBRM1 predisposes to renal cell carcinoma. J Med Genet 2015;52(6):426–30.
26. Maher ER, Kaelin WG Jr. von Hippel-Lindau disease. Medicine (Baltim) 1997; 76(6):381–91.
27. Kaelin WG Jr. Von Hippel-Lindau disease: insights into oxygen sensing, protein degradation, and cancer. J Clin Invest 2022;132(18).

28. Kaelin WG. Von Hippel-Lindau disease. Annu Rev Pathol 2007;2:145–73.
29. Seizinger BR, et al. Von Hippel-Lindau disease maps to the region of chromosome 3 associated with renal cell carcinoma. Nature 1988;332(6161):268–9.
30. Latif F, et al. Identification of the von Hippel-Lindau disease tumor suppressor gene. Science 1993;260(5112):1317–20.
31. Herman JG, et al. Silencing of the VHL tumor-suppressor gene by DNA methylation in renal carcinoma. Proc Natl Acad Sci U S A 1994;91(21):9700–4.
32. Kim WY, Kaelin WG. Role of VHL gene mutation in human cancer. J Clin Oncol 2004;22(24):4991–5004.
33. Crossey PA, et al. Identification of intragenic mutations in the von Hippel-Lindau disease tumour suppressor gene and correlation with disease phenotype. Hum Mol Genet 1994;3(8):1303–8.
34. Chen F, et al. Germline mutations in the von Hippel-Lindau disease tumor suppressor gene: correlations with phenotype. Hum Mutat 1995;5(1):66–75.
35. Choyke PL, et al. The natural history of renal lesions in von Hippel-Lindau disease: a serial CT study in 28 patients. AJR Am J Roentgenol 1992;159(6):1229–34.
36. Gerlinger M, et al. Genomic architecture and evolution of clear cell renal cell carcinomas defined by multiregion sequencing. Nat Genet 2014;46(3):225–33.
37. Xu X, et al. Single-cell exome sequencing reveals single-nucleotide mutation characteristics of a kidney tumor. Cell 2012;148(5):886–95.
38. Fisher R, et al. Development of synchronous VHL syndrome tumors reveals contingencies and constraints to tumor evolution. Genome Biol 2014;15(8):433.
39. Sankin A, et al. The impact of genetic heterogeneity on biomarker development in kidney cancer assessed by multiregional sampling. Cancer Med 2014;3(6):1485–92.
40. Gnarra JR, et al. Mutations of the VHL tumour suppressor gene in renal carcinoma. Nat Genet 1994;7(1):85–90.
41. Banks RE, et al. Genetic and epigenetic analysis of von Hippel-Lindau (VHL) gene alterations and relationship with clinical variables in sporadic renal cancer. Cancer Res 2006;66(4):2000–11.
42. Nickerson ML, et al. Improved identification of von Hippel-Lindau gene alterations in clear cell renal tumors. Clin Cancer Res 2008;14(15):4726–34.
43. Cho H, Kaelin WG. Targeting HIF2 in Clear Cell Renal Cell Carcinoma. Cold Spring Harb Symp Quant Biol 2016;81:113–21.
44. Beroukhim R, et al. Patterns of gene expression and copy-number alterations in von-hippel lindau disease-associated and sporadic clear cell carcinoma of the kidney. Cancer Res 2009;69(11):4674–81.
45. Walther MM, et al. Prevalence of microscopic lesions in grossly normal renal parenchyma from patients with von Hippel-Lindau disease, sporadic renal cell carcinoma and no renal disease: clinical implications. J Urol 1995;154(6):2010–4, discussion 2014-5.
46. Lubensky IA, et al. Allelic deletions of the VHL gene detected in multiple microscopic clear cell renal lesions in von Hippel-Lindau disease patients. Am J Pathol 1996;149(6):2089–94.
47. Montani M, et al. VHL-gene deletion in single renal tubular epithelial cells and renal tubular cysts: further evidence for a cyst-dependent progression pathway of clear cell renal carcinoma in von Hippel-Lindau disease. Am J Surg Pathol 2010;34(6):806–15.
48. Sato Y, et al. Integrated molecular analysis of clear-cell renal cell carcinoma. Nat Genet 2013;45(8):860–7.

49. Guo G, et al. Frequent mutations of genes encoding ubiquitin-mediated proteolysis pathway components in clear cell renal cell carcinoma. Nat Genet 2011;44(1):17–9.
50. Varela I, et al. Exome sequencing identifies frequent mutation of the SWI/SNF complex gene PBRM1 in renal carcinoma. Nature 2011;469(7331):539–42.
51. Pena-Llopis S, et al. BAP1 loss defines a new class of renal cell carcinoma. Nat Genet 2012;44(7):751–9.
52. Dalgliesh GL, et al. Systematic sequencing of renal carcinoma reveals inactivation of histone modifying genes. Nature 2010;463(7279):360–3.
53. Kibel A, et al. Binding of the von Hippel-Lindau tumor suppressor protein to Elongin B and C. Science 1995;269(5229):1444–6.
54. Kamura T, et al. Rbx1, a component of the VHL tumor suppressor complex and SCF ubiquitin ligase. Science 1999;284(5414):657–61.
55. Duan DR, et al. Inhibition of transcription elongation by the VHL tumor suppressor protein. Science 1995;269(5229):1402–6.
56. Pause A, et al. The von Hippel-Lindau tumor-suppressor gene product forms a stable complex with human CUL-2, a member of the Cdc53 family of proteins. Proc Natl Acad Sci U S A 1997;94(6):2156–61.
57. Lonergan KM, et al. Regulation of hypoxia-inducible mRNAs by the von Hippel-Lindau tumor suppressor protein requires binding to complexes containing elongins B/C and Cul2. Mol Cell Biol 1998;18(2):732–41.
58. Iwai K, et al. Identification of the von Hippel-lindau tumor-suppressor protein as part of an active E3 ubiquitin ligase complex. Proc Natl Acad Sci U S A 1999; 96(22):12436–41.
59. Cockman ME, et al. Hypoxia inducible factor-alpha binding and ubiquitylation by the von Hippel-Lindau tumor suppressor protein. J Biol Chem 2000; 275(33):25733–41.
60. Tanimoto K, et al. Mechanism of regulation of the hypoxia-inducible factor-1 alpha by the von Hippel-Lindau tumor suppressor protein. EMBO J 2000; 19(16):4298–309.
61. Kamura T, et al. Activation of HIF1alpha ubiquitination by a reconstituted von Hippel-Lindau (VHL) tumor suppressor complex. Proc Natl Acad Sci U S A 2000;97(19):10430–5.
62. Ohh M, et al. Ubiquitination of hypoxia-inducible factor requires direct binding to the beta-domain of the von Hippel-Lindau protein. Nat Cell Biol 2000;2(7):423–7.
63. Stebbins CE, Kaelin WG Jr, Pavletich NP. Structure of the VHL-ElonginC-ElonginB complex: implications for VHL tumor suppressor function. Science 1999;284(5413):455–61.
64. Kaelin WG Jr, Ratcliffe PJ. Oxygen sensing by metazoans: the central role of the HIF hydroxylase pathway. Mol Cell 2008;30(4):393–402.
65. Semenza GL. Oxygen sensing, homeostasis, and disease. N Engl J Med 2011; 365(6):537–47.
66. Kewley RJ, Whitelaw ML, Chapman-Smith A. The mammalian basic helix-loop-helix/PAS family of transcriptional regulators. Int J Biochem Cell Biol 2004; 36(2):189–204.
67. Bersten DC, et al. bHLH-PAS proteins in cancer. Nat Rev Cancer 2013;13(12): 827–41.
68. Harris AL. Hypoxia–a key regulatory factor in tumour growth. Nat Rev Cancer 2002;2(1):38–47.
69. Ivan M, et al. HIFalpha targeted for VHL-mediated destruction by proline hydroxylation: implications for O2 sensing. Science 2001;292(5516):464–8.

70. Jaakkola P, et al. Targeting of HIF-alpha to the von Hippel-Lindau ubiquitylation complex by O2-regulated prolyl hydroxylation. Science 2001;292(5516):468–72.

71. Yu F, et al. HIF-1alpha binding to VHL is regulated by stimulus-sensitive proline hydroxylation. Proc Natl Acad Sci U S A 2001;98(17):9630–5.

72. Keith B, Johnson RS, Simon MC. HIF1alpha and HIF2alpha: sibling rivalry in hypoxic tumour growth and progression. Nat Rev Cancer 2011;12(1):9–22.

73. Ivan M, Kaelin WG Jr. The EGLN-HIF O(2)-Sensing System: Multiple Inputs and Feedbacks. Mol Cell 2017;66(6):772–9.

74. Hu CJ, et al. Differential roles of hypoxia-inducible factor 1alpha (HIF-1alpha) and HIF-2alpha in hypoxic gene regulation. Mol Cell Biol 2003;23(24):9361–74.

75. Hu CJ, et al. The N-terminal transactivation domain confers target gene specificity of hypoxia-inducible factors HIF-1alpha and HIF-2alpha. Mol Biol Cell 2007;18(11):4528–42.

76. Warnecke C, et al. Differentiating the functional role of hypoxia-inducible factor (HIF)-1alpha and HIF-2alpha (EPAS-1) by the use of RNA interference: erythropoietin is a HIF-2alpha target gene in Hep3B and Kelly cells. FASEB J 2004; 18(12):1462–4.

77. Rankin EB, et al. Hypoxia-inducible factor-2 (HIF-2) regulates hepatic erythropoietin in vivo. J Clin Invest 2007;117(4):1068–77.

78. Minamishima YA, et al. A feedback loop involving the Phd3 prolyl hydroxylase tunes the mammalian hypoxic response in vivo. Mol Cell Biol 2009;29(21): 5729–41.

79. Dengler VL, Galbraith M, Espinosa JM. Transcriptional regulation by hypoxia inducible factors. Crit Rev Biochem Mol Biol 2014;49(1):1–15.

80. Bracken CP, et al. Cell-specific regulation of hypoxia-inducible factor (HIF)-1alpha and HIF-2alpha stabilization and transactivation in a graded oxygen environment. J Biol Chem 2006;281(32):22575–85.

81. Yan Q, et al. The hypoxia-inducible factor 2alpha N-terminal and C-terminal transactivation domains cooperate to promote renal tumorigenesis in vivo. Mol Cell Biol 2007;27(6):2092–102.

82. Kaelin WG Jr. Common pitfalls in preclinical cancer target validation. Nat Rev Cancer 2017;17(7):425–40.

83. DeYoung MP, et al. Hypoxia regulates TSC1/2-mTOR signaling and tumor suppression through REDD1-mediated 14-3-3 shuttling. Genes Dev 2008;22(2): 239–51.

84. Brugarolas J, et al. Regulation of mTOR function in response to hypoxia by REDD1 and the TSC1/TSC2 tumor suppressor complex. Genes Dev 2004; 18(23):2893–904.

85. Reiling JH, Hafen E. The hypoxia-induced paralogs Scylla and Charybdis inhibit growth by down-regulating S6K activity upstream of TSC in Drosophila. Genes Dev 2004;18(23):2879–92.

86. Li Y, et al. Bnip3 mediates the hypoxia-induced inhibition on mammalian target of rapamycin by interacting with Rheb. J Biol Chem 2007;282(49):35803–13.

87. Gordan JD, et al. HIF-alpha effects on c-Myc distinguish two subtypes of sporadic VHL-deficient clear cell renal carcinoma. Cancer Cell 2008;14(6):435–46.

88. Blouw B, et al. The hypoxic response of tumors is dependent on their microenvironment. Cancer Cell 2003;4(2):133–46.

89. Carmeliet P, et al. Role of HIF-1alpha in hypoxia-mediated apoptosis, cell proliferation and tumour angiogenesis. Nature 1998;394(6692):485–90.

90. Velasco-Hernandez T, et al. HIF-1alpha can act as a tumor suppressor gene in murine acute myeloid leukemia. Blood 2014;124(24):3597–607.

91. Andrysik Z, et al. Multi-omics analysis reveals contextual tumor suppressive and oncogenic gene modules within the acute hypoxic response. Nat Commun 2021;12(1):1375.
92. Iliopoulos O, et al. Tumour suppression by the human von Hippel-Lindau gene product. Nat Med 1995;1(8):822–6.
93. Kondo K, et al. Inhibition of HIF2alpha is sufficient to suppress pVHL-defective tumor growth. PLoS Biol 2003;1(3):E83.
94. Zimmer M, et al. Inhibition of hypoxia-inducible factor is sufficient for growth suppression of VHL-/- tumors. Mol Cancer Res 2004;2(2):89–95.
95. Kondo K, et al. Inhibition of HIF is necessary for tumor suppression by the von Hippel-Lindau protein. Cancer Cell 2002;1(3):237–46.
96. Raval RR, et al. Contrasting properties of hypoxia-inducible factor 1 (HIF-1) and HIF-2 in von Hippel-Lindau-associated renal cell carcinoma. Mol Cell Biol 2005;25(13):5675–86.
97. Maranchie JK, et al. The contribution of VHL substrate binding and HIF1-alpha to the phenotype of VHL loss in renal cell carcinoma. Cancer Cell 2002;1(3):247–55.
98. Shen C, et al. Genetic and functional studies implicate HIF1alpha as a 14q kidney cancer suppressor gene. Cancer Discov 2011;1(3):222–35.
99. Morris MR, et al. Mutation analysis of hypoxia-inducible factors HIF1A and HIF2A in renal cell carcinoma. Anticancer Res 2009;29(11):4337–43.
100. Chen W, et al. Targeting renal cell carcinoma with a HIF-2 antagonist. Nature 2016;539(7627):112–7.
101. Cho H, et al. On-target efficacy of a HIF-2alpha antagonist in preclinical kidney cancer models. Nature 2016;539(7627):107–11.
102. Stransky LA, et al. Sensitivity of VHL mutant kidney cancers to HIF2 inhibitors does not require an intact p53 pathway. Proc Natl Acad Sci U S A 2022;119(14). e2120403119.
103. Mandriota SJ, et al. HIF activation identifies early lesions in VHL kidneys: evidence for site-specific tumor suppressor function in the nephron. Cancer Cell 2002;1(5):459–68.
104. Schletke RE, et al. Renal tubular HIF-2alpha expression requires VHL inactivation and causes fibrosis and cysts. PLoS One 2012;7(1):e31034.
105. Gao W, et al. Inactivation of the PBRM1 tumor suppressor gene amplifies the HIF-response in VHL-/- clear cell renal carcinoma. Proc Natl Acad Sci U S A 2017;114(5):1027–32.
106. Nargund AM, et al. The SWI/SNF Protein PBRM1 Restrains VHL-Loss-Driven Clear Cell Renal Cell Carcinoma. Cell Rep 2017;18(12):2893–906.
107. Zhou M, et al. PBRM1 Inactivation Promotes Upregulation of Human Endogenous Retroviruses in a HIF-Dependent Manner. Cancer Immunol Res 2022;10(3):285–90.
108. Purdue MP, et al. Genome-wide association study of renal cell carcinoma identifies two susceptibility loci on 2p21 and 11q13.3. Nat Genet 2011;43(1):60–5.
109. Jubb AM, et al. Expression of vascular endothelial growth factor, hypoxia inducible factor 1alpha, and carbonic anhydrase IX in human tumours. J Clin Pathol 2004;57(5):504–12.
110. Choueiri TK, Kaelin WG Jr. Targeting the HIF2-VEGF axis in renal cell carcinoma. Nat Med 2020;26(10):1519–30.
111. Baba M, et al. Loss of von Hippel-Lindau protein causes cell density dependent deregulation of CyclinD1 expression through hypoxia-inducible factor. Oncogene 2003;22(18):2728–38.

112. Zatyka M, et al. Identification of cyclin D1 and other novel targets for the von Hippel-Lindau tumor suppressor gene by expression array analysis and investigation of cyclin D1 genotype as a modifier in von Hippel-Lindau disease. Cancer Res 2002;62(13):3803–11.

113. Bindra RS, et al. VHL-mediated hypoxia regulation of cyclin D1 in renal carcinoma cells. Cancer Res 2002;62(11):3014–9.

114. Wykoff CC, et al. Gene array of VHL mutation and hypoxia shows novel hypoxia-induced genes and that cyclin D1 is a VHL target gene. Br J Cancer 2004;90(6): 1235–43.

115. Kitagawa M, et al. The consensus motif for phosphorylation by cyclin D1-Cdk4 is different from that for phosphorylation by cyclin A/E-Cdk2. EMBO J 1996;15(24): 7060–9.

116. Ewen ME, et al. Functional interactions of the retinoblastoma protein with mammalian D-type cyclins. Cell 1993;73(3):487–97.

117. Zhang T, et al. The contributions of HIF-target genes to tumor growth in RCC. PLoS One 2013;8(11):e80544.

118. Bommi-Reddy A, et al. Kinase requirements in human cells: III. Altered kinase requirements in VHL-/- cancer cells detected in a pilot synthetic lethal screen. Proc Natl Acad Sci U S A 2008;105(43):16484–9.

119. Nicholson HE, et al. HIF-independent synthetic lethality between CDK4/6 inhibition and VHL loss across species. Sci Signal 2019;12(601).

120. de Paulsen N, et al. Role of transforming growth factor-alpha in von Hippel–Lindau (VHL)(-/-) clear cell renal carcinoma cell proliferation: a possible mechanism coupling VHL tumor suppressor inactivation and tumorigenesis. Proc Natl Acad Sci U S A 2001;98(4):1387–92.

121. Zhou L, Yang H. The von Hippel-Lindau tumor suppressor protein promotes c-Cbl-independent poly-ubiquitylation and degradation of the activated EGFR. PLoS One 2011;6(9):e23936.

122. Wang Y, et al. Hypoxia promotes ligand-independent EGF receptor signaling via hypoxia-inducible factor-mediated upregulation of caveolin-1. Proc Natl Acad Sci U S A 2012;109(13):4892–7.

123. Smith K, et al. Silencing of epidermal growth factor receptor suppresses hypoxia-inducible factor-2-driven VHL-/- renal cancer. Cancer Res 2005; 65(12):5221–30.

124. Franovic A, et al. Human cancers converge at the HIF-2alpha oncogenic axis. Proc Natl Acad Sci U S A 2009;106(50):21306–11.

125. Zhang YW, et al. Enhanced growth of human met-expressing xenografts in a new strain of immunocompromised mice transgenic for human hepatocyte growth factor/scatter factor. Oncogene 2005;24(1):101–6.

126. Yakes FM, et al. Cabozantinib (XL184), a novel MET and VEGFR2 inhibitor, simultaneously suppresses metastasis, angiogenesis, and tumor growth. Mol Cancer Ther 2011;10(12):2298–308.

127. Choueiri TK, et al. A phase I study of cabozantinib (XL184) in patients with renal cell cancer. Ann Oncol 2014;25(8):1603–8.

128. Scheuermann TH, et al. Allosteric inhibition of hypoxia inducible factor-2 with small molecules. Nat Chem Biol 2013;9(4):271–6.

129. Scheuermann TH, et al. Artificial ligand binding within the HIF2alpha PAS-B domain of the HIF2 transcription factor. Proc Natl Acad Sci U S A 2009; 106(2):450–5.

130. Rogers JL, et al. Development of inhibitors of the PAS-B domain of the HIF-2alpha transcription factor. J Med Chem 2013;56(4):1739–47.

131. Courtney KD, et al. HIF-2 Complex Dissociation, Target Inhibition, and Acquired Resistance with PT2385, a First-in-Class HIF-2 Inhibitor, in Patients with Clear Cell Renal Cell Carcinoma. Clin Cancer Res 2020;26(4):793–803.
132. Wehn PM, et al. Design and Activity of Specific Hypoxia-Inducible Factor-2alpha (HIF-2alpha) Inhibitors for the Treatment of Clear Cell Renal Cell Carcinoma: Discovery of Clinical Candidate (S)-3-((2,2-Difluoro-1-hydroxy-7-(methylsulfonyl)-2,3-dihydro-1 H-inden-4-yl)oxy)-5-fluorobenzonitrile (PT2385). J Med Chem 2018;61(21):9691–721.
133. Wallace EM, et al. A Small-Molecule Antagonist of HIF2alpha Is Efficacious in Preclinical Models of Renal Cell Carcinoma. Cancer Res 2016;76(18):5491–500.
134. Xu R, et al. 3-[(1S,2S,3R)-2,3-Difluoro-1-hydroxy-7-methylsulfonylindan-4-yl]oxy-5-fluorobenzonitrile (PT2977), a Hypoxia-Inducible Factor 2alpha (HIF-2alpha) Inhibitor for the Treatment of Clear Cell Renal Cell Carcinoma. J Med Chem 2019;62(15):6876–93.
135. Courtney KD, et al. Phase I Dose-Escalation Trial of PT2385, a First-in-Class Hypoxia-Inducible Factor-2alpha Antagonist in Patients With Previously Treated Advanced Clear Cell Renal Cell Carcinoma. J Clin Oncol 2018;36(9):867–74.
136. Choueiri TK, et al. Inhibition of hypoxia-inducible factor-2alpha in renal cell carcinoma with belzutifan: a phase 1 trial and biomarker analysis. Nat Med 2021; 27(5):802–5.
137. Jonasch E, et al. Belzutifan for Renal Cell Carcinoma in von Hippel-Lindau Disease. N Engl J Med 2021;385(22):2036–46.
138. Hasanov E, Jonasch E. MK-6482 as a potential treatment for von Hippel-Lindau disease-associated clear cell renal cell carcinoma. Expert Opin Investig Drugs 2021;30(5):495–504.
139. Toledo RA, et al. Hypoxia Inducible factor 2 alpha (HIF2alpha) inhibitors: targeting genetically driven tumor hypoxia. Endocr Rev 2022;44(2):312–22.
140. Ma Y, et al. HIF2 Inactivation and Tumor Suppression with a Tumor-Directed RNA-Silencing Drug in Mice and Humans. Clin Cancer Res 2022;28(24): 5405–18.
141. Sourbier C, et al. Targeting HIF2alpha translation with Tempol in VHL deficient clear cell renal cell carcinoma. Oncotarget 2012;3(11):1472–82.

Immunobiology and Metabolic Pathways of Renal Cell Carcinoma

David A. Braun, MD, PhD[a],*, Abhishek A. Chakraborty, PhD[b,c,*]

KEYWORDS

- Immune checkpoint inhibitor • Tumor microenvironment • Metabolic dysregulation
- Metabolic dependencies • Renal cell carcinoma

KEY POINTS

- Clear cell renal cell carcinoma (ccRCC) is a historically and contemporarily immunotherapy-responsive cancer, but its immunobiology differs substantially from other solid tumors.
- ccRCC has only a modest number of mutations, and unlike other solid tumors, a high tumor mutation burden or neoantigen load does not correlate with improved immunotherapy response.
- There is an abundant T-cell infiltration in ccRCC, but they are often dysfunctional (or "exhausted"), in part due to inhibitory interactions with tumor-associated macrophages.
- Chronic Hypoxia Inducible Factor activation, a hallmark of ccRCC, is associated with altered central carbon, lipid, and amino acid metabolism.
- Metabolic dysregulation in ccRCC may create tumor-specific dependencies that can be exploited as therapeutic targets.

INTRODUCTION

The management of advanced renal cell carcinoma (RCC), and particularly the most common histology clear cell RCC (ccRCC), has changed dramatically over the past few decades. However, most patients with advanced ccRCC do not have long-term clinical responses to currently available therapies and will ultimately pass away from their disease. The development of novel therapies capable of delivering durable clinical benefit will require an improved understanding of the biology of this disease. In this review, we discuss the unique immunobiologic and metabolic dysregulation in ccRCC,

[a] Center of Molecular and Cellular Oncology, Yale Cancer Center, Yale School of Medicine, 300 George Street (Suite 6400), New Haven, CT 06511, USA; [b] Department of Cancer Biology, Lerner Research Institute, Cleveland Clinical, 9500 Euclid Avenue (NB40), Cleveland, OH 44195, USA; [c] Case Comprehensive Cancer Center, Case Western Reserve University, Cleveland, OH 44106, USA
* Corresponding authors.
E-mail addresses: david.braun@yale.edu (D.A.B.); chakraa@ccf.org (A.A.C.)

Hematol Oncol Clin N Am 37 (2023) 827–840
https://doi.org/10.1016/j.hoc.2023.04.012
0889-8588/23/© 2023 Elsevier Inc. All rights reserved.

with implications for understanding response and resistance to current systemic treatments and for the development of new therapeutic approaches.

IMMUNOBIOLOGY OF RENAL CELL CARCINOMA

The immunogenic nature of ccRCC is reflected in the success of numerous immunotherapy approaches. Historically, ccRCC was one of the few tumor types responsive to cytokines, including high-dose interleukin-2 (IL-2) and interferon alfa-2a.[1] Importantly, a small percentage of patients with advanced ccRCC had durable complete responses with high-dose IL-2,[2,3] and this provided an early proof of concept that immunotherapies could lead to long-term survival in this disease. Contemporarily, immune checkpoint inhibitors (ICIs) targeting the programmed cell death protein 1 (PD-1) pathway are the backbone of first-line therapy for advanced ccRCC, either in combination with another ICI targeting the cytotoxic T-lymphocyte-associated protein 4 (CTLA-4) inhibitory receptor,[4] or with anti-angiogenic tyrosine kinase inhibitors targeting the vascular endothelial growth factor receptors (VEGFRs).[5-8]

Although ccRCC is considered highly immunogenic, it is immunobiologically distinct from other immunotherapy-responsive solid tumors. Most other ICI-responsive tumors, such as melanoma, non-small cell lung cancer, microsatellite instability-high colorectal cancer, and urothelial carcinoma, typically have a high number of somatic mutations,[9] and the total mutation burden (TMB) correlates with immunotherapy response.[10] In contrast, ccRCC has only a low-to-modest number of mutations and there is no association between TMB and response to ICIs.[11] Further, whereas a high infiltration of CD8+ T cells (a primary effector of anti-tumor immune responses) is typically associated with an improved prognosis across most solid tumors,[12] the converse is true in ccRCC where an abundant CD8+ T-cell infiltration was associated with worse survival in ccRCC.[13-15] These data highlight the need to account for the distinct immunobiology of ccRCC while investigating current and future immunotherapies.

Renal Cell Carcinoma Immunophenotype

ccRCC tumors are typically among the most highly immune infiltrated. In a pan-cancer transcriptomic analysis of 18 tumor types, ccRCC had the highest expression of a signature of immune cytolytic activity (specifically, expression of the genes encoding granzyme A and perforin).[16] Similarly, a second pan-cancer transcriptomic analysis using a distinct T-cell infiltration score identified ccRCC as the most highly T-cell infiltrated tumor across 19 tumor types.[17] In other tumor types, resistance to ICI therapy has, in part, been associated with a lack of T-cell infiltration into the tumor. This was either due to a complete paucity of CD8+ T cells in the tumor microenvironment (TME) or the apparent "exclusion" of T cells, whereby T cells may be abundant at the tumor margin but are unable to infiltrate the tumor center to carry out effector function.[18] In fact, this "immune excluded" phenotype may be seen in nearly 50% of metastatic urothelial carcinomas and is associated with resistance to anti-PD-L1 therapy in that disease.[19] In contrast, an immunofluorescence analysis of over 200 advanced ccRCC tumors demonstrated that immune exclusion is uncommon (only 5% of tumors), and that the far majority (73%) are highly infiltrated by CD8+ T cells.[11]

Lymphoid Cell Infiltration and Phenotype in Renal Cell Carcinoma

Although ccRCC is highly infiltrated by T cells, in contrast to most tumors paradoxically there has historically been an inverse correlation between CD8+ T-cell infiltration and prognosis. This may be due to (i) high T-cell infiltration being associated with a more aggressive disease biology, such as higher grade disease[13] or the presence of clinically aggressive sarcomatoid and/or rhabdoid differentiation[20]; (ii) T cells having a dysfunctional or terminally exhausted phenotype incapable of proper effector function[21,22]; (iii) high T-cell infiltration being correlated with the presence of other immunosuppressive populations, such as tumor-associated macrophages (TAMs)[22,23]; and (iv) tumor-infiltrating T cells lacking an anti-tumor specificity (ie, the presence of "bystander" T cells), which has been described in other solid tumor types.[24,25]

The development of high-dimensional single-cell analytic tools has enabled the detailed dissection of T-cell phenotypes in ccRCC. These studies have revealed tremendous phenotypic heterogeneity in the tumor-infiltrating T-cell compartment, including terminally exhausted CD8+ T-cell populations. These populations express additional inhibitory checkpoint receptors such as T-cell immunoglobulin, mucin-domain containing-3 (TIM-3), and lymphocyte-activation gene 3 (LAG-3).[22,23]These terminally exhausted CD8+ T cells are enriched in more advanced disease stages.[22] Further, in situ analysis of ccRCC tumors by multiplex immunofluorescence has demonstrated that infiltration by CD8+ T cells that express PD-1 (which also can serve as a marker of prior antigen experience) but the lack expression of TIM-3 and LAG-3 (markers of more terminal T-cell exhaustion) are associated with improved response and survival with anti-PD-1 ICI therapy.[26,27]

Beyond T-cell infiltration, other lymphoid populations almost certainly play a role in effective anti-tumor immunity in ccRCC. High infiltration by natural killer (NK) cells is associated with an improved prognosis in ccRCC,[28] and numerous clinical trials are exploring NK cell-based immunotherapies in this disease.[29] A higher number of B-cell containing tertiary lymphoid structures (TLSs) are associated with improved clinical outcomes in RCC, and infiltrating plasma cells within TLS+ tumors produce antibodies capable of binding ccRCC tumor cells, suggesting possible anti-tumor activity.[30] More work is needed to understand these additional lymphoid populations, and how they interact with other cell populations in the ccRCC TME.

Targeting Immune Checkpoints

ICIs are now a standard component of the therapeutic armamentarium in ccRCC, with combined anti-PD-1 and anti-CTLA-4 antibodies leading to durable survival in a subset of patients.[31] However, numerous other inhibitory and stimulatory immune checkpoints may play a role in modulating anti-tumor immune responses in ccRCC.[32] Both TIM-3 and LAG-3 are expressed on tumor-infiltrating T cells, though less frequently than PD-1.[27] The in vitro inhibition of TIM-3 on ccRCC patient tumor-infiltrating lymphocytes (TILs; both CD4+ and CD8+) partially restored T-cell function, as measured by increased proliferation and production of the effector cytokine IFNγ.[33] In ccRCC TILs, the in vitro dual inhibition of PD-1 and LAG-3 led to the greatest increase in T-cell function (as measured by IFNγ).[34] Other inhibitory checkpoints, including TIGIT,[22] VISTA,[35] and HHLA2,[36] are under active investigation in ccRCC.

Antigen Specificity

The T-cell receptor (TCR) repertoire can be notably restricted in ccRCC, with tremendous expansion of a single T-cell clonotype (T cells that share the same TCR sequence and therefore recognize the same target antigen) that may account for up to 20% to 40% of all tumor-infiltrating T cells.[22] Further, expansion of T-cell clonotypes is associated with improved response to anti-PD-1 therapy.[37] Although there are numerous classes of potential tumor antigens (**Fig. 1**), the specific T-cell targets in ccRCC remain largely unknown. Although numerous tumor-associated antigens (TAAs; peptides derived from proteins overexpressed in tumor relative to normal tissue) have been identified in ccRCC, it has been difficult to therapeutically target them effectively.[38] The

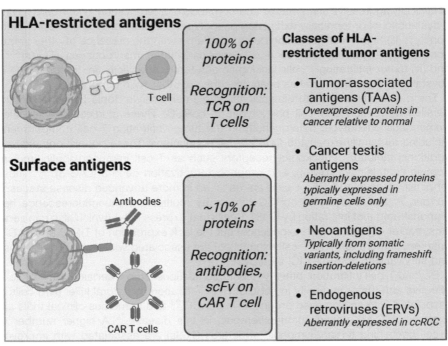

Fig. 1. Overview of antigen classes. Tumor antigens can be either cell surface proteins, recognized by antibodies, or CAR T cells, and HLA-restricted antigens, presented to T cells through their TCR. Types of HLA-restricted tumor antigens include overexpressed proteins (TAAs), cancer testis antigens, neoantigens, and antigens from ERVs. Other possible classes include antigens derived from aberrant splicing, and viral antigens.

phase II IMPRINT study of a TAA vaccine plus sunitinib versus sunitinib alone showed no benefit with the addition of the vaccine.[39] More recently, next generation sequencing technologies have enabled the rapid identification of tumor neoantigens–altered peptides derived from nonsynonymous somatic mutations. However, neoantigens can be immunogenic in ccRCC[40] and are being actively targeted in phase I personalized vaccine trial (NCT02950766) in patients with localized disease following resection.

One antigen class of particular interest derives from endogenous retroviruses (ERVs), fragments of retroviruses that integrated into the human genome millions of years ago, and may be aberrantly expressed in a variety of pathologic states, including cancer. Early evidence for ERV-derived antigens came from nonmyeloablative allogeneic stem cell transplantation in ccRCC, which produced tumor regression in some patients.[41] Through the investigation of expanded circulating expanded CD8$^+$ T cells in a long-term responder to allogeneic stem cell transplant, a 10-amino-acid peptide derived from aberrant expression of an ERV (ERVE-4) was identified as an antigenic cell target in ccRCC.[42] More recent transcriptomic studies have uncovered the broader expression of multiple ERVs in ccRCC and have identified a general correlation between high ERV expression and signatures of immune activation.[16,43] Interestingly, numerous studies have identified associations between the expression of specific ERVs and improved response to or survival with ICIs, including hERV4700,[43] ERV3-2,[44] and ERVE-4.[26] However, it is worth noting that this association is not always consistent between studies, and that tumor-infiltrating immune cells can also express ERVs,[37] which may complicate their therapeutic targeting. Ultimately, broader antigen discovery efforts are needed to fully understand the targets of T-cell-mediated immunity in ccRCC and open the door to novel antigen-directed therapies.

Tumor-Associated Macrophages and Other Infiltrating Myeloid Cells

TAMs are abundant in ccRCC and exhibit substantial phenotypic diversity between patients.[23] The phenotype of TAMs changes with advanced disease stage (ie, stage III/IV vs stage I/II), and the proportion of certain TAM populations correlates with infiltration by terminally exhausted CD8[+] T cells.[22,23] These TAMs express C1Q, TREM2, and APOE, and are associated with an increased risk of recurrence after nephrectomy[45] and were found to be enriched in a tumor resistant to ICI.[46] In addition, they expressed ligands for inhibitory receptors that support T-cell dysfunction, including ligands for PD-1, CTLA-4, TIM-3, and TIGIT. Of note, this interaction appeared to be bi-directional, with those enriched exhausted CD8[+] T cells also producing factors that support a more anti-inflammatory or protumorigenic phenotypes (sometimes referred to as "M2-like"), including colony stimulating factor 1 (CSF-1) and macrophage migration inhibitory factor (MIF).[22] This interaction does appear to be functional, as in vivo depletion of TAMs in pre-clinical models reduced the exhaustion phenotype in tumor-infiltrating CD8[+] T cells.[47] Overall then, these TAMs and exhausted CD8[+] T cells appear to form a bidirectional "immune dysfunction circuit" (**Fig. 2**), and work is ongoing to target additional cell–cell interactions in this circuit to restore immune function.

The optimal approach to modulating the infiltration of TAMs and other potentially immunosuppressive myeloid populations (such as myeloid-derived suppressor cells, MDSCs) remains unknown. Preclinical modeling has shown that blockade of the inflammatory cytokine interleukin-1 beta (IL-1β) can reduce infiltration of "M2-like" TAMs and MDSCs into the TME,[48] and this has led to early phase clinical trials of IL-1β in ccRCC (NCT04028245). In patient samples from multiple clinical trials in ccRCC and other solid tumors,[49,50] high levels of interleukin-8 (IL-8) from circulating and intratumoral myeloid cells were associated with worse response to ICI, which prompt further exploration of this target in kidney cancer.

Although certain infiltrating myeloid subsets inhibit effective immune responses, other myeloid cell types, including antigen presenting cells (APCs) like dendritic cells, could positively impact antigen-specific T-cell-mediated immunity in the local TME. Within the RCC TME, APCs (marked by the expression of HLA class II molecules) form "niches" that support stem-like CD8[+] T cells and may be associated with improved response to ICI.[51] Moving forward, additional efforts are needed to understand how to best modulate the myeloid compartment to foster an effective anti-tumor immune response.

METABOLIC DYSREGULATION IN RENAL CELL CARCINOMA

Much of our understanding of dysregulated tumor metabolism in RCCs comes from studies in ccRCCs. This is in part because ccRCCs, by virtue of their genetics (eg, loss of the von-Hippel Lindau protein [pVHL] and consequent chronic hypoxia inducible factor [HIF] activation unlinked from oxygen status, described below), are perhaps exemplars of dysregulated tumor metabolism. However, this is also in part because of our relative inattention to metabolic dysregulation in other RCC subtypes—representing an area that deserves careful future examination.

Aberrant Central Carbon Metabolism in Tumor Cells

Profound metabolic differences in carbon utilization exist between normal cells and their transformed cancerous counterparts. Whereas normal cells teeter toward maximal energy utilization and thus burn sugars (eg, glucose) using aerobic respiration, cancer cells

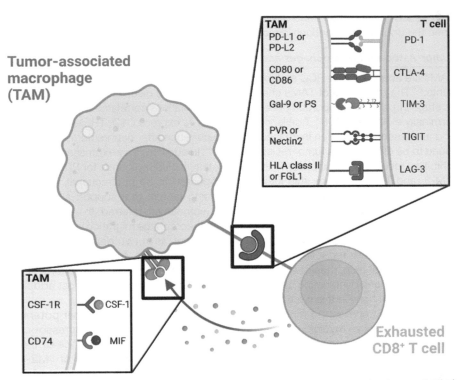

Fig. 2. A bidirectional "immune dysfunction circuit" in ccRCC. TAMs and exhausted CD8⁺ T cells form bidirectional interactions that inhibit effective anti-tumor immunity, with TAMs providing ligands for T-cell inhibitory receptors (*top right*), and CD8⁺ T cells producing ligands that support an immunosuppressive, "M2-like" TAM polarization (*bottom left*). TAM, tumor-associated macrophage.

dampen mitochondrial respiration, and instead use glycolytic and the tricarboxylic acid (TCA) cycle intermediates for biosynthetic processes. This switch, called the "Warburg effect" in honor of Nobel laureate Dr Otto Warburg, for his seminal observations describing this phenomenon in the 1950s,[52] is believed to support the cancer cell's perpetual need for basic building blocks. This model has exceptions, and recent data have not only suggested metabolic differences in primary versus metastatic tumors,[53] but also highlighted how the "landing-site" could impact the metabolic rewiring of tumors.[54] Thus, both the "seed" and the "soil" play a critical role in determining the metabolic state of tumor cells. The "Warburg effect," however, continues to inform our understanding of tumor metabolism and is supported by experimental evidence, including recent studies in ccRCC, using steady-state metabolomics and isotope-labeling strategies directly in patients,[55] which demonstrated that ccRCCs are glycolysis-avid solid tumors and display metabolic features consistent with the "Warburg effect."

Hypoxia Inducible Factor-Dependent Alterations in Central Carbon Metabolism

Mechanistically, the Warburg effect is strongly supported by HIF activation (**Fig. 3**A). Increased HIF activity promotes the uptake of glucose (via transporters, such as SLC2A1/GLUT1), increases glycolytic flux (via glycolytic enzymes, such as HK2, GAPDH, etc), produces reducing cofactors to sustain glycolysis (via conversion of pyruvate to lactate by LDH), and dampens mitochondrial respiration (via inhibition of

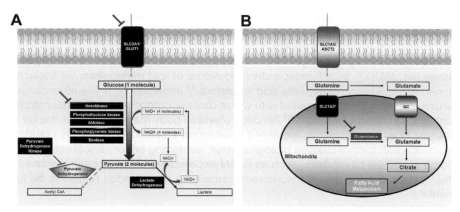

Fig. 3. Metabolic dependencies in kidney cancer. (*A*) Glucose uptake, mediated by glucose transporters (eg, SLC2A1/GLUT1), produces pyruvate and glycolytic intermediates that are precursors for other biomolecules and reducing equivalents (NADH). Conversion of pyruvate into lactate recycles NADH to its oxidized form, NAD+. HIF target genes (*black boxes*) act at various steps to channel metabolites into the cell and then into the appropriate pathways, which include an inhibition of pyruvate's conversion into acetyl-CoA. (*B*) Glutamine uptake into the cell and then into the mitochondria (*gray oval*) is mediated by 2 different variants of the SLC1A5 transporter (*mitochondrial variant). Glutaminase converts glutamine into glutamate and provides the precursors for citrate and fatty acids, via the reductive carboxylation pathway. In both (*A*) and (*B*), red inhibitory hammers mark potential nodes of therapeutic intervention.

mitochondrial pyruvate uptake).[56,57] Consistent with these findings, pVHL-deficient ccRCC cells exhibit increased glycolytic dependency. Inhibiting glycolysis, either by targeting glucose uptake[58] or glucose utilization via glycolysis, causes growth defects in ccRCC. Unfortunately, the biochemical/pharmacological properties of these molecules and, perhaps, their unintended impact on immune cells in the tumor microenvironment have limited their translation into effective drugs in renal cancer.

Nutrient Sensing as an Actionable Target in Kidney Cancer

Nutrient sensing pathways have been interrogated as an actionable dependency in kidney cancer. The mammalian target of rapamycin (mTOR), which is possibly the best known nutrient sensor in mammalian cells, is activated by a number of mechanisms in ccRCC, including (i) activating mutations in mTOR and PI3 kinase[59]; (ii) inactivating mutations in mTOR inhibitory proteins, including the phosphatase and tensin homologue lipid phosphatase and the tuberous sclerosis complex 1/2 (TSC1/2); (iii) elevated mTOR function via activating mutations in AKT1/2 (albeit at a low frequency in RCC); and, finally, (iv) activation of AKT1 in pVHL-deficient cells via hydroxylation-dependent signal-transduction cascade.[60] In summary, there is strong biological rationale to target mTOR in kidney cancer, and this continues to be deployed in treatment-refractory conditions for the clinical management of advanced ccRCC.

Fat Storage and the "Obesity Paradox"

"Clear cell" RCCs owe their name to the copious amounts of lipid deposition because of dysregulated lipid metabolism. Importantly, both HIF-dependent and independent processes have been implicated in this altered lipid metabolism. These include the HIF2α-dependent activation of the lipogenic protein perilipin 2 (PLIN2), which promotes intracellular lipid droplet accumulation,[61] and the HIF-dependent repression of the mitochondrial fatty acid transporter carnitine palmitoyltransferase 1A (CPT1A), which diminishes fatty acid transport into the mitochondria promoting the redirection of fatty acids into lipid storage.[62] However, recent studies have also pinned dioxygenases (eg, JMJD6), as HIF-independent regulators of lipid metabolism, via transcriptional reprogramming of key fatty acid regulators.[63] Interestingly, unlike other cancers where obesity is often associated with worse disease outcomes, renal cancer studies highlight an "obesity paradox."[64] Although elevated body mass index (as a marker for obesity) does associate with increased renal tumor incidence, obesity also tends to associate with a more indolent biological state, conferring better clinical outcomes.[65] Some molecular biomarkers, such as FASN expression,[64,65] have been identified in this context, but the overall mechanisms underlying this paradox remain to be fully clarified.

Dysregulated Amino Acid Metabolism in pVHL-Deficient Tumors

Amino acid dependencies are also altered in kidney cancer cells. Comparisons between isogenic pVHL-proficient and pVHL-deficient ccRCC cells (and more broadly HIF-activated hypoxic cells) have shown that unlike the standard "oxidative" TCA cycle, which drives conversion of 2-oxo-glutarate (2-OG) to succinate, HIF-activated cells shuttle 2-OG backwards (in the reductive direction) to form citrate, which is then utilized as a biosynthetic precursor to synthesize lipids.[66,67] This "reductive carboxylation" process confers actionable weaknesses in ccRCCs (**Fig. 3B**).

Biosynthesis of 2-OG occurs via conversion of glutamine (Gln) into glutamate (Glu) by the enzyme glutaminase, and then the conversion of glu to 2-OG. Blocking glutaminase activity diminishes 2-OG and intracellular citrate pools,[66] and thereby causes profound fitness defects in pVHL-deficient cells, thus rationalizing the use of glutaminase inhibitors in the clinic.[68] Unfortunately, although glutaminase inhibition appeared to have modest benefit in an early phase II trial (ENTRATA),[69] it failed to show benefit in a large phase III trial (CANTATA).[70] Some likely reasons of this failure could be (1) an inadvertent deleterious impact of glutaminase inhibitors on cells in the tumor microenvironment; or (2) the presence of alternative metabolic redundancies that overcome the functional consequences of glutaminase loss. Indeed, recent studies have found increased dependence of glutaminase-deficient cancers on cellular amido-transferases, suggesting that combined glutaminase/aminotransferase blockade could be feasible strategy to target renal cancer.[71]

Linking Epigenetic and Metabolic Dysfunction in Renal Cancer

Chromatin dysregulation is a recurrent feature of ccRCC. Somatic alterations in SWI/SNF regulators (eg, PBRM1)[72] or histone modifying enzymes (eg, KDM5C, KDM6A, etc.)[73] have all been reported. Interestingly, these JumonjiC-family histone demethylases (KDMs) are 2-OG-dependent enzymes, which can be competitively inhibited by the 2-OG analog 2-hydroxyglutarate (2-HG), a natural byproduct of certain metabolic enzymes. The R-enantiomer of 2-HG (R-2-HG) is now a well-studied oncometabolite, synthesized by cancer-associated mutants of the isocitrate dehydrogenase (IDH) enzyme.[74,75] S-2-HG (also called L-2-HG), however, is typically associated with metabolic perturbations triggered by environmental changes, especially hypoxia.[76–78] Interestingly, cellular clearance of L-2-HG is mediated by L-2-HG dehydrogenase (L2HGDH), which resides on 14q, a site of recurrent chromosomal loss in ccRCCs.[79] The consequent accumulation of L-2-HG in L2HGDH-deficient cells has been shown to drive oncogenesis by inactivating 2-OG-dependent tumor suppressors in ccRCC (eg, KDM6A).[79,80] Targeting the biochemical and consequent epigenetic perturbations triggered by excessive L-2-HG production in ccRCC could be an area of future therapeutic intervention.

Metabolic Dysregulation in the Tumor Microenvironment

The impact of genetic and epigenetic perturbations on metabolic pathways has been largely studied in cancer cells; however, the metabolic conditions within the TME can impact T-cell function (reviewed in ref.[81]). In ccRCC, nutrient uptake is partitioned, with infiltrating immune cells predominantly consuming glucose (highest in myeloid cells) and the tumor cells predominantly using glutamine.[82] Although bulk T cells may import more glucose than tumor cells, tumor-infiltrating CD8$^+$ T cells have impaired glucose uptake and diminished glycolysis upon activation, perhaps contributing to their dysfunctional state.[83] Further, the presence of other metabolites such as high kynurenine (relative to tryptophan), likely related to the expression of indoleamine 2,3 deoxygenase (IDO1), has been associated with ICI resistance in ccRCC.[84] Other immune metabolic pathways, such as the adenosine signaling pathway, may also play a role in immune cell function and clinical outcomes in ccRCC.[85] Additional studies are needed to link dysregulated metabolism to altered immune function in the TME, especially given the inherent differences in HIF function in tumor cells versus immune cells[86]; and, the role of 2-HG in regulating immune cell fate.[87] Ideal pharmacological agents would preferentially target oncogenic features in tumors, without having deleterious effects on immune cells in the microenvironment.

SUMMARY

A knowledge of RCC-specific immunobiology and metabolic dysregulation will be critical for the development of future therapeutics. Although RCC is historically and contemporarily immunogenic, conventional biomarkers of ICI response (eg, TMB, CD8$^+$ T-cell infiltration) are not predictive. ccRCC is a highly CD8$^+$ T-cell infiltrated tumor; yet, the specificity of these T cells is largely unknown. Further, in advanced disease, infiltrating T cells are typically exhausted, in part due to interactions with immunosuppressive TAMs. Metabolically, HIF-dependent and independent changes impact central carbon, amino acid, and lipid metabolism pathways. Unfortunately, strategies to pharmacologically target these metabolic changes have thus far failed in the clinic. The successful targeting of metabolic dependencies in ccRCC will not only require increased understanding of metabolic dependencies in tumor cells but also require an understanding of the impact of metabolic changes on the infiltrating immune cells and the TME.

CLINICS CARE POINTS

- In contrast to other tumors, TMB is not associated with improved ICI response in ccRCC.
- ccRCC has an abundant CD8$^+$ T-cell infiltration, but this alone is not predictive of ICI response.
- ccRCC has a heterogeneous microenvironment; future immunotherapy efforts will likely need to target additional immune components such as TAMs.
- Chronic HIF activation is a hallmark feature of ccRCC, and contributes to metabolic dysregulation.
- Numerous metabolic alterations in ccRCC, such as a reliance on glycolysis, lipid accumulation, and glutamine metabolism, may create opportunities for therapeutically targeting such dependencies.

DISCLOSURE

D.A. Braun reports honoraria from LM Education/Exchange Services, advisory board fees from Exelixis and AVEO, personal fees from Schlesinger Associates, Cancer Expert Now, Adnovate Strategies, MDedge, CancerNetwork, Catenion, OncLive, Cello Health BioConsulting, PWW Consulting, Haymarket Medical Network, Aptitude Health, ASCO Post/Harborside, Targeted Oncology, AbbVie, and research support from Exelixis, United States and AstraZeneca, United Kingdom, outside of the submitted work. A.A. Chakraborty reports no conflict of interest.

ACKNOWLEDGMENTS

D.A. Braun acknowledges support from the Dept of Defense Early Career Investigator grant (KCRP AKCI-ECI, W81XWH-20-1-0882), the Louis Goodman and Alfred Gilman Yale Scholar Fund, and the Yale Cancer Center, United States (supported by NIH, United States/NCI research grant P30CA016359). A.A. Chakraborty is supported by seed money from the Cleveland Clinic Foundation, United States, the V Foundation Scholar award (V2020–011), a Dept of Defense Early Career Investigator grant (KCRP AKCI-ECI, W81XWH-20-1-0804), an NCCN Young Investigator Award (2022), and an American Cancer Society Research Scholar Grant (RSG-22-067-01-TBE). **Figs. 1** and **2** were created using BioRender.com.

REFERENCES

1. Negrier S, Escudier B, Lasset C, et al. Recombinant human interleukin-2, recombinant human interferon alfa-2a, or both in metastatic renal-cell carcinoma. Groupe Francais d'Immunotherapie. N Engl J Med 1998;338:1272–8.

2. Atkins MB, Kunkel L, Sznol M, et al. High-dose recombinant interleukin-2 therapy in patients with metastatic melanoma: long-term survival update. Cancer J Sci Am 2000;6(Suppl 1):S11–4.

3. McDermott DF, Cheng SC, Signoretti S, et al. The high-dose aldesleukin "select" trial: a trial to prospectively validate predictive models of response to treatment in patients with metastatic renal cell carcinoma. Clin Cancer Res 2015;21:561–8.

4. Motzer RJ, Tannir NM, McDermott DF, et al. Nivolumab plus Ipilimumab versus Sunitinib in Advanced Renal-Cell Carcinoma. N Engl J Med 2018;378:1277–90.

5. Rini BI, Plimack ER, Stus V, et al. Pembrolizumab plus Axitinib versus Sunitinib for Advanced Renal-Cell Carcinoma. N Engl J Med 2019;380:1116–27.

6. Choueiri TK, Powles T, Burotto M, et al. Nivolumab plus Cabozantinib versus Sunitinib for Advanced Renal-Cell Carcinoma. N Engl J Med 2021;384:829–41.

7. Motzer R, Alekseev B, Rha SY, et al. Lenvatinib plus Pembrolizumab or Everolimus for Advanced Renal Cell Carcinoma. N Engl J Med 2021;384:1289–300.

8. Motzer RJ, Penkov K, Haanen J, et al. Avelumab plus Axitinib versus Sunitinib for Advanced Renal-Cell Carcinoma. N Engl J Med 2019;380:1103–15.

9. Lawrence MS, Stojanov P, Polak P, et al. Mutational heterogeneity in cancer and the search for new cancer-associated genes. Nature 2013;499:214–8.

10. Samstein RM, Lee CH, Shoushtari AN, et al. Tumor mutational load predicts survival after immunotherapy across multiple cancer types. Nat Genet 2019;51:202–6.

11. Braun DA, Hou Y, Bakouny Z, et al. Interplay of somatic alterations and immune infiltration modulates response to PD-1 blockade in advanced clear cell renal cell carcinoma. Nat Med 2020;26:909–18.

12. Fridman WH, Zitvogel L, Sautes-Fridman C, et al. The immune contexture in cancer prognosis and treatment. Nat Rev Clin Oncol 2017;14:717–34.
13. Giraldo NA, Becht E, Pages F, et al. Orchestration and Prognostic Significance of Immune Checkpoints in the Microenvironment of Primary and Metastatic Renal Cell Cancer. Clin Cancer Res 2015;21:3031–40.
14. Geissler K, Fornara P, Lautenschlager C, et al. Immune signature of tumor infiltrating immune cells in renal cancer. OncoImmunology 2015;4:e985082.
15. Nakano O, Sato M, Naito Y, et al. Proliferative activity of intratumoral CD8(+) T-lymphocytes as a prognostic factor in human renal cell carcinoma: clinicopathologic demonstration of antitumor immunity. Cancer Res 2001;61:5132–6.
16. Rooney MS, Shukla SA, Wu CJ, et al. Molecular and genetic properties of tumors associated with local immune cytolytic activity. Cell 2015;160:48–61.
17. Senbabaoglu Y, Gejman RS, Winer AG, et al. Tumor immune microenvironment characterization in clear cell renal cell carcinoma identifies prognostic and immunotherapeutically relevant messenger RNA signatures. Genome Biol 2016; 17:231.
18. Chen DS, Mellman I. Elements of cancer immunity and the cancer-immune set point. Nature 2017;541:321–30.
19. Mariathasan S, Turley SJ, Nickles D, et al. TGFbeta attenuates tumour response to PD-L1 blockade by contributing to exclusion of T cells. Nature 2018;554:544–8.
20. Bakouny Z, Braun DA, Shukla SA, et al. Integrative molecular characterization of sarcomatoid and rhabdoid renal cell carcinoma. Nat Commun 2021;12:808.
21. Giraldo NA, Becht E, Vano Y, et al. Tumor-Infiltrating and Peripheral Blood T-cell Immunophenotypes Predict Early Relapse in Localized Clear Cell Renal Cell Carcinoma. Clin Cancer Res 2017;23:4416–28.
22. Braun DA, Street K, Burke KP, et al. Progressive immune dysfunction with advancing disease stage in renal cell carcinoma. Cancer Cell 2021;39: 632–48.e8.
23. Chevrier S, Levine JH, Zanotelli VRT, et al. An Immune Atlas of Clear Cell Renal Cell Carcinoma. Cell 2017;169:736–749 e18.
24. Scheper W, Kelderman S, Fanchi LF, et al. Low and variable tumor reactivity of the intratumoral TCR repertoire in human cancers. Nat Med 2019;25:89–94.
25. Simoni Y, Becht E, Fehlings M, et al. Bystander CD8(+) T cells are abundant and phenotypically distinct in human tumour infiltrates. Nature 2018;557:575–9.
26. Ficial M, Jegede OA, Sant'Angelo M, et al. Expression of T-Cell Exhaustion Molecules and Human Endogenous Retroviruses as Predictive Biomarkers for Response to Nivolumab in Metastatic Clear Cell Renal Cell Carcinoma. Clin Cancer Res 2021;27:1371–80.
27. Pignon JC, Jegede O, Shukla SA, et al. irRECIST for the Evaluation of Candidate Biomarkers of Response to Nivolumab in Metastatic Clear Cell Renal Cell Carcinoma: Analysis of a Phase II Prospective Clinical Trial. Clin Cancer Res 2019;25: 2174–84.
28. Remark R, Alifano M, Cremer I, et al. Characteristics and clinical impacts of the immune environments in colorectal and renal cell carcinoma lung metastases: influence of tumor origin. Clin Cancer Res 2013;19:4079–91.
29. Terren I, Orrantia A, Mikelez-Alonso I, et al. NK Cell-Based Immunotherapy in Renal Cell Carcinoma. Cancers 2020;12.
30. Meylan M, Petitprez F, Becht E, et al. Tertiary lymphoid structures generate and propagate anti-tumor antibody-producing plasma cells in renal cell cancer. Immunity 2022;55:527–541 e5.

31. Albiges L, Tannir NM, Burotto M, et al. Nivolumab plus ipilimumab versus sunitinib for first-line treatment of advanced renal cell carcinoma: extended 4-year follow-up of the phase III CheckMate 214 trial. ESMO Open 2020;5:e001079.

32. Braun DA, Bakouny Z, Hirsch L, et al. Beyond conventional immune-checkpoint inhibition - novel immunotherapies for renal cell carcinoma. Nat Rev Clin Oncol 2021;18:199–214.

33. Cai C, Xu YF, Wu ZJ, et al. Tim-3 expression represents dysfunctional tumor infiltrating T cells in renal cell carcinoma. World J Urol 2016;34:561–7.

34. Zelba H, Bedke J, Hennenlotter J, et al. PD-1 and LAG-3 Dominate Checkpoint Receptor-Mediated T-cell Inhibition in Renal Cell Carcinoma. Cancer Immunol Res 2019;7:1891–9.

35. Hong S, Yuan Q, Xia H, et al. Analysis of VISTA expression and function in renal cell carcinoma highlights VISTA as a potential target for immunotherapy. Protein Cell 2019;10:840–5.

36. Chen D, Chen W, Xu Y, et al. Upregulated immune checkpoint HHLA2 in clear cell renal cell carcinoma: a novel prognostic biomarker and potential therapeutic target. J Med Genet 2019;56:43–9.

37. Au L, Hatipoglu E, Robert de Massy M, et al. Determinants of anti-PD-1 response and resistance in clear cell renal cell carcinoma. Cancer Cell 2021;39: 1497–518.e11.

38. Walter S, Weinschenk T, Stenzl A, et al. Multipeptide immune response to cancer vaccine IMA901 after single-dose cyclophosphamide associates with longer patient survival. Nat Med 2012;18:1254–61.

39. Rini BI, Stenzl A, Zdrojowy R, et al. IMA901, a multipeptide cancer vaccine, plus sunitinib versus sunitinib alone, as first-line therapy for advanced or metastatic renal cell carcinoma (IMPRINT): a multicentre, open-label, randomised, controlled, phase 3 trial. Lancet Oncol 2016;17:1599–611.

40. Hansen UK, Ramskov S, Bjerregaard AM, et al. Tumor-Infiltrating T Cells From Clear Cell Renal Cell Carcinoma Patients Recognize Neoepitopes Derived From Point and Frameshift Mutations. Front Immunol 2020;11:373.

41. Childs R, Chernoff A, Contentin N, et al. Regression of metastatic renal-cell carcinoma after nonmyeloablative allogeneic peripheral-blood stem-cell transplantation. N Engl J Med 2000;343:750–8.

42. Takahashi Y, Harashima N, Kajigaya S, et al. Regression of human kidney cancer following allogeneic stem cell transplantation is associated with recognition of an HERV-E antigen by T cells. J Clin Invest 2008;118:1099–109.

43. Smith CC, Beckermann KE, Bortone DS, et al. Endogenous retroviral signatures predict immunotherapy response in clear cell renal cell carcinoma. J Clin Invest 2018;128:4804–20.

44. Panda A, de Cubas AA, Stein M, et al. Endogenous retrovirus expression is associated with response to immune checkpoint blockade in clear cell renal cell carcinoma. JCI Insight 2018;3.

45. Obradovic A, Chowdhury N, Haake SM, et al. Single-cell protein activity analysis identifies recurrence-associated renal tumor macrophages. Cell 2021;184: 2988–3005.e16.

46. Krishna C, DiNatale RG, Kuo F, et al. Single-cell sequencing links multiregional immune landscapes and tissue-resident T cells in ccRCC to tumor topology and therapy efficacy. Cancer Cell 2021;39:662–77.e6.

47. Kersten K, Hu KH, Combes AJ, et al. Spatiotemporal co-dependency between macrophages and exhausted CD8(+) T cells in cancer. Cancer Cell 2022;40: 624–38.e9.

48. Aggen DH, Ager CR, Obradovic AZ, et al. Blocking IL1 Beta Promotes Tumor Regression and Remodeling of the Myeloid Compartment in a Renal Cell Carcinoma Model: Multidimensional Analyses. Clin Cancer Res 2021;27:608–21.
49. Yuen KC, Liu LF, Gupta V, et al. High systemic and tumor-associated IL-8 correlates with reduced clinical benefit of PD-L1 blockade. Nat Med 2020;26:693–8.
50. Schalper KA, Carleton M, Zhou M, et al. Elevated serum interleukin-8 is associated with enhanced intratumor neutrophils and reduced clinical benefit of immune-checkpoint inhibitors. Nat Med 2020;26:688–92.
51. Jansen CS, Prokhnevska N, Master VA, et al. An intra-tumoral niche maintains and differentiates stem-like CD8 T cells. Nature 2019;576:465–70.
52. Warburg O. On respiratory impairment in cancer cells. Science 1956;124:269–70.
53. Bartman CR, Weilandt DR, Shen Y, et al. Slow TCA flux and ATP production in primary solid tumours but not metastases. Nature 2023;614(7947):349–57.
54. Sullivan MR, Danai LV, Lewis CA, et al. Quantification of microenvironmental metabolites in murine cancers reveals determinants of tumor nutrient availability. Elife 2019;8.
55. Courtney KD, Bezwada D, Mashimo T, et al. Isotope Tracing of Human Clear Cell Renal Cell Carcinomas Demonstrates Suppressed Glucose Oxidation In Vivo. Cell Metab 2018;28:793–800 e2.
56. Kim JW, Tchernyshyov I, Semenza GL, et al. HIF-1-mediated expression of pyruvate dehydrogenase kinase: a metabolic switch required for cellular adaptation to hypoxia. Cell Metab 2006;3:177–85.
57. Papandreou I, Cairns RA, Fontana L, et al. HIF-1 mediates adaptation to hypoxia by actively downregulating mitochondrial oxygen consumption. Cell Metab 2006; 3:187–97.
58. Chan DA, Sutphin PD, Nguyen P, et al. Targeting GLUT1 and the Warburg effect in renal cell carcinoma by chemical synthetic lethality. Sci Transl Med 2011;3: 94ra70.
59. Cancer Genome Atlas Research N. Comprehensive molecular characterization of clear cell renal cell carcinoma. Nature 2013;499:43–9.
60. Guo J, Chakraborty AA, Liu P, et al. pVHL suppresses kinase activity of Akt in a proline-hydroxylation-dependent manner. Science 2016;353:929–32.
61. Qiu B, Ackerman D, Sanchez DJ, et al. HIF2alpha-Dependent Lipid Storage Promotes Endoplasmic Reticulum Homeostasis in Clear-Cell Renal Cell Carcinoma. Cancer Discov 2015;5:652–67.
62. Du W, Zhang L, Brett-Morris A, et al. HIF drives lipid deposition and cancer in ccRCC via repression of fatty acid metabolism. Nat Commun 2017;8:1769.
63. Zhou J, Simon JM, Liao C, et al. An oncogenic JMJD6-DGAT1 axis tunes the epigenetic regulation of lipid droplet formation in clear cell renal cell carcinoma. Mol Cell 2022;82:3030–44.e8.
64. Albiges L, Hakimi AA, Xie W, et al. Body Mass Index and Metastatic Renal Cell Carcinoma: Clinical and Biological Correlations. J Clin Oncol 2016;34:3655–63.
65. Hakimi AA, Furberg H, Zabor EC, et al. An epidemiologic and genomic investigation into the obesity paradox in renal cell carcinoma. J Natl Cancer Inst 2013;105: 1862–70.
66. Gameiro PA, Yang J, Metelo AM, et al. In vivo HIF-mediated reductive carboxylation is regulated by citrate levels and sensitizes VHL-deficient cells to glutamine deprivation. Cell Metab 2013;17:372–85.
67. Metallo CM, Gameiro PA, Bell EL, et al. Reductive glutamine metabolism by IDH1 mediates lipogenesis under hypoxia. Nature 2011;481:380–4.

68. Meric-Bernstam F, Tannir NM, Iliopoulos O, et al. Telaglenastat Plus Cabozantinib or Everolimus for Advanced or Metastatic Renal Cell Carcinoma: An Open-Label Phase I Trial. Clin Cancer Res 2022;28:1540–8.

69. Lee CH, Motzer R, Emamekhoo H, et al. Telaglenastat plus Everolimus in Advanced Renal Cell Carcinoma: A Randomized, Double-Blinded, Placebo-Controlled, Phase II ENTRATA Trial. Clin Cancer Res 2022;28:3248–55.

70. Tannir NM, Agarwal N, Porta C, et al. Efficacy and Safety of Telaglenastat Plus Cabozantinib vs Placebo Plus Cabozantinib in Patients With Advanced Renal Cell Carcinoma: The CANTATA Randomized Clinical Trial. JAMA Oncol 2022;8: 1411–8.

71. Kaushik AK, Tarangelo A, Boroughs LK, et al. In vivo characterization of glutamine metabolism identifies therapeutic targets in clear cell renal cell carcinoma. Sci Adv 2022;8:eabp8293.

72. Varela I, Tarpey P, Raine K, et al. Exome sequencing identifies frequent mutation of the SWI/SNF complex gene PBRM1 in renal carcinoma. Nature 2011;469: 539–42.

73. Dalgliesh GL, Furge K, Greenman C, et al. Systematic sequencing of renal carcinoma reveals inactivation of histone modifying genes. Nature 2010;463:360–3.

74. Dang L, White DW, Gross S, et al. Cancer-associated IDH1 mutations produce 2-hydroxyglutarate. Nature 2009;462:739–44.

75. Figueroa ME, Abdel-Wahab O, Lu C, et al. Leukemic IDH1 and IDH2 mutations result in a hypermethylation phenotype, disrupt TET2 function, and impair hematopoietic differentiation. Cancer Cell 2010;18:553–67.

76. Intlekofer AM, Dematteo RG, Venneti S, et al. Hypoxia Induces Production of L-2-Hydroxyglutarate. Cell Metab 2015;22:304–11.

77. Oldham WM, Clish CB, Yang Y, et al. Hypoxia-Mediated Increases in L-2-hydroxyglutarate Coordinate the Metabolic Response to Reductive Stress. Cell Metab 2015;22:291–303.

78. Intlekofer AM, Wang B, Liu H, et al. L-2-Hydroxyglutarate production arises from noncanonical enzyme function at acidic pH. Nat Chem Biol 2017;13:494–500.

79. Shim EH, Livi CB, Rakheja D, et al. L-2-Hydroxyglutarate: an epigenetic modifier and putative oncometabolite in renal cancer. Cancer Discov 2014;4:1290–8.

80. Shelar S, Shim EH, Brinkley GJ, et al. Biochemical and Epigenetic Insights into L-2-Hydroxyglutarate, a Potential Therapeutic Target in Renal Cancer. Clin Cancer Res 2018;24:6433–46.

81. Chang CH, Pearce EL. Emerging concepts of T cell metabolism as a target of immunotherapy. Nat Immunol 2016;17:364–8.

82. Reinfeld BI, Madden MZ, Wolf MM, et al. Cell-programmed nutrient partitioning in the tumour microenvironment. Nature 2021;593:282–8.

83. Siska PJ, Beckermann KE, Mason FM, et al. Mitochondrial dysregulation and glycolytic insufficiency functionally impair CD8 T cells infiltrating human renal cell carcinoma. JCI Insight 2017;2.

84. Li H, Bullock K, Gurjao C, et al. Metabolomic adaptations and correlates of survival to immune checkpoint blockade. Nat Commun 2019;10:4346.

85. Song L, Ye W, Cui Y, et al. Ecto-5'-nucleotidase (CD73) is a biomarker for clear cell renal carcinoma stem-like cells. Oncotarget 2017;8:31977–92.

86. Cowman SJ, Fuja DG, Liu XD, et al. Macrophage HIF-1alpha Is an Independent Prognostic Indicator in Kidney Cancer. Clin Cancer Res 2020;26:4970–82.

87. Tyrakis PA, Palazon A, Macias D, et al. S-2-hydroxyglutarate regulates CD8+ T-lymphocyte fate. Nature 2016;540:236–41.

Hereditary Renal Cell Carcinoma Syndromes

Maria I. Carlo, MD

KEYWORDS

- Genetic testing • Genetic risk • Hereditary renal cell carcinoma • Von hippel-lindau
- Hereditary leiomyomatosis and renal cell carcinoma • Fumarate hydratase
- BAP1-Tumor predisposition syndrome • Birt–Hogg–Dubé

KEY POINTS

- Hereditary renal cell carcinoma (RCC) syndromes have variable clinical characteristics and a spectrum of risk for RCC.
- Several expert consensus guidelines recommend genetic evaluation for individuals with RCC and early age of onset, family history of RCC, or multifocal disease.
- Renal imaging, preferably MRI, is recommended for early detection in individuals diagnosed with RCC syndromes.

INTRODUCTION

Approximately 5% of renal cell carcinomas (RCCs) are associated with a known hereditary RCC syndrome.[1] In the last 2 decades, several new RCC hereditary syndromes have been described, and our knowledge of the clinical phenotype of these syndromes has expanded. Still, most of the familial RCC likely remains unexplained. Most of the established RCC syndromes are inherited in an autosomal dominant fashion. With the exception of hereditary papillary RCC syndrome (caused by activating mutations in the *MET* oncogene), the RCC syndromes are caused by mutations in tumor suppressor genes and thought to require a "second-hit" in the wild-type allele to lead to disease. What follows is a discussion of germline genetic evaluation for patients with RCC, a summary of the known and emerging hereditary RCC syndromes, and their clinical implications.

CRITERIA FOR GENETIC EVALUATION OF PATIENTS WITH RENAL CELL CARCINOMA

There are several consensus guidelines that delineate which clinical features should prompt referral for genetic evaluation. The National Comprehensive Cancer Network (NCCN) and American Urologic Association both recommend genetic evaluation for

Genitourinary Oncology Service, Clinical Genetics Service, Memorial Sloan Kettering Cancer Center, 353 East 68th Street. New York, NY 10065, USA
E-mail address: carlom@mskcc.org

Hematol Oncol Clin N Am 37 (2023) 841–848
https://doi.org/10.1016/j.hoc.2023.04.013
0889-8588/23/© 2023 Elsevier Inc. All rights reserved.

hemonc.theclinics.com

individuals diagnosed with RCC (1) at early onset, defined as age 46 years and under, (2) with a family history of RCC, (3) with multifocal or bilateral renal masses, or (4) suspicious histologies.[2,3] Suspicious histologies can include fumarate hydratase (FH)-deficient RCC, succinate dehydrogenase (SDH)-deficient RCC, or hybrid oncocytic/chromophobe, which are associated with germline variants in the *FH*, *SDHB*, and *FLCN* genes, respectively. Testing is also recommended for individuals with additional clinical features of a known hereditary syndrome. Although some syndromes can be highly penetrant with very apparent clinical features, such as Von Hippel–Lindau (VHL) syndrome, others can have a more subtle clinical presentation and keeping a high index of suspicion is important.

ESTABLISHED RENAL CELL CARCINOMA HEREDITARY SYNDROMES AND CLINICAL PRESENTATION

Fumarate Hydratase-Tumor Predisposition Syndrome (Previously Known as Hereditary Leiomyomatosis and Renal Cell Carcinoma Syndrome)

FH-tumor predisposition syndrome is caused by germline variants in the *fumarate hydratase* gene, which encodes for the Krebs cycle enzyme of the same name. Individuals have an increased risk of a type of RCC known as FH-deficient RCC, cutaneous leiomyomas, and uterine leiomyomas (fibroids) in women. The estimated lifetime risk of RCC is unclear, but more recent studies suggest an approximately 15% risk.[4] Nevertheless, these tumors can be aggressive even at a small size, so radical nephrectomy should be considered. There also seems to be an increased risk of pheochromocytoma/paraganglioma in carriers of certain *FH* variants.[5] Of note, the common FH c.1431_1433dupAAA (*P.Lys477dup*) variant has not associated with cancer in the heterozygous state.[6]

Von Hippel–Lindau Syndrome

VHL syndrome is a highly penetrant tumor predisposition syndrome caused by germline variants in the *VHL* gene. VHL acts as an E3 ubiquitin ligase that in normal oxygen states targets the alpha subunit of hypoxia-inducible factor (HIF) for degradation. VHL syndrome is characterized by hemangioblastomas of the central nervous system, pheochromocytomas, renal and pancreatic cysts, pancreatic neuroendocrine tumors, and clear cell RCC. Other rare tumors include endolymphatic sac tumors and epididymal and broad ligament cysts. *De novo* variants are not uncommon, so patients may lack a family history of VHL-associated disease. The care of patients with VHL syndrome is multidisciplinary and requires careful follow-up of multiple organs (The VHL Alliance: https://www.vhl.org/ Accessed on January 30, 2023). The care of patients with VHL has been revolutionized with the Food and Drug Administration (FDA)-approval of belzutifan, an HIF2alpha inhibitor. The landmark LITESPARK-004 study led to the approval of this agent in patients with RCC and other tumors associated with VHL disease that require therapy, but not immediate surgery.[7] This was a single-arm, phase 2 study, in which patients with RCC and VHL disease were given belzutifan 120 mg daily. The objective response was 49%, with responses also observed in patients with pancreatic lesions, central nervous system hemangioblastomas, and retinal hemangioblastomas. Most common adverse events include anemia, fatigue, and headaches. An updated analysis with more extended follow-up showed a response rate of 64% in RCC lesions.[8]

Birt–Hogg–Dubé Syndrome

Birt–Hogg–Dubé (BHD) syndrome is caused by germline variants in the *folliculin* (*FLCN*) gene. Patients with BHD have a high prevalence of pulmonary cysts, which are mostly in the basal lung regions in the intrapulmonary and subpleural areas, and are at higher risk of pneumothorax. They can have characteristic facial fibrofolliculomas, which can be subtle, and the lack of apparent lesions should not exclude BHD. The full phenotypic spectrum and cancer prevalences in *FLCN* germline carriers remain to be clarified. For example, case series have reported colon polyps and other cancers in *FLCN* carriers, but it remains to be seen whether these are linked to *FLCN* or sporadic.[9]

BAP1-Tumor Predisposition Syndrome

BAP1-tumor predisposition syndrome is caused by germline variants in the *BAP1* gene, which codes for a deubiquitinating enzyme and acts as a tumor suppressor. Individuals with germline BRCA1 associated protein-1 (BAP1) mutations are at increased risk of melanoma, uveal melanoma, mesothelioma (both peritoneal and pleural), and RCC. Individuals also are predisposed to skin lesions called BAP1-inactivated melanocytic tumors, and these can be the first sign of the syndrome.[10] The penetrance of *BAP1* has not been well established, but from described case series, it seems to be relatively high for having at least one of the related cancers.[11]

Hereditary Paraganglioma–Pheochromocytoma Syndrome

Hereditary paraganglioma–pheochromocytoma syndrome is caused by germline variants in *SDHB, SDHC, SDHD, SDHA, SDHAF2, MAX,* or *TMEM127.* In particular, carriers of *SDHB* germline variants are also at an increased risk of a type of RCC known as SDH-deficient RCC. SDH-deficient RCC can have unique histologic features, and the diagnosis is confirmed by the lack of SDHB staining on immunohistochemistry.[12] The association between germline *SDHB* mutations and increased RCC risk has been well established with an estimated lifetime risk of RCC of 5%.[13] SDHB-deficient RCCs can occur at young ages and can be aggressive warranting careful surveillance.

The association of other SDH complex genes (*SDHA, SDHC, SDHD,* and *SDHAF2*) with RCC is not well established. There are case reports of patients with one of these germline mutations and RCC, but not, to our knowledge, any reported SDH-deficient RCCs in carriers of non-SDHB variants.[14,15] Nevertheless, these variants still predispose to hereditary pheochromocytomas/paragangliomas and gastrointestinal stromal tumor (GISTs), so there is a presumed increased risk of RCC as well, and expert consensus recommend screening with a similar protocol to SDHB.[16]

Hereditary Papillary Renal Cell Carcinoma

Hereditary papillary RCC is a very rare syndrome that predisposes to multifocal papillary RCCs and is caused by germline *MET* activating mutations.[17] There are no known extrarenal manifestations. Agents that target the MET pathway in hereditary and sporadic RCC have substantial activity. In a phase 2 trial testing foretinib, a multikinase MET inhibitor, in papillary RCC with *MET* alterations, the ORR was 13.5%, but germline *MET* mutations were highly predictive of response (50% vs 9%).[18] The role of MET alterations as a biomarker is being further studied in clinical trials.

PTEN Hamartoma Tumor Syndrome (Cowden)

Individuals with PTEN Hamartoma Tumor syndrome, caused by loss-of-function variants in *PTEN,* are at an increased risk of RCC. The major clinical characteristics are macrocephaly, breast, endometrial, and thyroid cancer, but RCC is a minor criterion in the clinical diagnosis. This syndrome is rare, and the precise lifetime RCC risk estimates are unknown with reported ranges from 2% to 24%.[19,20] Multiple RCC

Table 1
Additional selected genes with possible increased renal cell carcinoma risk

Gene	Evidence
MITF	• The *MITF* E318 K variant has been associated with a fivefold increased risk of developing melanoma and/or RCC; no evidence for other mutations.[28] • The histology of *MITF* E318 K mutated RCCs has been variable with papillary type 1 and clear cell histology noted in case series.[9,29] • The *MITF* E318 K is not frequent in patients with sporadic RCC; in one retrospective series of 403 RCCs, there was only one tumor with the variant.[29]
CDC73	• Associated with hyperparathyroidism-jaw tumor syndrome, which predisposes to hyperparathyroidism from adenomas, or rarely, carcinomas, and ossifying fibromas of the mandible or maxilla; about 20% of individuals can have renal lesions, mainly cysts.[30] • There are reported cases of renal malignancies include a family with mixed epithelial and stromal tumor of the kidney (MEST).[31,32]
TMEM127	• Associated with hereditary pheochromocytomas and paragangliomas, but reports have also identified potential increased risk of RCC.[33]
PBRM1	• One report from Benusuglio et al described a proband with a strong family history of RCC and a germline frameshift variant that co-segregated to those with RCC.[34] • *PBRM1* germline variants have not been systematically analyzed in large cohorts, so it remains to be seen whether this is a recurrent cause of unexplained familial RCC.
Elongin C (ELOC)/ TCEB	• One report on a novel germline *ELOC* (also known as *TCEB1*) variant in an individual with bilateral RCC, retinal angiomas, and multiple hemangioblastomas.[35] • ELOC-mutated RCC was recognized in the 2022 World Health Classification of renal tumors and these can have morphologies similar to clear cell RCC, but lack the typical VHL mutations and 3p loss, and instead have chromosome 8p loss in addition to the ELOC mutations.[36]
CDKN2B	• In an exome sequencing study of a proband with unexplained familial RCC, a germline truncating variant in *CDKN2B* was identified, with co-segregation in affected relatives.[37] Additional missense *CDKN2B* variants were identified in a cohort of individuals with non-syndromic, familial RCC.

histologies have been reported, but mostly chromophobe and papillary RCC.[21,22] Currently, NCCN criteria recommend screening renal imaging starting at age 40 years; however, some have suggested starting screening earlier given several reports of early-onset RCC.[20,23,24]

Tuberous Sclerosis Complex

Tuberous sclerosis complex (TSC) is a hereditary syndrome caused by loss-of-function variants in *TSC1* or *TSC2* and can affect multiple organs, including brain, skin, heart, and kidneys.[25] Most patients with TSC will develop renal angiomyolipomas during their lifetime, and they can start in childhood. There seems to be an increased risk of RCC, with an estimated 2% to 3% lifetime incidence, and more recently, distinct morphologic spectrums of TSC-associated RCC have been described (**Table 1**).[26,27]

Table 2
Screening interval for lindividuals with RCC syndromes without personal history of RCC

Syndrome	Gene	Imaging Interval[3]	Age to Start Screening[a]
HLRCC	FH	Yearly	8–10
VHL	VHL	Every 2 y	15
Birt–Hogg–Dubé	FLCN	Every 3 y	20
BAP1-tumor predisposition	BAP1	Every 2 y	20
Hereditary pheochromocytoma/ paraganglioma syndrome	SDHB and other SDHx genes	Every 4–6[b] years	12
Hereditary papillary RCC	MET	Every 1–2 y	30
Cowden	PTEN	Every 1–2 y	40 (consider starting earlier)
Tuberous sclerosis	TSC1/2	Every 3–5 y	12

[a] Or 10 y before earliest age of diagnosis in a family member, whichever comes first.
[b] Patients with SDHB and other SDH genes are recommended to undergo more frequent abdominal screening for pheochromocytomas/paragangliomas, which also include the abdominal imaging.

SCREENING GUIDELINES

The NCCN and other expert consensus statements have suggested imaging intervals for screening for RCC in unaffected individuals diagnosed with an RCC syndrome (**Table 2**). For all syndromes, MRI is the preferred modality to minimize lifetime radiation exposure but preserve resolution. Other modalities such as CT and ultrasound can be considered on an individual basis.

SUMMARY

In the last few years, progress has been made in the characterization of hereditary RCC syndromes, development of targeted treatments, and establishment of guidelines on who should be referred for genetic evaluation and what screening should be done. Still, much work is needed—guidelines are still mostly based on expert opinion and the role of emerging genetic associations needs to be clarified.

FUNDING

NCI P30 Cancer Center Support Grant (CCSG) (P30 CA008748). Robert Wood Johnson Harold Amos Faculty Development Award.

CLINICS CARE POINTS

- The National Comprehensive Cancer Network and American Urologic Association recommend genetic evaluation for individuals diagnosed with renal cell carcinoma (RCC) (1) at early onset, defined as age 46 years and under, (2) with a family history of RCC, (3) with multifocal or bilateral renal masses, or (4) suspicious histologies.
- Individuals with hereditary RCC syndromes, unaffected by cancer, should be referred for renal imaging for early detection.

- Most hereditary RCC syndromes have multiorgan manifestations and should be managed by multidisciplinary groups.
- There are multiple emerging RCC risk alleles, including *MITF* E318 K variant.

REFERENCES

1. Huang K, Mashl RJ, Wu Y, et al. Pathogenic germline variants in 10,389 adult cancers. Cell 2018;173(2):355–70.e14.
2. Campbell SC, Clark PE, Chang SS, et al. Renal Mass and Localized Renal Cancer: Evaluation, Management, and Follow-Up: AUA Guideline: Part I. J Urol 2021; 206(2):199–208.
3. Motzer RJ, Jonasch E, Agarwal N, et al. Kidney Cancer, Version 3.2022, NCCN Clinical Practice Guidelines in Oncology. J Natl Compr Cancer Netw JNCCN 2022;20(1):71–90.
4. Muller M, Ferlicot S, Guillaud-Bataille M, et al. Reassessing the clinical spectrum associated with hereditary leiomyomatosis and renal cell carcinoma syndrome in French FH mutation carriers. Clin Genet 2017;92(6):606–15.
5. Zavoshi S, Lu E, Boutros PC, et al. Fumarate Hydratase Variants and their Association with Paraganglioma/Pheochromocytoma. Urology 2023;S0090-4295(23): 00054-7.
6. Zhang L, Walsh MF, Jairam S, et al. Fumarate hydratase FH c.1431_1433dupAAA (p.Lys477dup) variant is not associated with cancer including renal cell carcinoma. Hum Mutat 2020;41(1):103–9.
7. Jonasch E, Donskov F, Iliopoulos O, et al. Belzutifan for Renal Cell Carcinoma in von Hippel-Lindau Disease. N Engl J Med 2021;385(22):2036–46.
8. Srinivasan R, Iliopoulos O, Rathmell WK, et al. LBA69 - Belzutifan, a HIF-2α Inhibitor, for von Hippel-Lindau (VHL) disease-associated neoplasms: 36 months of follow-up of the phase II LITESPARK-004 study. Ann Oncol 2022;33(Suppl7): S808–69, 101016annoncannonc1089.
9. Gupta S, Erickson LA, Lohse CM, et al. Assessment of risk of hereditary predisposition in patients with melanoma and/or mesothelioma and renal neoplasia. JAMA Netw Open 2021;4(11):e2132615.
10. Haugh AM, Njauw CN, Bubley JA, et al. Genotypic and Phenotypic Features of BAP1 Cancer Syndrome: A Report of 8 New Families and Review of Cases in the Literature. JAMA Dermatol 2017;153(10):999–1006.
11. Walpole S, Pritchard AL, Cebulla CM, et al. Comprehensive Study of the Clinical Phenotype of Germline *BAP1* Variant-Carrying Families Worldwide. JNCI J Natl Cancer Inst 2018;110(12):1328–41.
12. Williamson SR, Eble JN, Amin MB, et al. Succinate dehydrogenase-deficient renal cell carcinoma: detailed characterization of 11 tumors defining a unique subtype of renal cell carcinoma. Mod Pathol 2015;28(1):80–94.
13. Andrews KA, Ascher DB, Pires DEV, et al. Tumour risks and genotype–phenotype correlations associated with germline variants in succinate dehydrogenase subunit genes *SDHB* , *SDHC* and *SDHD*. J Med Genet 2018;55(6):384–94.
14. Dubard Gault M, Mandelker D, DeLair D, et al. Germline SDHA mutations in children and adults with cancer. Cold Spring Harb Mol Case Stud 2018;4(4): a002584.
15. Jiang Q, Zhang Y, Zhou YH, et al. A novel germline mutation in SDHA identified in a rare case of gastrointestinal stromal tumor complicated with renal cell carcinoma. Int J Clin Exp Pathol 2015;8(10):12188–97.

16. Amar L, Pacak K, Steichen O, et al. International consensus on initial screening and follow-up of asymptomatic SDHx mutation carriers. Nat Rev Endocrinol 2021;17(7):435–44.

17. Schmidt L, Duh FM, Chen F, et al. Germline and somatic mutations in the tyrosine kinase domain of the MET proto-oncogene in papillary renal carcinomas. Nat Genet 1997;16(1):68–73.

18. Choueiri TK, Vaishampayan U, Rosenberg JE, et al. Phase II and Biomarker Study of the Dual MET/VEGFR2 Inhibitor Foretinib in Patients With Papillary Renal Cell Carcinoma. J Clin Oncol 2013;31(2):181–6.

19. Tan MH, Mester JL, Ngeow J, et al. Lifetime cancer risks in individuals with germline PTEN mutations. Clin Cancer Res 2012;18(2):400–7.

20. Hendricks LAJ, Hoogerbrugge N, Schuurs-Hoeijmakers JHM, et al. A review on age-related cancer risks in PTEN hamartoma tumor syndrome. Clin Genet 2021;99(2):219–25.

21. Shuch B, Ricketts CJ, Vocke CD, et al. Germline PTEN Mutation Cowden Syndrome: An Under-Appreciated Form of Hereditary Kidney Cancer. J Urol 2013; 190(6):1990–8.

22. Mester JL, Zhou M, Prescott N, et al. Papillary renal cell carcinoma is associated with PTEN hamartoma tumor syndrome. Urology 2012;79(5):1187.e1–7.

23. Kim RH, Wang X, Evans AJ, et al. Early-onset renal cell carcinoma in PTEN harmatoma tumour syndrome. Npj Genomic Med 2020;5(1):1–5.

24. Ramkumar RR, Murthy PB, Nguyen JK, et al. PTEN Hamartoma Tumor Syndrome: A Case of Renal Cell Carcinoma in a Young Female. Urology 2021;148:113–7.

25. Henske EP, Jóźwiak S, Kingswood JC, et al. Tuberous sclerosis complex. Nat Rev Dis Primer 2016;2(1):16035.

26. Yang P, Cornejo KM, Sadow PM, et al. Renal Cell Carcinoma in Tuberous Sclerosis Complex. Am J Surg Pathol 2014;38(7):895–909.

27. Argani P, Mehra R. Renal cell carcinoma associated with tuberous sclerosis complex (TSC)/mammalian target of rapamycin (MTOR) genetic alterations. Mod Pathol 2022;35(3):296–7.

28. Bertolotto C, Lesueur F, Giuliano S, et al. A SUMOylation-defective MITF germline mutation predisposes to melanoma and renal carcinoma. Nature 2011; 480(7375):94–8.

29. Stoehr CG, Walter B, Denzinger S, et al. The Microphthalmia-Associated Transcription Factor p.E318K Mutation Does Not Play a Major Role in Sporadic Renal Cell Tumors from Caucasian Patients. Pathobiol J Immunopathol Mol Cell Biol 2016;83(4):165–9.

30. Hyde SM, Rich TA, Waguespack SG, et al. CDC73-Related Disorders. In: Adam MP, Everman DB, Mirzaa GM, et al, editors. GeneReviews®. Seattle: University of Washington; 1993. Available at: http://www.ncbi.nlm.nih.gov/books/NBK3789/. Accessed 30 January, 2023.

31. Haven CJ, Wong FK, van Dam EW, et al. A genotypic and histopathological study of a large Dutch kindred with hyperparathyroidism-jaw tumor syndrome. J Clin Endocrinol Metab 2000;85(4):1449–54.

32. Vocke CD, Ricketts CJ, Ball MW, et al. CDC73 germline mutation in a family with mixed epithelial and stromal tumors. Urology 2019;124:91–7.

33. Qin Y, Deng Y, Ricketts CJ, et al. The tumor susceptibility gene TMEM127 is mutated in renal cell carcinomas and modulates endolysosomal function. Hum Mol Genet 2014;23(9):2428–39.

34. Benusiglio PR, Couvé S, Gilbert-Dussardier B, et al. A germline mutation in PBRM1 predisposes to renal cell carcinoma. J Med Genet 2015;52(6):426–30.

35. Andreou A, Yngvadottir B, Bassaganyas L, et al. Elongin C (*ELOC/TCEB1*)-associated von Hippel–Lindau disease. Hum Mol Genet 2022;31(16):2728–37.

36. Moch H, Amin MB, Berney DM, et al. The 2022 World Health Organization Classification of Tumours of the Urinary System and Male Genital Organs-Part A: Renal, Penile, and Testicular Tumours. Eur Urol 2022;82(5):458–68.

37. Jafri M, Wake NC, Ascher DB, et al. Germline Mutations in the CDKN2B Tumor Suppressor Gene Predispose to Renal Cell Carcinoma. Cancer Discov 2015; 5(7):723–9.

The Role of the Pathologist in Renal Cell Carcinoma Management

Sayed Matar, MD[a,b], Nourhan El Ahmar, MD[a,b],
Yasmin Nabil Laimon, MD[a,b], Fatme Ghandour, MD[a,b],
Sabina Signoretti, MD[a,b,c,d],*

KEYWORDS

- Renal cell carcinoma • Classification • Pathology • Immunohistochemistry • PD-L1
- PD-1 • Immune checkpoints • Biomarker

KEY POINTS

- The pathologic assessment of surgical and biopsy specimens plays a central role in the diagnosis and treatment of patients with renal cell carcinoma (RCC).
- RCC is a heterogeneous disease that comprises different tumor types with distinct histologic, immunohistochemical/molecular and clinical features.
- The classification of renal cell tumors has evolved significantly throughout the years due to our increasing understanding of the molecular drivers of specific RCC types.
- Although no biomarkers are currently approved for the management of patients with RCC, pathologist-driven research efforts have the potential of developing predictive models that can guide treatment selection in clinical practice.

INTRODUCTION

Renal cell carcinoma (RCC) accounts for the vast majority of kidney cancers.[1] Similar to other malignancies, the management of RCC needs a multidisciplinary approach that involves multiple specialties, including pathology.[2] RCC is often initially diagnosed by imaging studies, either in patients undergoing workup for symptoms suspicious of RCC or as renal masses incidentally found during evaluation for unrelated medical problems.[3] The initial diagnosis is usually followed by surgical resection of

[a] Department of Pathology, Brigham and Women's Hospital, 75 Francis Street, Boston, MA 02115, USA; [b] Harvard Medical School, 25 Shattuck Street, Boston, MA 02115, USA; [c] Broad Institute of MIT and Harvard, Merkin Building, 415 Main Street, Cambridge, MA 02142, USA; [d] Department of Oncologic Pathology, Dana-Farber Cancer Institute, 450 Brookline Avenue, Boston, MA 02215, USA
* Corresponding author. Brigham and Women's Hospital, Thorn Building 504A, 75 Francis Street, Boston, MA 02115.
E-mail address: ssignoretti@bwh.harvard.edu

Hematol Oncol Clin N Am 37 (2023) 849–862
https://doi.org/10.1016/j.hoc.2023.04.014
0889-8588/23/© 2023 Elsevier Inc. All rights reserved.

the primary tumor and pathologic analysis.[3] The pathologic evaluation of the specimens includes confirming the diagnosis of malignancy and determining the histologic type of RCC, the extent of the local tumor, the involvement of regional lymph nodes, the grade of the tumor, and the status of other prognostic parameters. Tumor tissue for pathologic evaluation can alternatively be obtained from a biopsy. However, the routine use of biopsy in RCC diagnosis is most frequently used for establishing the diagnosis of small renal masses, unresectable tumors, or extrarenal lesions suspicious for metastatic RCC.[4–6]

In more recent years, with the implementation of targeted therapies and immunotherapy for advanced RCC, pathologists have been, and continue to be, instrumental in translational research aimed at developing tissue-based predictive biomarkers that can aid in the selection of optimal treatment of individual patients. Here, the authors discuss the evolving role of pathologists both in patient care and in the development of precision medicine strategies for RCC.

CLASSIFICATION OF RENAL CELL TUMORS: RECENT UPDATES

RCC is a heterogeneous disease and consists of distinct tumor types that originate from the epithelial cells of renal tubules. The pathologic classification of RCC has changed significantly throughout the years, due to our increasing understanding of the molecular alterations based on specific tumor entities. Of note, the 2022 World health Organization (WHO) classification of renal tumors includes a new category of molecularly defined renal carcinomas that cannot be identified by morphologic analysis but are diagnosed based on unique molecular changes (**Box 1**).[7]

The molecularly defined RCC subtypes are relatively uncommon and include ELOC-mutated RCC, TFE3-rearranged RCC, TFEB-altered RCC, fumarate hydratase (FH)-deficient RCC, succinate dehydrogenase–deficient RCC, ALK-rearranged RCC, and SMARCB1-deficient renal medullary carcinoma.[7] These subtypes do not show specific pathologic features, and although they may have morphologic similarities to other RCC subtypes, they have a different clinical behavior and may require different therapeutic strategies. Although the inclusion of molecularly defined RCC subtypes is an important step toward the development of a molecular classification of renal tumors, it should be noted that most RCC entities are still identified based on morphologic and immunophenotypic features (see **Box 1**). Future investigations aimed at discovering additional key drivers of RCC development and progression will hopefully lead to a more biologically relevant classification of RCC with improved clinical utility.[8]

The most common RCC subtype is clear cell renal cell carcinoma (ccRCC) (~70%–80%), followed by papillary renal cell carcinoma (PRCC) (10%–15%), and chromophobe renal cell carcinoma (CHRCC) (3%–5%).[9,10]

ccRCC typically consists of cells with clear cytoplasm that are surrounded by a complex vascular network and arranged in nests, tubules, or alveoli. High-grade tumors may contain cells with eosinophilic cytoplasm or hyaline globules. Molecularly, biallelic inactivation of the *Von Hippel-Lindau (VHL)* gene is the main driver of both sporadic and VHL-associated ccRCC, and this alteration is detected in the vast majority (ie, greater than 90%) of sporadic cases, when using optimized sequencing protocols and promoter methylation assays.[11–13] Other recurrently mutated genes include *PBRM1*, *BAP1*, and *SETD2*.[11] By immunohistochemistry, the tumor cells of ccRCC are typically positive for vimentin, cytokeratin (CAM5.2, AE1/AE3), and carbonic anhydrase-IX (CAIX) and negative for CK7.[14–16]

PRCC was first recognized as a separate entity over 4 decades ago.[17] In recent years, it has become evident that a papillary pattern of growth is not diagnostic of

> **Box 1**
> **Histologic types of renal cell tumors according to the 2022 WHO classification of urinary and male genital tumors (fifth edition)**
>
> Clear cell renal tumors
>   Clear cell renal cell carcinoma
>   Multilocular cystic renal neoplasm of low malignant potential
>
> Papillary renal tumors
>   Renal papillary adenoma
>   Papillary renal cell carcinoma
>
> Oncocytic and chromophobe renal tumors
>   Oncocytoma of the kidney
>   Chromophobe renal cell carcinoma
>   Other oncocytic tumors of the kidney
>
> Collecting duct tumors
>   Collecting duct carcinoma
>
> Other renal tumors
>   Clear cell papillary renal cell tumor
>   Mucinous tubular and spindle cell carcinoma
>   Tubulocystic renal cell carcinoma
>   Acquired cystic disease–associated renal cell carcinoma
>   Eosinophilic solid and cystic renal cell carcinoma
>   Renal cell carcinoma, NOS
>
> Molecularly defined renal carcinomas
>   TFE3-rearranged renal cell carcinomas
>   TFEB-altered renal cell carcinomas
>   ELOC (formerly TCEB1)-mutated renal cell carcinoma
>   Fumarate hydratase–deficient renal cell carcinoma
>   Succinate dehydrogenase–deficient renal cell carcinoma
>   ALK-rearranged renal cell carcinomas
>   SMARCB1-deficient renal medullary carcinoma
>
> *Abbreviation:* NOS, not otherwise specified.

PRCC, and some RCC types that were previously included in this category (eg, FH-deficient RCC, TFE3-rearranged RCC, and others) are now recognized as separate entities.[18,19] Historically, PRCC has been morphologically subclassified into 2 different groups, type 1 and type 2, although this classification has now fallen out of favor.[20–22] Classically, type 1 PRCC was characterized by well-defined papillary or tubular structures lined by a single layer of cuboidal cells with scant cytoplasm and low-grade nuclear features that typically show strong positivity for CK7 and alpha-methyl-cyl-CoA racemase (AMACR). In contrast, in what was formerly type 2 PRCC, the neoplastic cells lining the papillary and tubular structures are pseudostratified, have abundant eosinophilic cytoplasm and high-grade nuclear features, and are less consistently positive for CK7 and AMACR. Although this subclassification has been used for many years, it is problematic for several reasons.

First, many PRCC cases have overlapping or mixed features of type 1 and type 2 and cannot be properly categorized.[23] Second, molecular studies have shown that both sporadic and hereditary type 1 PRCC represent a relatively well-defined entity characterized by activating alteration in the *MET* oncogene.[24–26] On the other hand, type 2 PRCC is molecularly heterogeneous, with subsets of tumors showing various alterations (eg, *CDKN2A* inactivation, mutations in NRF2 pathway genes, *SETD2* mutations, and amplification of chromosome 8q involving *MYC*).[25,27] Importantly, there is evidence that in PRCC with mixed histologic features, both the type 1 and type 2 areas harbor genetic alterations characteristic of type 1 RCC, further challenging the concept that type 2 PRCC is a separate entity.[23] Finally, recent studies have shown that the subclassification in type 1 and type 2 PRCC is not an independent prognostic factor.[28,29] For the aforementioned reasons, in the 2022 WHO classification of renal cell tumors the distinction into PRCC type 1 and type 2 is no longer recommended. It is acknowledged that PRCCs are heterogeneous, ranging from low-grade to high-grade tumors. Moreover, the former type 1 PRCC is now considered the classic form of PRCC. It is also recognized that *MET* alterations are more common in low-grade PRCC.[7] Therapeutic clinical trials dedicated to papillary RCC are now selecting patients based on MET pathways dependence.[30]

CHRCC is characterized by tumor cells with pale cytoplasm, wrinkled nuclei, coarse chromatin, and prominent plantlike cell membranes that can display multiple architectural patterns, including nested, trabecular, cystic, tubulocystic, or tubular.[31,32] It is well established that a subset of CHRCCs mostly consists of cells with eosinophilic/oncocytic cytoplasm and resemble renal oncocytoma on histologic examination.[33] A molecular feature that can be of diagnostic utility in CHRCC is the loss of whole chromosomes (most commonly chromosomes 1, 2, 6, 10, 13, 17, and 21),[34,35] although a recent analysis revealed that a significant proportion of the eosinophilic cases does not harbor copy number alterations.[36] *PTEN and TP53* are the most commonly mutated genes in CHRCC, and mutations in these genes are more frequently seen in tumors that metastasize.[36,37] By immunohistochemistry, CHRCC tumors are usually positive for CK7 and KIT (CD117) and negative for CAIX.[14,38]

Although eosinophilic CHRCC and renal oncocytoma can be distinguished by histologic examination (and ancillary studies), the existence of oncocytic tumors that have borderline features between the 2 entities have long been recognized. Most of these neoplasms are sporadic but some of them arise in patients with Birt-Hogg-Dubé or tuberous sclerosis syndrome. In past years, these difficult-to-diagnose tumors have been frequently designated as hybrid tumors but in 2021, the Genitourinary Pathology Society proposed a new definition for sporadic cases: "oncocytic renal neoplasm of low malignant potential, not further classified."[39] More recently, the 2022 WHO classification introduced a new category called "other oncocytic tumors of the kidney" (see **Box 1**), which includes neoplasms that cannot be classified as oncocytoma, CHRCC, or other tumor types with eosinophilic features; these tumors are typically low-grade and indolent and need to be differentiated from high-grade unclassified RCC, which is associated with aggressive behavior.[40]

STAGING, GRADING, AND OTHER PROGNOSTIC FACTORS REPORTED BY PATHOLOGISTS

The pathologic stage of RCC tumors is an important prognostic factor that guides patient management.[41] Regardless of the subtype of the RCC, the tumor, node and metastasis (TNM) system is used to stage the tumors.[42] Pathologic evaluation of nephrectomy specimens provides information about the extent of the tumor (T) and the involvement of regional lymph nodes (N).[43] The International Society of Urologic Pathology (ISUP) published recommendations on handling and sampling nephrectomy specimens to guide pathologists in the assessment of T and N staging.[43]

Grading tumors based on their nuclear features is an important component of the pathologic assessment of RCC. The Fuhrman grade has been used for decades because of its utility in predicting tumor progression and metastasis after nephrectomy.[44,45] In 2012, the ISUP introduced a new grading system, which is more reproducible and clinically applicable than the Fuhrman grade and is recommended for use by the WHO.[46] In the WHO/ISUP grading system, grades 1 to 3 are determined solely based on nucleolar prominence/eosinophilia, whereas grade 4 is defined by nuclear pleomorphism and/or the identification of sarcomatoid or rhabdoid features.[46] The WHO/ISUP grade is associated with survival in patients with ccRCC and PRCC,[47,48] but it does not predict the survival of patients with CHRCC.[49] Thus, it is recommended that CHRCC not be graded. The prognostic significance of WHO/ISUP grading has not been validated in other RCC types.

Other important prognostic factors based on the pathologic evaluation of RCC samples include the presence of sarcomatoid or rhabdoid features, tumor necrosis, microvascular invasion, and the status of the surgical margins.[46]

Sarcomatoid dedifferentiation can occur in any RCC type, is more frequently observed in advanced stage disease, and is associated with poor prognosis.[46,50] Of note, it has treatment implications, as it has been recently shown that RCC tumors with sarcomatoid dedifferentiation respond to systemic therapy with immune checkpoint inhibitors.[51–55] Although there is no consensus on the definition of sarcomatoid dedifferentiation, it is usually reported when any component of spindled tumor cells reminiscent of sarcoma is detected.[50,56] The percentage of sarcomatoid component can also be noted, as it has been shown to have prognostic significance.[57] However, it should be noted that detecting sarcomatoid dedifferentiation and accurately measuring the percentage of the sarcomatoid component in patients with RCC require a thorough evaluation of nephrectomy specimens. Indeed, the assessment of sarcomatoid dedifferentiation in biopsy specimens (especially of primary RCC tumors) has a very low sensitivity and is thus unreliable.[56,58]

The presence of rhabdoid differentiation defined as high-grade tumor cells with rhabdoid morphology is associated with more aggressive disease, extrarenal extension, and distant metastases.[46] Although the ISUP recommends reporting the presence or absence of rhabdoid features, there is, currently, no support for reporting the percentage of the rhabdoid component. Rhabdoid features frequently cooccur with sarcomatoid features although tumors harboring rhabdoid features alone are also possible. One study found that the molecular features of tumors with sarcomatoid and rhabdoid components are not significantly different.[55]

THE ROLE OF PATHOLOGISTS IN THE DEVELOPMENT OF PERSONALIZED MEDICINE STRATEGIES FOR RENAL CELL CARCINOMA

In recent years, immune checkpoint inhibitors (ICI) have revolutionized the treatment of kidney cancer, and several ICI-based combinations are now standard of care as first-line therapy in advanced ccRCC. These regimens include anti-PD-1 plus anti-CTLA4 therapy as well as anti-PD-1/anti-PD-L1 treatment in combination with vascular endothelial growth factor receptor (VEGFR) tyrosine kinase inhibitors (TKI).[59] In spite of this progress, patient stratification for treatment selection is still solely based on clinical criteria, as there are currently no Food and Drug Administration (FDA)-approved biomarkers that can guide the treatment of patients with kidney cancer. Large-scale multidisciplinary investigations of clinical trial cohorts aimed at discovering genomic and transcriptomic predictors of response to ICI-based treatment have been conducted, and some candidate biomarkers have recently emerged.[54,60–62] In parallel studies, pathologists have used their unique expertise in in situ tissue analyses (eg, immunohistochemistry [IHC] and multiplex immunofluorescence [mIF]) to define tumor features that can predict the clinical outcome of patients with RCC receiving immunotherapy. Some of these pathology-based efforts are discussed later.

Programmed Cell Death Ligand 1 as a Biomarker of Response to Immune Check Point Inhibitor Therapy in Clear Cell Renal Cell Carcinoma

Quantification of programmed cell death ligand 1 (PD-L1) expression by tumor cells (TC) and/or tumor-infiltrating immune cells in IHC-stained formalin-fixed-paraffin-embedded (FFPE) slides is clinically implemented in multiple solid tumors as a predictive biomarker to select patients for treatment with ICI.[63] A variety of assays are used to immunostain tissues for PD-L1, each developed and FDA-approved for particular ICI agents.[63,64] In addition, different measurement criteria are used to score PD-L1 expression in different tumor types. For instance, in non–small cell lung carcinoma, the tumor proportion score, defined as the percentage of tumor cells positive for PD-L1, is used. In contrast, in urothelial carcinoma, PD-L1 status is determined based on a combined positivity score, defined as the sum of PD-L1 positive tumor cells and PD-L1 positive intratumor immune cells over the total number of tumor cells multiplied by 100 (with a maximum of 100).[63]

In clinical trials evaluating ICI agents for RCC, different assays and scoring criteria were used to define PD-L1 positivity and that variation was reflected in the different proportions of patients who were determined to have PD-L1 positive tumors in these studies. Unfortunately, the association between PD-L1 expression and clinical benefit in this tumor type remains unclear, as these trials have generated inconsistent results.

In the randomized CheckMate 025 clinical trial of patients with metastatic ccRCC previously treated with VEGFR-TKI, PD-L1 expression in TC was not associated with benefit from nivolumab (anti-PD-L1) monotherapy.[65,66] On the other hand, in the HCRN GU16-260 clinical trial that evaluated nivolumab and salvage nivolumab/ipilimumab in the first-line setting, patients with ccRCC with PD-L1–positive TC experienced significantly higher objective response rate (ORR) on nivolumab.[67] Similar results were observed in the KEYNOTE-427 trial of first-line pembrolizumab (anti-PD-1) in advanced ccRCC, where a PD-L1 combined positive score (tumor cells and immune cells) was associated with improved ORR.[68] The lack of association between PD-L1 expression and clinical outcome in VEGFR-TKI–pretreated patients from the CheckMate 025 trial might be explained, at least in part, by the fact that PD-L1 analysis was mostly conducted on nephrectomy samples obtained before the beginning of the initial systemic therapy; therefore, PD-L1 expression assessed in baseline primary tumors might have not reflected PD-L1 levels in the VEGFR-TKI–resistant metastases that were the target of the nivolumab therapy.

With regard to first-line ICI-based combination therapies, a recent meta-analysis of data from several clinical trials (IMmotion 150, IMmotion 151, JAVELIN Renal 101, KEYNOTE-426, CheckMate-214) suggested that, compared with sunitinib, treatment with ICI was associated with higher ORR and longer progression-free survival (PFS) in patients with PD-L1–positive tumors but not in patients with PD-L1–negative tumors. Of note, the improved outcome in patients with PD-L1–positive tumors was most evident with nivolumab and ipilimumab (anti-CTLA4) but was questionable with VEGFR-TKI.[69,70] Moreover, a separate analysis of the CheckMate 9ER trial demonstrated that nivolumab plus the TKI cabozantinib had significantly longer PFS compared with sunitinib regardless of tumor PD-L1 expression.[71]

Taken together, current data seem to indicate that PD-L1 expression is associated with responses in patients treated with frontline anti-PD-1 therapy either as single agent or in combination with anti-CTLA4 (although anti-PD-1 monotherapy is currently not approved for treatment-naïve patients with ccRCC). In contrast, PD-L1 expression does not play a clear role in predicting outcome to ICI in combination with VEGFR-TKI treatment; this is not entirely surprising, as patients with PD-L1–positive tumors treated with VEGFR-TKI are known to experience worse clinical outcome.[72,73] In spite of these findings, it should be noted that the value of PD-L1 IHC assessment by itself in selecting patients with ccRCC for treatment with first-line anti-PD-1 plus anti-CTLA4 or anti-PD-1 alone is limited because many responses to these therapies are also observed in patients with PD-L1–negative tumors. Indeed, because PD-L1 is expressed only in a subset of patients with ccRCC, a large proportion of the responders actually have PD-L1–negative tumors. At this time, PD-L1 expression cannot be routinely recommended to guide treatment decisions in metastatic RCC, and the identification of additional predictors of response to ICI, which can be potentially combined with PD-L1 status to create an integrated predictive model, is needed to develop more clinically relevant biomarkers for RCC.

Candidate Biomarkers for Immune Checkpoint Inhibitor Therapy Identified by Multiplex Immunofluorescence

Many factors other than PD-L1 expression may affect the response to ICI-based therapies; these include key features of the tumor microenvironment (TME) such as infiltration by effector T cells, B cells, and immune suppressive cell populations. Pathologists are uniquely positioned to investigate the composition of the TME in FFPE tissue samples using mIF staining coupled with spectral imaging and image analysis software.[74] This methodology allows to quantify tumor-infiltrating immune cell populations and determines their functional state in intact tissue sections by measuring, at the cellular level, the coexpression of immune molecules on cell types of interest (**Fig. 1**). In addition, this in situ imaging technique can be used to evaluate spatial relationships between different types of cells, which might be clinically relevant.

mIF studies of tissues from patients with ccRCC treated with nivolumab within 2 independent clinical trials (ChechMate-010 and ChechMate-025) have recently demonstrated that high levels of CD8-positive tumor-infiltrating lymphocytes (TIL) expressing PD-1 but negative for the expression of the immune checkpoint molecules TIM-3 and LAG-3 are associated with longer PFS and higher ORR (see **Fig. 1**).[65,75] These results suggest that the expression of PD-1 (ie, the target of the therapy) on CD8-positive TIL that is negative for other inhibitory receptors identifies a population of antigen-experienced but nonterminally exhausted T cells that can be effectively rejuvenated by anti-PD-1 monotherapy. Of note, in both clinical trials, combining the levels of CD8-positive TIL-expressing PD-1 (but not TIM-3 or LAG-3) with TC PD-L1 status further separated clinical outcomes and identified a subset of patients with high likelihood of experiencing durable responses to anti-PD-1 therapy.[65,75]

Tertiary lymphoid structures (TLS) are organized aggregates of B cells and T cells that resemble lymphoid follicles in secondary lymphoid organs and are found in many cancer types, where they may contribute to antitumor immunity.[76] Recent studies have implicated TLS as predictors of ICI efficacy in solid tumors, including RCC.[77,78] As the number of patients with RCC analyzed to date is relatively low, future mIF analyses of tumor tissues from large clinical trial cohorts will be helpful in further assessing the role of TLS as predictive biomarker for ICI therapy in RCC.

Although IHC-based assays are already widely used to direct patient care, translating mIF-based biomarkers into clinical practice requires additional investigations aimed at developing a robust, standardized, and validated workflow that can be implemented in the clinic. Of note, encouraging data from a recent multiinstitutional study

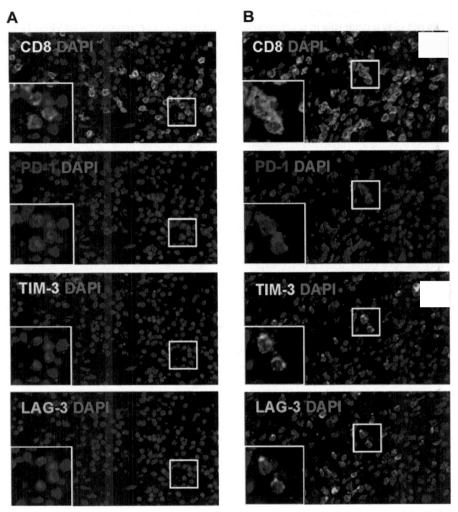

Fig. 1. Multiplex immunofluorescence assay to quantify expression of PD-1, TIM-3, and LAG-3 on CD8-positive cells in FFPE ccRCC tissues. (*A*) Representative image of a ccRCC tissue sample with high percentage of CD8-positive cells expressing PD-1, but not TIM-3 or LAG-3. (*B*) Representative image of a ccRCC sample with high percentage of CD8-positive cells expressing PD-1, TIM-3, and LAG-3.

showed that an optimized mIF assay produced highly reproducible staining results in tumor samples when performed at 6 independent laboratories.[79]

SUMMARY

Pathologists play a central role in RCC patient care by confirming the diagnosis of malignancy, determining the histologic type of RCC, and assessing many important prognostic factors such as the pathologic stage, nuclear grade, presence of sarcomatoid or rhabdoid features, and others. In recent years, our increased understanding of the molecular alterations driving specific RCC types has led to an improved classification scheme that better informs patient prognosis and treatment. In spite of this progress, no predictive biomarkers are currently approved for the management of patients with RCC. Pathologists are uniquely positioned to move the field forward by developing IHC-/mIF-based predictors of outcome to ICI-based therapy that could be used in the clinic.

CLINICS CARE POINTS

- The 2022 WHO Classification of renal tumors introduced several changes, including a new class of "molecularly defined renal carcinomas" and a new category of oncocytic neoplasms called "other oncocytic tumors of the kidney." Moreover, the subclassification of PRCC into type 1 and type 2 is no longer recommended.

- Sarcomatoid dedifferentiation in RCC tumors is a poor prognostic factor, which is associated with poor response to targeted therapies but sensitivity to ICI-based therapies.

- Although an association between PD-L1 expression and improved response is observed in ccRCC patients with ccRCC treated with frontline ICI therapy, the clinical utility of PD-L1 status as a predictive biomarker is limited.

- Pathologist-driven research efforts focused on the characterization of the TME using mIF staining of tumor tissues coupled with spectral imaging have identified new promising predictive biomarkers that have the potential to provide guidance for personalized treatment of patients with RCC.

ACKNOWLEDGMENTS

Acknowledgments of research support for the study: this work was supported in part by the NCI (Dana-Farber/Harvard Cancer Center Kidney Cancer SPORE: P50-CA101942–12, Dana-Farber/Harvard Cancer Center Kidney Program: P30 CA06516, 1R01CA266424–01A1), and DOD CDMRP (W81XWH2210523). N. El Ahmar is supported by a DOD CDMRP Postdoctoral Fellowship Award (W81XWH2110808).

The authors thank Jean-Christophe Pignon for the assistance with figure preparation and Destiny Jasmine West, Varunika Savla, and Aseman Bagheri for their critical reading of the manuscript.

DISCLOSURES

S. Signoretti reports receiving commercial research grants from Bristol-Myers Squibb, AstraZeneca, Exelixis, and Novartis; is a consultant/advisory board member for Merck, AstraZeneca, Bristol-Myers Squibb, CRISPR Therapeutics AG, AACR, and NCI; receives royalties from Biogenex; and mentored several non-US citizens on research projects with potential funding (in part) from non-US sources/Foreign Components.

REFERENCES

1. Bukavina L., Bensalah K., Bray F., et al., Epidemiology of Renal Cell Carcinoma: 2022 Update, *Eur Urol*, 82, 2022, 529–542.
2. Selby P, Popescu R, Lawler M, et al. The Value and Future Developments of Multidisciplinary Team Cancer Care. Am Soc Clin Oncol Educ Book 2022. https://doi.org/10.1200/EDBK.
3. Campbell S, Uzzo RG, Allaf ME, et al. Renal Mass and Localized Renal Cancer: AUA Guideline. J Urol 2017;198:520–9.
4. Sahni VA, Silverman SG. Biopsy of renal masses: when and why. Cancer Imag 2009;9:44–55.

5. Shah RB, Bakshi N, Hafez KS, et al. Image-guided biopsy in the evaluation of renal mass lesions in contemporary urological practice: Indications, adequacy, clinical impact, and limitations of the pathological diagnosis. Hum Pathol 2005; 36:1309–15.

6. Lim CS, Schieda N, Silverman SG. Update on Indications for Percutaneous Renal Mass Biopsy in the Era of Advanced CT and MRI. AJR Am J Roentgenol 2019;1–10. https://doi.org/10.2214/AJR.19.21093.

7. Raspollini M., Moch H., Tan P., et al., Renal cell tumours: introduction, In: Tumours Editorial Board, *Urinary and male genital tumours, WHO classification of tumours*, vol. 8, 5th edition [Internet] , 2022, Lyon (France): International Agency for Research on Cancer, https://tumourclassification.iarc.who.int/chaptercontent/36/4.

8. Manley BJ, Hakimi AA. Molecular profiling of renal cell carcinoma: Building a bridge toward clinical impact. Curr Opin Urol 2016;26:383–7.

9. Warren AY, Harrison D. WHO/ISUP classification, grading and pathological staging of renal cell carcinoma: standards and controversies. World J Urol 2018;36: 1913–26.

10. WHO Classification of Tumours Editorial Board, *Urinary and male genital tumours*, vol. 8, 2022, Lyon (France): International Agency for Research on Cancer.

11. Cancer Genome Atlas Research Network. Comprehensive molecular characterization of clear cell renal cell carcinoma. Nature 2013;499:43–9.

12. Beroukhim R, Brunet JP, Di Napoli A, et al. Patterns of gene expression and copy-number alterations in von-hippel lindau disease-associated and sporadic clear cell carcinoma of the kidney. Cancer Res 2009;69:4674–81.

13. Nickerson ML, Jaeger E, Shi Y, et al. Improved identification of von Hippel-Lindau gene alterations in clear cell renal tumors. Clin Cancer Res 2008;14:4726–34.

14. Mathers ME, Pollock AM, Marsh C, et al. Cytokeratin 7: A useful adjunct in the diagnosis of chromophobe renal cell carcinoma. Histopathology 2002;40:563–7.

15. Skinnider BF, Folpe AL, Hennigar RA, et al. Distribution of Cytokeratins and Vimentin in Adult Renal Neoplasms and Normal Renal Tissue Potential Utility of a Cytokeratin Antibody Panel in the Differential Diagnosis of Renal Tumors. Am J Surg Pathol 2005;29:747–54.

16. Kim M, Joo JW, Lee SJ, et al. Comprehensive immunoprofiles of renal cell carcinoma subtypes. Cancers 2020;12.

17. Mancilla-Jimenez R, Stanley RJ, Blath RA. Papillary renal cell carcinoma: a clinical, radiologic, and pathologic study of 34 cases. Cancer 1976;38:2469–80.

18. Lobo J., Ohashi R., Amin M.B., et al., WHO 2022 landscape of papillary and chromophobe renal cell carcinoma, Histopathology, 81, 2022, 426–438.

19. Lobo J, Ohashi R, Helmchen BM, et al. The Morphological Spectrum of Papillary Renal Cell Carcinoma and Prevalence of Provisional/Emerging Renal Tumor Entities with Papillary Growth. Biomedicines 2021;9.

20. Delahunt B, Eble JN. Papillary renal cell carcinoma: a clinicopathologic and immunohistochemical study of 105 tumors. Mod Pathol 1997;10:537–44.

21. Eble JN, Sauter G, Epstein J & Sesterhenn I. Pathology and Genetics of Tumours of the Urinary System and Male Genital Organs. vol. 7 (International Agency for Research on Cancer, 2004).

22. Moch H, Humphrey PA, Ulbright TM & Reuter VE. WHO Classification of Tumours of the Urinary System and Male Genital Organs. vol. 8 (International Agency for Research on Cancer, 2016).

23. Murugan P., Jia L., Dinatale R.G., et al., Papillary renal cell carcinoma: a single institutional study of 199 cases addressing classification, clinicopathologic and molecular features, and treatment outcome, *Mod Pathol*, 35, 2022, 825–835.

24. Pitra T, Pivovarcikova K, Alaghehbandan R, et al. Chromosomal numerical aberration pattern in papillary renal cell carcinoma: Review article. Ann Diagn Pathol 2019. https://doi.org/10.1016/j.anndiagpath.2017.11.004.

25. The Cancer Genome Atlas Research Network. Comprehensive Molecular Characterization of Papillary Renal-Cell Carcinoma. N Engl J Med 2016;374:135–45.

26. Zbar B, Tory K, Merino M, et al. Hereditary papillary renal cell carcinoma. J Urol 1994;151:561–6.

27. Furge KA, Chen J, Koeman J, et al. Detection of DNA copy number changes and oncogenic signaling abnormalities from gene expression data reveals MYC activation in high-grade papillary renal cell carcinoma. Cancer Res 2007;67:3171–6.

28. Le X, Wang X-B, Zhao H, et al. Comparison of clinicopathologic parameters and oncologic outcomes between type 1 and type 2 papillary renal cell carcinoma. BMC Urol 2020;20:148.

29. Pan H, Ye L, Zhu Q, et al. The effect of the papillary renal cell carcinoma subtype on oncological outcomes. Sci Rep 2020;10:21073.

30. Choueiri TK, Xu W, Poole L, et al. SAMETA: An open-label, three-arm, multicenter, phase III study of savolitinib + durvalumab versus sunitinib and durvalumab monotherapy in patients with MET-driven, unresectable, locally advanced/metastatic papillary renal cell carcinoma (PRCC). J Clin Oncol 2022;40:TPS4601.

31. Amin MB, Paner GP, Alvarado-Cabrero I, et al. Chromophobe Renal Cell Carcinoma: Histomorphologic Characteristics and Evaluation of Conventional Pathologic Prognostic Parameters in 145 Cases. Am J Surg Pathol 2008;32.

32. Przybycin, C. G. et al. Chromophobe Renal Cell Carcinoma: A Clinicopathologic Study of 203 Tumors in 200 Patients With Primary Resection at a Single Institution. Available at: www.ajsp.com (2011).

33. Thoenes W, Störkel S, Rumpelt HJ, et al. Chromophobe cell renal carcinoma and its variants–a report on 32 cases. J Pathol 1988;155:277–87.

34. Speicher M.R., Schoell B., du Manoir S., et al., Specific loss of chromosomes 1, 2, 6, 10, 13, 17, and 21 in chromophobe renal cell carcinomas revealed by comparative genomic hybridization, Am J Pathol, 145, 1994, 356–364.

35. Brunelli M, Eble JN, Zhang S, et al. Eosinophilic and classic chromophobe renal cell carcinomas have similar frequent losses of multiple chromosomes from among chromosomes 1, 2, 6, 10, and 17, and this pattern of genetic abnormality is not present in renal oncocytoma. Mod Pathol 2005;18:161–9.

36. Davis CF, Ricketts CJ, Wang M, et al. The somatic genomic landscape of chromophobe renal cell carcinoma. Cancer Cell 2014;26:319–30.

37. Casuscelli J, Weinhold N, Gundem G, et al. Genomic landscape and evolution of metastatic chromophobe renal cell carcinoma. JCI Insight 2017;2.

38. Yamazaki K, Sakamoto M, Ohta T, et al. Overexpression of KIT in chromophobe renal cell carcinoma. Oncogene 2003;22:847–52.

39. Trpkov K, Hes O, Williamson SR, et al. New developments in existing WHO entities and evolving molecular concepts: The Genitourinary Pathology Society (GUPS) update on renal neoplasia. Mod Pathol 2021;34:1392–424.

40. Chen YB, Xu J, Skanderup AJ, et al. Molecular analysis of aggressive renal cell carcinoma with unclassified histology reveals distinct subsets. Nat Commun 2016;7:13131.

41. Moch H, Gasser T, Amin MB, et al. Prognostic utility of the recently recommended histologic classification and revised TNM staging system of renal cell carcinoma: A swiss experience with 588 tumors. Cancer 2000;89:604–14.
42. Rini BI, McKiernan JM, Chang SS, et al. Kidney. In: Amin MB, Edge SB, Greene FL, et al, editors. AJCC cancer staging manual. 8th edition. New York: Springer; 2017. p. 739.
43. Trpkov K, Grignon DJ, Bonsib SM, et al. Handling and staging of renal cell carcinoma: the International Society of Urological Pathology Consensus (ISUP) conference recommendations. Am J Surg Pathol 2013;37:1505–17.
44. Fuhrman SA, Lasky LC, Limas C. Prognostic significance of morphologic parameters in renal cell carcinoma. Am J Surg Pathol 1982;6:655–64.
45. Novara G, Martignoni G, Artibani W, et al. Grading Systems in Renal Cell Carcinoma. J Urol 2007. https://doi.org/10.1016/j.juro.2006.09.034.
46. Delahunt B., Cheville J.C., Martignoni G., et al., The International Society of Urological Pathology (ISUP) Grading System for Renal Cell Carcinoma and Other Prognostic Parameters The Members of the ISUP Renal Tumor Panel, Am J Surg Pathol, 37, 2013, Available at: www.ajsp.com.
47. Dagher J, Delahunt B, Rioux-Leclercq N, et al. Clear cell renal cell carcinoma: validation of World Health Organization/International Society of Urological Pathology grading. Histopathology 2017;71:918–25.
48. Sika-Paotonu D, Bethwaite PB, Mccredie MRE, et al. Nucleolar Grade But Not Fuhrman Grade is Applicable to Papillary Renal Cell Carcinoma. For Pathol 2006;30.
49. Delahunt B, Sika-Paotonu D, Bethwaite PB, et al. Fuhrman grading is not appropriate for chromophobe renal cell carcinoma. Am J Surg Pathol 2007;31:957–60.
50. Hahn AW, Lebenthal J, Genovese G, et al. The significance of sarcomatoid and rhabdoid dedifferentiation in renal cell carcinoma. Cancer Treat Res Commun 2022;33.
51. Janisch F, Kienapfel C, Fühner C, et al. Treatment and Outcome of Metastatic Renal Cell Carcinoma With Sarcomatoid Differentiation: A Single-Center, Real-World Analysis of Retrospective Data. Front Surg 2021;8.
52. Iacovelli R, Ciccarese C, Bria E, et al. Patients with sarcomatoid renal cell carcinoma – re-defining the first-line of treatment: A meta-analysis of randomised clinical trials with immune checkpoint inhibitors. Eur J Cancer 2020;136:195–203.
53. Tannir NM, Signoretti S, Choueiri TK, et al. Efficacy and Safety of Nivolumab Plus Ipilimumab versus Sunitinib in First-line Treatment of Patients with Advanced Sarcomatoid Renal Cell Carcinoma. Clin Cancer Res 2021;27:78–86.
54. Motzer R.J., Banchereau R., Hamidi H., et al., Molecular Subsets in Renal Cancer Determine Outcome to Checkpoint and Angiogenesis Blockade, Cancer Cell, 38, 2020, 803–817.e4.
55. Bakouny Z, Braun DA, Shukla SA, et al. Integrative molecular characterization of sarcomatoid and rhabdoid renal cell carcinoma. Nat Commun 2021;12:808.
56. Blum KA, Gupta S, Tickoo SK, et al. Sarcomatoid renal cell carcinoma: biology, natural history and management. Nat Rev Urol 2020. https://doi.org/10.1038/s41585-020-00382-9.
57. Adibi M, Thomas AZ, Borregales LD, et al. Percentage of sarcomatoid component as a prognostic indicator for survival in renal cell carcinoma with sarcomatoid dedifferentiation. Urol Oncol 2015;33:427.e17–23.
58. Abel EJ, Carrasco A, Culp SH, et al. Limitations of preoperative biopsy in patients with metastatic renal cell carcinoma: comparison to surgical pathology in 405 cases. BJU Int 2012;110:1742–6.

59. Motzer RJ, Jonasch E, Agarwal N, et al. Kidney Cancer, Version 3.2022, NCCN Clinical Practice Guidelines in Oncology. JNCCN 2022. https://doi.org/10.6004/jnccn.2022.0001.
60. McDermott D.F., Huseni M.A., Atkins M.B., et al., Clinical activity and molecular correlates of response to atezolizumab alone or in combination with bevacizumab versus sunitinib in renal cell carcinoma, Nat Med, 24, 2018, 749–757.
61. Braun D.A., Hou Y., Bakouny Z., et al., Interplay of somatic alterations and immune infiltration modulates response to PD-1 blockade in advanced clear cell renal cell carcinoma, Nat Med, 26, 2020, 909–918.
62. Denize T, Hou Y, Pignon JC, et al. Transcriptomic Correlates of Tumor Cell PD-L1 Expression and Response to Nivolumab Monotherapy in Metastatic Clear Cell Renal Cell Carcinoma. Clin Cancer Res 2022;28:4045–55.
63. Paver E.C., Cooper W.A., Colebatch A.J., et al., Programmed death ligand-1 (PD-L1) as a predictive marker for immunotherapy in solid tumours: a guide to immunohistochemistry implementation and interpretation, Pathology, 53, 2021, 141–156.
64. Koomen BM, Badrising SK, van den Heuvel MM, et al. Comparability of PD-L1 immunohistochemistry assays for non-small-cell lung cancer: a systematic review. Histopathology 2020;76:793–802.
65. Ficial M, Jegede OA, Sant'Angelo M, et al. Expression of T-Cell Exhaustion Molecules and Human Endogenous Retroviruses as Predictive Biomarkers for Response to Nivolumab in Metastatic Clear Cell Renal Cell Carcinoma. Clin Cancer Res 2021;27:1371–80.
66. Motzer RJ, Escudier B, McDermott DF, et al. Nivolumab versus Everolimus in Advanced Renal-Cell Carcinoma. N Engl J Med 2015;373:1803–13.
67. Atkins MB, Jegede OA, Haas NB, et al. Phase II Study of Nivolumab and Salvage Nivolumab/Ipilimumab in Treatment-Naive Patients With Advanced Clear Cell Renal Cell Carcinoma (HCRN GU16-260-Cohort A). J Clin Oncol 2022;40.
68. McDermott DF, Lee JL, Bjarnason GA, et al. Open-Label, Single-Arm Phase II Study of Pembrolizumab Monotherapy as First-Line Therapy in Patients With Advanced Clear Cell Renal Cell Carcinoma. J Clin Oncol 2021;39:1020–8.
69. Albiges L, Flippot R, Escudier B. Immune Checkpoint Inhibitors in Metastatic Clear-cell Renal Cell Carcinoma: Is PD-L1 Expression Useful? Eur Urol 2021;79:793–5.
70. Mori K, Abufaraj M, Mostafaei H, et al. The Predictive Value of Programmed Death Ligand 1 in Patients with Metastatic Renal Cell Carcinoma Treated with Immune-checkpoint Inhibitors: A Systematic Review and Meta-analysis. Eur Urol 2021;79. https://doi.org/10.1016/j.eururo.2020.10.006.
71. Choueiri T.K., Powles T., Burotto M., et al., Nivolumab plus Cabozantinib versus Sunitinib for Advanced Renal-Cell Carcinoma, N Engl J Med, 384, 2021, 829–841.
72. Choueiri TK, Figueroa DJ, Fay AP, et al. Correlation of PD-L1 tumor expression and treatment outcomes in patients with renal cell carcinoma receiving sunitinib or pazopanib: results from COMPARZ, a randomized controlled trial. Clin Cancer Res 2015;21:1071–7.
73. Flaifel A, Xie W, Braun DA, et al. PD-L1 expression and clinical outcomes to cabozantinib, everolimus, and sunitinib in patients with metastatic renal cell carcinoma: Analysis of the randomized clinical trials Meteor and Cabosun. Clin Cancer Res 2019;25:6080–8.

74. Hoyt CC. Multiplex Immunofluorescence and Multispectral Imaging: Forming the Basis of a Clinical Test Platform for Immuno-Oncology. Front Mol Biosci 2021;8. https://doi.org/10.3389/fmolb.2021.674747.

75. Pignon JC, Jegede O, Shukla SA, et al. Irrecist for the evaluation of candidate biomarkers of response to nivolumab in metastatic clear cell renal cell carcinoma: Analysis of a phase II prospective clinical trial. Clin Cancer Res 2019;25:2174–84.

76. Schumacher TN, Thommen DS. Tertiary lymphoid structures in cancer. Science 2022;375. eabf9419.

77. Vanhersecke L, Brunet M, Guégan JP, et al. Mature tertiary lymphoid structures predict immune checkpoint inhibitor efficacy in solid tumors independently of PD-L1 expression. Nat Cancer 2021;2:794–802.

78. Helmink B.A., Reddy S.M., Gao J., et al., B cells and tertiary lymphoid structures promote immunotherapy response, *Nature*, 577, 2020, 549–555.

79. Taube JM, Roman K, Engle EL, et al. Multi-institutional TSA-amplified Multiplexed Immunofluorescence Reproducibility Evaluation (MITRE) Study. J Immunother Cancer 2021;9.

Insights into Renal Cell Carcinoma with Novel Imaging Approaches

Khoschy Schawkat, MD, PhD[a,b], Katherine M. Krajewski, MD[a,b,c],*

KEYWORDS

- Renal cell carcinoma • Bosniak classification version 2019
- Clear cell likelihood score version 2.0 • Contrast-enhanced ultrasound
- Dual-energy CT • Girentuximab PET/CT
- Prostate-specific membrane antigen (PSMA) PET/CT • Radiomics

KEY POINTS

- The updated Bosniak classification, version 2019, predicts the likelihood of malignancy in cystic renal masses, with improved specificity of the higher risk categories, thereby expanding the number of masses that can be monitored.
- In the clear cell likelihood score, version 2.0, multiparametric MRI features of small renal masses without macroscopic fat are sequentially analyzed to determine the likelihood of clear cell renal cell carcinoma.
- Contrast-enhanced ultrasound and dual energy computed tomography are useful in the identification and characterization of solid and cystic renal masses.
- Several radiopharmaceuticals may contribute to the characterization of renal masses, such as [99m]-technetium sestamibi, radiolabeled girentuximab and ^{68}Ga-prostate-specific membrane antigen.
- In the future, RCC may be diagnosed, managed, and treated more effectively using radiomics and artificial intelligence.

INTRODUCTION

Renal masses are commonly encountered in abdominal imaging performed for a wide variety of indications.[1] Although it is necessary to diagnose renal cell carcinoma (RCC), the most common solid tumor of the kidney,[2] incidental renal mass characterization typically involves efforts to differentiate cystic from solid masses and to discriminate benign and indolent renal masses from the aggressive ones, without

[a] Brigham and Women's Hospital, 75 Francis Street, Boston, MA 02115, USA; [b] Harvard Medical School; [c] Dana-Farber Cancer Institute, 440 Brookline Avenue, Building MA Floor L1 Room 04AC, Boston, MA 02215, USA
* Corresponding author.
E-mail address: kmkrajewski@bwh.harvard.edu

Hematol Oncol Clin N Am 37 (2023) 863–875
https://doi.org/10.1016/j.hoc.2023.05.002
0889-8588/23/© 2023 Elsevier Inc. All rights reserved.

the need for tissue diagnosis. In the last few decades, an extensive body of literature has been dedicated to renal mass radiologic-pathologic correlation, yet diagnostic challenges remain in daily clinical practice.

Newer imaging algorithms have been developed to improve and standardize radiologists' approach to renal mass and RCC characterization with conventional computed tomography (CT) and MRI. Novel imaging techniques have also been studied to help resolve remaining diagnostic uncertainty, using contrast-enhanced ultrasound, dual-energy CT, molecular imaging, radiomics/genomics and machine learning. Radiologic indicators of tumor aggressiveness and imaging correlates of underlying genetic features continue to be defined. Current diagnostic algorithms combined with new imaging techniques have the potential to optimize comprehensive noninvasive renal mass characterization, termed "virtual biopsy."[3]

Renal mass management strategies have evolved in concert with better understanding of cancer biology and advanced imaging technology to provide patients personalized options based their individual tumor features and clinical situation. To guide patients to the most appropriate management, contemporary efforts in renal mass imaging have centered on improved noninvasive mass characterization to risk stratify patients. In this literature review, we provide an overview of novel imaging approaches in RCC which show the most promise.

New Imaging Algorithms Using Established Imaging Techniques

In the last few years, diagnostic algorithms aimed at cystic and solid renal mass characterization have been refined via the Bosniak classification, version 2019, and the clear cell likelihood score (ccLS), version 2.0, respectively.[3,4] The Bosniak classification, version 2019 incorporates both CT and MRI imaging features to determine the likelihood of malignancy in cystic renal masses, defined as one in which less than approximately 25% of the mass is composed of enhancing tissue.[5] As in the original Bosniak classification, category I-II lesions may be ignored, category IIF lesions are observed, and category III-IV may be considered for resection/ablation (**Fig. 1**). Refinements in the updated Bosniak classification are aimed at improving specificity of the higher risk categories, thereby increasing the number of masses that are amenable to surveillance, with quantitative criteria to improve characterization. Interreader agreement is slightly improved using the Bosniak classification, version 2019, compared with the original version.[6] Bosniak version 2019 definitions for wall/septa thickness and protrusions were associated with malignancy in one report[6] and another study showed higher diagnostic specificity for malignancy using version 2019.[7]

Solid renal mass characterization has been recently standardized using the ccLS, version 2.0.[8] In this algorithm, multiparametric MRI features of small renal masses without macroscopic fat are sequentially analyzed to determine the likelihood of clear cell RCC, the most aggressive form of RCC, with ccLS scores of 1 to 5 indicating clear cell RCC is very unlikely to very likely, which could inform management (**Fig. 2**). The unique advantages of MRI over CT are brought to bear in this system, including characterization of microscopic and macroscopic fat elements, superior soft tissue contrast, and corticomedullary enhancement features. In a retrospective cohort study, positive predictive value (PPV) for detecting clear cell RCC correlated with ccLS score, wherein PPV of ccLS1 was 5%, ccLS2 was 6%, ccLS3 was 35%, ccLS4 was 78%, and in ccLS5 was 93%.[4] Sensitivity of ccLS of 4 or greater and specificity of ccLS of 2 or lesser were 91% and 56%, respectively. ccLS scoring has been validated in an external cohort of cT1a and cT1b solid renal masses with high-interobserver agreement.[9] Growth in small renal masses has been associated with ccLS, with higher ccLS correlating with faster growth.[10] This algorithm has

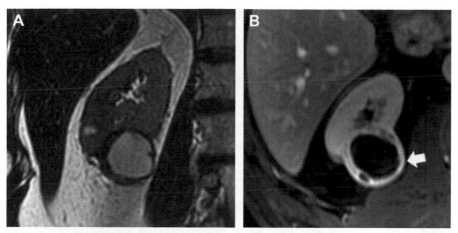

Fig. 1. A 65-year-old man with multiple myeloma and cystic renal mass detected on PET/CT (not shown). Coronal T2-weighted half-Fourier single-shot fast-spin echo image (*A*) and axial gadolinium-enhanced T1-weighted 3D fat-saturated spoiled gradient echo image (*B*) show a 3.9 cm cystic renal mass with peripheral thick enhancing rim measuring 4.5 mm in thickness (*arrow* in B), representing a Bosniak III cystic mass according to the Bosniak Classification version 2019. The patient opted for partial nephrectomy; pathology showed pT1a clear cell RCC, Fuhrman grade 2 of 4. Approximately 50% of Bosniak III masses are malignant.

not yet been widely adopted into radiologic reporting for renal mass characterization but may be in the near future.

Novel Modalities

Contrast-enhanced US

Contrast-enhanced US (CEUS) has great potential and usefulness in identification and characterization of solid and cystic renal masses. Contrast agents used in ultrasound are not nephrotoxic or hepatotoxic. Furthermore, they have a short half-life (5 minutes) and elimination takes place via the lungs by exhalation.[11] CEUS has an advantage over contrast-enhanced CT for visualization of hypovascular renal lesions due to excellent background tissue suppression (**Fig. 3**). CEUS may be of special utility in characterization of indeterminate masses on CT/MRI or in patients with renal insufficiency or contraindications to CT/MRI contrast agents. CEUS has been designated "usually appropriate" in the American College of Radiology Appropriateness Criteria of evaluation of indeterminate renal masses in the latter circumstance.[12] At present, CEUS in the kidney is an off-label indication but can be reimbursable by insurance.[13] A 2022 meta-analysis showed a pooled sensitivity and specificity of CEUS for characterization of solid lesions (331 patients; 341 lesions) of 98% (95% CI 95%, 100%) and 78% (95% CI 68%, 88%), respectively.[13] Pooled sensitivity and specificity of CEUS for the characterization of complex cystic renal lesions (419 patients; 436 lesions) was 95% (95% CI 91%, 99%) and 84% (95% CI 77%, 90%), respectively. CEUS has been associated with high specificity and PPV to diagnose RCC in small indeterminate solid renal masses (sSRMs) on CT or MRI. Once lipid-rich angiomyolipoma (AML) was excluded by the other modalities, sSRM arterial phase hypoenhancement relative to renal cortex on CEUS yielded high specificity (97.4%) and PPV (98.2%) to diagnose RCC.[14] CEUS also contributed to cystic renal mass characterization in this study. However, complete subtyping of renal masses is not currently known, and knowledge

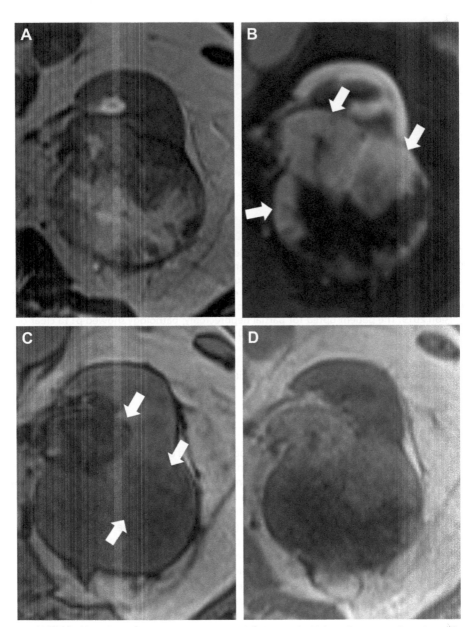

Fig. 2. A 52-year-old man with back pain and incidental left renal mass on imaging. The mass did not contain macroscopic fat and was greater than 25% enhancing, thus the ccLS could be assigned. Axial T2-weighted half-Fourier single-shot fast-spin echo image (*A*) shows a 9.5 cm renal mass with T2 isointensity to renal cortex within the enhancing components (demonstrated in *B*). Axial T1-weighted, fat-saturated postcontrast MRI performed during the corticomedullary phase (*B*) shows heterogeneous, intense peripheral enhancement within the renal mass (*arrows*). An axial out-of-phase image (*C*) shows areas of signal loss (*arrows*) compared with signal on the in-phase image at the same anatomic level (*D*), representing microscopic fat elements. The features result in a ccLS score of 5 in this mass, which was subsequently resected and shown to represent clear cell RCC.

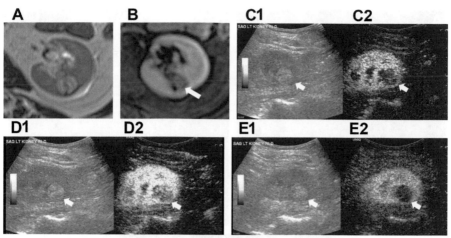

Fig. 3. A 78-year-old man with incidentally detected left renal mass. Axial T2-weighted half-Fourier single-shot fast-spin echo image (*A*) shows a 2.0 cm predominately markedly hyperintense left renal mass. Axial T1-weighted, fat-saturated postcontrast subtraction MRI (nephrographic phase-precontrast imaging) (*B*) shows heterogeneous, mild-to-moderate enhancement of internal components occupying at least 25% of the entire mass (*arrow*). The patient and his physician elected active surveillance of this mass. Nine months later, CEUS was performed. Gray scale imaging (C1, D1, and E1) shows an echogenic 2 cm left renal mass (*arrow*), with little CEUS contrast enhancement on the earliest corticomedullary imaging (C2, *arrow*) but diffuse CEUS contrast enhancement is shown slightly later in the arterial phase (D2, *arrow*), confirming solid enhancing elements. There is near complete washout in the mass in the delayed phase (E2, *arrow*). There is delayed washout of contrast from the background renal parenchyma related to underlying renal parenchymal disease. This mass has not been biopsied; the patient continues in active surveillance. Case courtesy of Jessie Chai, MD and Elizabeth Asch, MD.

of this modality is still increasing.[15] Pilot studies have proposed a CEUS Bosniak classification or adjunct CEUS measures to further risk stratify complex cystic renal masses.[14,16]

Dual energy CT

Dual energy CT (DECT) is another modality that contributes to renal mass detection and characterization. Dual energy CT uses 2 different x-ray photon energy spectra to interrogate materials with different attenuation properties at different energies. Several implementations are currently available, including sequential scanning DECT, split filter DECT, rapid kilovoltage-peak switching DECT, dual source DECT and dual layer DECT.[17] All these modalities are based on variations in CT. Postprocessing permits the characterization of tissues, including iodine content from administered intravenous contrast, enabling the differentiation of enhancing and nonenhancing components of renal masses and iodine quantification, although limitations exist (**Fig. 4**). DECT has special relevance in the setting of an incidentally encountered renal mass on abdominal imaging because a substantial proportion of incidental indeterminate renal lesions can be characterized as nonenhancing benign Bosniak II cysts using this technology (which would not require additional follow-up), including more than half of the encountered indeterminate lesions in one cohort.[18]

Once a renal mass is characterized as a solid enhancing mass, the role of DECT is not as well defined. Diagnostic accuracy of DECT using quantitative iodine concentration for

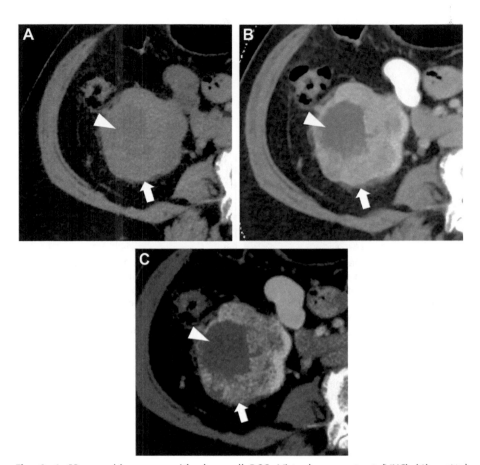

Fig. 4. A 68-year-old woman with clear cell RCC. Virtual noncontrast (VNC) (*A*), portal venous phase contrast-enhanced dual-energy (*B*) and iodine overlay map (*C*) images show a heterogeneous right renal mass representing known clear cell RCC. The VNC image (*A*) shows peripheral tissue attenuation (*arrow*) and central hypoattenuation (*arrowhead*), corresponding to enhancing soft tissue (*arrow*) and central necrosis (*arrowhead*) on the contrast-enhanced image (*B*). Iodine content is seen within the peripheral enhancing component (*arrow*) on the iodine overlay map (*C*), and iodine is absent centrally within the necrotic component (*arrowhead*).

the evaluation of renal masses was assessed in a couple of recent meta-analyses. One meta-analysis showed pooled sensitivity and specificity for characterizing solid renal masses with DECT of 96.6% and 95.1%, respectively.[19] However, no difference in accuracy was identified in renal mass evaluation using DECT with iodine quantification and conventional single-energy CT and further large multicenter studies would be needed to assess incremental DECT value. Another meta-analysis showed high-pooled sensitivity and specificity of iodine quantification in distinguishing nonenhancing and enhancing renal masses.[20] A recent single-center study to assess the influence of DECT compared with single-energy CT (using unenhanced and contrast-enhanced nephrographic phase imaging) on renal lesion characterization revealed higher confidence in lesion characterization with DECT and lower requests for additional imaging follow-up, using contrast-enhanced MRI as a reference standard.[21]

Several reports correlating DECT measures to histologic subtypes of RCC have been published, including iodine quantification differences between clear cell and papillary subtypes.[22–24] Whether iodine concentration correlates to tumor grade is controversial.[22,24] Importantly, evidence to support a role for DECT in differentiating benign from malignant solid renal masses is lacking, to date.

Molecular imaging

Diagnostic and therapeutic applications of radiopharmaceuticals in oncology have exponentially increased in recent years. Several radiopharmaceuticals are poised to contribute to renal mass characterization, including [99m]-technetium sestamibi, radio-labeled girentuximab and ^{68}Ga-prostate-specific membrane antigen (PSMA).[25]

Sestamibi

[99m]Tc-sestamibi is a radiopharmaceutical already in widespread use and approved by the US Food and Drug Administration (FDA) for myocardial and parathyroid imaging. ^{99m}Tc-sestamibi accumulates in tissues with high mitochondrial content and low multidrug resistance pump expression; masses with ^{99m}Tc-sestamibi uptake include oncocytomas, rare hybrid oncocytic/chromophobe tumors (HOCT) and some lipid poor angiomyolipomas.[26] One meta-analysis showed single photon emission computed tomography imaging with ^{99m}Tc-sestamibi has high sensitivity and specificity for differentiating benign renal lesions from malignant ones, 86% (95% CI 66%–95%) and 90% (95% CI 80%–95%), respectively (when considering HOCTs as malignant, although this is controversial[27]). There was lower pooled specificity for differentiating oncocytomas from chromophobe RCC (67%). Because masses with no uptake have been associated with a higher probability of malignancy, this modality could contribute to cost-effective risk stratification of patients with small renal masses considering active surveillance.[28,29]

Girentuximab

Radiolabeled girentuximab is a radionuclide-linked antibody that binds to carbonic anhydrase IX, a transmembrane glycoprotein expressed in clear cell RCC. Two large phase III trials have examined the role of girentuximab PET/CT in patients with renal masses; specifically [124]I-labeled girentuximab accurately and noninvasively identified clear cell RCC in the REnal Masses: Pivotal Study to DEteCT Clear Cell Renal Cell Carcinoma With Pre-Surgical PET/CT (REDECT) trial with sensitivity of 86.2% (95% CI 75.3%–97.1%) and 85.9% (95% CI 69.4 %–99.9%), respectively,[30] and [89]Zr-DFO-girentuximab evaluated in the Zirconium in Renal Cancer Oncology trial has recently met its coprimary endpoints, with 85.5% sensitivity and 87% specificity of the agent to detect clear cell RCC, and sensitivity and specificity thresholds were exceeded by 3 independent readers.[31] Even combined radiopharmaceutical imaging strategies have been proposed for indeterminate solid renal masses, using both sestamibi and girentuximab radiotracers for future study.

Prostate-Specific Membrane Antigen

[68]Gallium-labelled PSMA is another agent with potential application in suspected RCC. PSMA is overexpressed in several solid tumors including RCC, especially in tumor-associated neovasculature (**Fig. 5**).[32] In a retrospective analysis of 257 patients with RCC (including clear cell, papillary, and chromophobe subtypes) higher grade and more advanced tumors correlated with stronger PSMA expression, which predicted overall poorer survival[32] Interestingly, uptake was markedly lower in non-cc-RCC subtypes (papillary and chromophobe) as compared with cc-RCC, which also

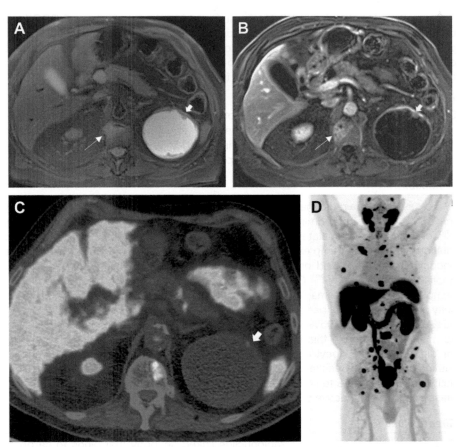

Fig. 5. 83-year-old man with a history of prostate cancer and cystic renal mass. Axial T2-weighted image with fat saturation (*A*) and axial gadolinium-enhanced T1-weighted 3D fat-saturated spoiled gradient echo subtraction image (postcontrast–precontrast; *B*) show an enhancing nodule within the predominately cystic left upper pole renal mass (*thick arrows*) representing a Bosniak 4 cystic renal mass. Bone metastasis in L1 is also present (*thin arrows*). Biopsy of a liver lesion (not shown) subsequently confirmed metastatic non-clear cell RCC, not further classified on the biopsy specimen. Fused PSMA PET/CT image (*C*) performed to assess the extent of prostate cancer demonstrated PSMA uptake in the enhancing nodules of the cystic left renal mass (*arrows*). Maximum Intensity Projection image from PSMA PET/CT (*D*) shows widespread metastatic disease.

may contribute to risk stratification.[33,34] However, primary RCCs have low-PSMA uptake in comparison to surrounding tissues,[33,35] limiting the usefulness of PSMA PET in localized RCC because of its low tumor-to-background ratio. RCC staging PSMA PET/CT could be an interesting staging tool; in early reports, PSMA PET/CT had higher sensitivity and PPV for metastases than conventional CT and could be used in patients with elevated creatinine and/or allergy to iodinated contrast.[35,36] In another more recent study of 61 patients undergoing PSMA PET/CT for restaging or suspected metastatic RCC, PSMA PET/CT findings lead to a change in management in 49% of patients.[37] Several molecular agents represent exciting new opportunities in RCC detection and risk stratification to be combined with the anatomic imaging approaches in future care algorithms.

Radiomics and Artificial Intelligence

Radiomics involves the use of machine learning algorithms to extract a large number of quantitative features from medical images, which are not perceivable by the human eye. The process of radiomics requires several steps, including CT, MRI, and/or PET/CT image acquisition, selection and segmentation of a volume of interest, and feature or quantitative value extraction for analysis and ultimate correlation to disease subtypes, genetic features, treatment response, and/or patient outcomes.[38] Radiomics features have been explored as complementary to tissue diagnosis and genomic analysis and one day may lend to an optimized "virtual biopsy." Radiomics is a field in its infancy, however, subject to many challenges including but not limited to its complexity, lack of widely accepted standards and guidelines, and the need for validation studies to support early findings.[38]

Radiomics features have been used to predict the risk of recurrence, metastasis, and overall survival in patients with RCC, with incremental value added to existing clinical factors.[39] In addition, radiomics have also been used to identify imaging biomarkers to better identify malignant renal masses, differentiate RCC subtypes, and predict RCC responses to various treatments.[40–43]

Artificial intelligence (AI) has the potential to transform the way that RCC is diagnosed and treated. There are various ways that radiomics and AI can potentially be applied in RCC, including (1) computer-aided diagnosis: AI algorithms can be used to analyze medical images to detect and diagnose RCC[44,45]; (2) predictive modeling: AI can be used to develop predictive models for postoperative progression free survival and overall survival.[39,46,47]; (3) treatment planning: AI can be used to help plan the most appropriate treatment strategy for patients with RCC, considering factors such as the stage and grade of the tumor, the patient's overall health, and the potential side effects of different treatment options[48–50]; and in; (4) drug development: AI can be used to analyze large datasets of patient information and drug responses to identify potential new therapies for RCC.[51] Radiomics and AI have the potential to revolutionize the way that RCC is diagnosed, managed, and treated but further research is needed before radiomics can be clinically implemented.

SUMMARY

The substantial body of literature focused on imaging examination of renal masses and RCC continues to increase. The Bosniak classification version 2019 and the ccLS are newer algorithms that improve and standardize cystic and solid mass characterization, respectively, but diagnostic uncertainty remains in certain instances, including Bosniak III lesions and ccLS score 3 lesions. When combined with the existing modalities, novel imaging techniques including CEUS, dual energy CT, molecular imaging and radiomics have the potential to truly optimize "virtual biopsy," RCC diagnosis and management.

Increasing evidence will ultimately determine which modality or combinations of modalities will provide better renal mass characterization than the current standard. Molecular agents are well positioned to enhance renal mass characterization in the near term, with some agents already FDA-approved for alternative indications. A new agent, ^{89}Zr-DFO-girentuximab, also showed high sensitivity and specificity for clear cell RCC in a recent phase III trial. It is likely molecular and anatomic imaging strategies will be combined into new renal mass characterization algorithms. In the more distant future, radiomics and AI are promising technologies, which may make "virtual biopsy" a reality.

CLINICS CARE POINTS

- The Bosniak classification, version 2019 incorporates CT and MRI imaging features to determine the likelihood of malignancy in cystic renal masses. Updates are aimed at improving specificity of the higher risk categories, thereby increasing the number of masses that are amenable to surveillance, with quantitative criteria to improve characterization.

- The ccLS is an imaging algorithm using multiparametric MRI features of small renal masses to determine the likelihood of clear cell RCC.

- Contrast-enhanced ultrasound is a modality, which can aid in characterization of indeterminate renal masses in patients with renal insufficiency or contraindications to CT/MRI contrast agents. It has been designated "usually appropriate" in the American College of Radiology Appropriateness Criteria for evaluation of indeterminate renal masses and can be reimbursable by insurance.

- Several molecular imaging agents are poised to contribute to renal mass characterization and RCC staging. For example, in a recent phase III trial, ^{89}Zr-DFO-girentuximab showed high sensitivity and specificity for clear cell RCC.

- In research settings, radiomics features have been used to predict the risk of recurrence, metastasis, and overall survival in patients with RCC, with incremental value added to existing clinical factors.

CONFLICTS OF INTEREST

K. Schawkat and K.M. Krajewski have no conflicts of interest to disclose.

REFERENCES

1. Capitanio U, Bensalah K, Bex A, et al. Epidemiology of Renal Cell Carcinoma. Eur Urol 2019;75(1):74–84.
2. Abou Elkassem AM, Lo SS, Gunn AJ, et al. Role of Imaging in Renal Cell Carcinoma: A Multidisciplinary Perspective. Radiographics 2021;41(5):1387–407.
3. Silverman SG, Pedrosa I, Ellis JH, et al. Bosniak Classification of Cystic Renal Masses, Version 2019: An Update Proposal and Needs Assessment. Radiology 2019;292(2):475–88.
4. Steinberg RL, Rasmussen RG, Johnson BA, et al. Prospective performance of clear cell likelihood scores (ccLS) in renal masses evaluated with multiparametric magnetic resonance imaging. Eur Radiol 2021;31(1):314–24.
5. Jhaveri K, Gupta P, Elmi A, et al. Cystic renal cell carcinomas: do they grow, metastasize, or recur? AJR Am J Roentgenol 2013;201(2):W292–6.
6. Yan JH, Chan J, Osman H, et al. Bosniak Classification version 2019: validation and comparison to original classification in pathologically confirmed cystic masses. Eur Radiol 2021;31(12):9579–87.
7. Park MY, Park KJ, Kim MH, et al. Bosniak Classification of Cystic Renal Masses Version 2019: Comparison With Version 2005 for Class Distribution, Diagnostic Performance, and Interreader Agreement Using CT and MRI. AJR Am J Roentgenol 2021;217(6):1367–76.
8. Pedrosa I, Cadeddu JA. How We Do It: Managing the Indeterminate Renal Mass with the MRI Clear Cell Likelihood Score. Radiology 2022;302(2):256–69.
9. Dunn M, Linehan V, Clarke SE, et al. Diagnostic Performance and Interreader Agreement of the MRI Clear Cell Likelihood Score for Characterization of cT1a

and cT1b Solid Renal Masses: An External Validation Study. AJR Am J Roentgenol 2022;219(5):793–803.

10. Rasmussen RG, Xi Y, Sibley RC 3rd, et al. Association of Clear Cell Likelihood Score on MRI and Growth Kinetics of Small Solid Renal Masses on Active Surveillance. AJR Am J Roentgenol 2022;218(1):101–10.

11. Barr RG, Wilson SR, Lyshchik A, et al. Contrast-enhanced Ultrasound-State of the Art in North America: Society of Radiologists in Ultrasound White Paper. Ultrasound Q 2020;36(4S Suppl 1):S1–39.

12. Expert Panel on Urologic I, Wang ZJ, Nikolaidis P, et al. ACR Appropriateness Criteria(R) Indeterminate Renal Mass. J Am Coll Radiol 2020;17(11S):S415–28.

13. Barr RG. Use of lumason/sonovue in contrast-enhanced ultrasound of the kidney for characterization of renal masses-a meta-analysis. Abdom Radiol (NY) 2022; 47(1):272–87.

14. Elbanna KY, Jang HJ, Kim TK, et al. The added value of contrast-enhanced ultrasound in evaluation of indeterminate small solid renal masses and risk stratification of cystic renal lesions. Eur Radiol 2021;31(11):8468–77.

15. King KG. Use of Contrast Ultrasound for Renal Mass Evaluation. Radiol Clin North Am 2020;58(5):935–49.

16. Chandrasekar T, Clark CB, Gomella A, et al. Volumetric Quantitative Contrast-enhanced Ultrasonography Evaluation of Complex Renal Cysts: An Adjunctive Metric to the Bosniak Classification System to Predict Malignancy. Eur Urol Focus 2022;9(2):336–44.

17. Thiravit S, Brunnquell C, Cai LM, et al. Use of dual-energy CT for renal mass assessment. Eur Radiol 2021;31(6):3721–33.

18. Wortman JR, Shyu JY, Fulwadhva UP, et al. Impact Analysis of the Routine Use of Dual-Energy Computed Tomography for Characterization of Incidental Renal Lesions. J Comput Assist Tomogr 2019;43(2):176–82.

19. Salameh JP, McInnes MDF, McGrath TA, et al. Diagnostic Accuracy of Dual-Energy CT for Evaluation of Renal Masses: Systematic Review and Meta-Analysis. AJR Am J Roentgenol 2019;212(4):W100–5.

20. Bellini D, Panvini N, Laghi A, et al. Systematic Review and Meta-Analysis Investigating the Diagnostic Yield of Dual-Energy CT for Renal Mass Assessment. AJR Am J Roentgenol 2019;212(5):1044–53.

21. Pourvaziri A, Mojtahed A, Hahn PF, et al. Renal lesion characterization: clinical utility of single-phase dual-energy CT compared to MRI and dual-phase single-energy CT. Eur Radiol 2022;33(2):1318–28.

22. Mileto A, Marin D, Alfaro-Cordoba M, et al. Iodine quantification to distinguish clear cell from papillary renal cell carcinoma at dual-energy multidetector CT: a multireader diagnostic performance study. Radiology 2014;273(3):813–20.

23. Dai C, Cao Y, Jia Y, et al. Differentiation of renal cell carcinoma subtypes with different iodine quantification methods using single-phase contrast-enhanced dual-energy CT: areal vs. volumetric analyses. Abdom Radiol (NY) 2018;43(3): 672–8.

24. Camlidag I, Nural MS, Danaci M, et al. Usefulness of rapid kV-switching dual energy CT in renal tumor characterization. Abdom Radiol (NY) 2019;44(5):1841–9.

25. Roussel E, Capitanio U, Kutikov A, et al. Novel Imaging Methods for Renal Mass Characterization: A Collaborative Review. Eur Urol 2022;81(5):476–88.

26. Rowe SP, Gorin MA, Solnes LB, et al. Correlation of (99m)Tc-sestamibi uptake in renal masses with mitochondrial content and multi-drug resistance pump expression. EJNMMI Res 2017;7(1):80.

27. Wilson MP, Katlariwala P, Murad MH, et al. Diagnostic accuracy of 99mTc-sesta-mibi SPECT/CT for detecting renal oncocytomas and other benign renal lesions: a systematic review and meta-analysis. Abdom Radiol (NY) 2020;45(8):2532–41.

28. Su ZT, Patel HD, Huang MM, et al. Cost-effectiveness Analysis of (99m)Tc-sesta-mibi SPECT/CT to Guide Management of Small Renal Masses. Eur Urol Focus 2021;7(4):827–34.

29. Asi T, Tuncali MC, Tuncel M, et al. The role of Tc-99m MIBI scintigraphy in clinical T1 renal mass assessment: Does it have a real benefit? Urol Oncol 2020;38(12): 937 e11–e17.

30. Divgi CR, Uzzo RG, Gatsonis C, et al. Positron emission tomography/computed tomography identification of clear cell renal cell carcinoma: results from the RE-DECT trial. J Clin Oncol 2013;31(2):187–94.

31. Mauro, Gina. Targeted Oncology, 19 Feb. 2023. Available at: www.targetedonc. com/view/phase-3-zircon-study-shows-high-sensitivity-specificity-with-89zr-dfo-girentuximab-in-ccrcc. Accessed Feb 25, 2023.

32. Spatz S, Tolkach Y, Jung K, et al. Comprehensive Evaluation of Prostate Specific Membrane Antigen Expression in the Vasculature of Renal Tumors: Implications for Imaging Studies and Prognostic Role. J Urol 2018;199(2):370–7.

33. Sawicki LM, Buchbender C, Boos J, et al. Diagnostic potential of PET/CT using a (68)Ga-labelled prostate-specific membrane antigen ligand in whole-body stag-ing of renal cell carcinoma: initial experience. Eur J Nucl Med Mol Imaging 2017; 44(1):102–7.

34. Raveenthiran S, Esler R, Yaxley J, et al. The use of (68)Ga-PET/CT PSMA in the staging of primary and suspected recurrent renal cell carcinoma. Eur J Nucl Med Mol Imaging 2019;46(11):2280–8.

35. Rhee H, Ng KL, Tse BW, et al. Using prostate specific membrane antigen (PSMA) expression in clear cell renal cell carcinoma for imaging advanced disease. Pa-thology 2016;48(6):613–6.

36. Rhee H, Blazak J, Tham CM, et al. Pilot study: use of gallium-68 PSMA PET for detection of metastatic lesions in patients with renal tumour. EJNMMI Res 2016;6(1):76.

37. Udovicich C, Callahan J, Bressel M, et al. Impact of Prostate-specific Membrane Antigen Positron Emission Tomography/Computed Tomography in the Manage-ment of Oligometastatic Renal Cell Carcinoma. Eur Urol Open Sci 2022;44:60–8.

38. Gillies RJ, Kinahan PE, Hricak H. Radiomics: Images Are More than Pictures, They Are Data. Radiology 2016;278(2):563–77.

39. Zhang H, Yin F, Chen M, et al. Development and Validation of a CT-Based Radio-mics Nomogram for Predicting Postoperative Progression-Free Survival in Stage I-III Renal Cell Carcinoma. Front Oncol 2021;11:742547.

40. Wang W, Cao K, Jin S, et al. Differentiation of renal cell carcinoma subtypes through MRI-based radiomics analysis. Eur Radiol 2020;30(10):5738–47.

41. Ursprung S, Beer L, Bruining A, et al. Radiomics of computed tomography and magnetic resonance imaging in renal cell carcinoma-a systematic review and meta-analysis. Eur Radiol 2020;30(6):3558–66.

42. Said D, Hectors SJ, Wilck E, et al. Characterization of solid renal neoplasms using MRI-based quantitative radiomics features. Abdom Radiol (NY) 2020;45(9): 2840–50.

43. Udayakumar D, Zhang Z, Xi Y, et al. Deciphering Intratumoral Molecular Hetero-geneity in Clear Cell Renal Cell Carcinoma with a Radiogenomics Platform. Clin Cancer Res 2021;27(17):4794–806.

44. Jian L, Liu Y, Xie Y, et al. MRI-Based Radiomics and Urine Creatinine for the Differentiation of Renal Angiomyolipoma With Minimal Fat From Renal Cell Carcinoma: A Preliminary Study. Front Oncol 2022;12:876664.
45. Campi R, Stewart GD, Staehler M, et al. Novel Liquid Biomarkers and Innovative Imaging for Kidney Cancer Diagnosis: What Can Be Implemented in Our Practice Today? A Systematic Review of the Literature. Eur Urol Oncol 2021;4(1):22–41.
46. Khodabakhshi Z, Amini M, Mostafaei S, et al. Overall Survival Prediction in Renal Cell Carcinoma Patients Using Computed Tomography Radiomic and Clinical Information. J Digit Imaging 2021;34(5):1086–98.
47. Khene ZE, Bigot P, Doumerc N, et al. Application of Machine Learning Models to Predict Recurrence After Surgical Resection of Nonmetastatic Renal Cell Carcinoma. Eur Urol Oncol 2022. S2588-9311(22)00137. PMID: 35987730.
48. Yang L, Gao L, Arefan D, et al. A CT-based radiomics model for predicting renal capsule invasion in renal cell carcinoma. BMC Med Imaging 2022;22(1):15.
49. Sun Z, Cui Y, Xu C, et al. Preoperative Prediction of Inferior Vena Cava Wall Invasion of Tumor Thrombus in Renal Cell Carcinoma: Radiomics Models Based on Magnetic Resonance Imaging. Front Oncol 2022;12:863534.
50. Liu J, Lin Z, Wang K, et al. A preliminary radiomics model for predicting perirenal fat invasion on renal cell carcinoma with contrast-enhanced CT images. Abdom Radiol (NY) 2022;48(2):649–58.
51. Rallis KS, Kleeman SO, Grant M, et al. Radiomics for Renal Cell Carcinoma: Predicting Outcomes from Immunotherapy and Targeted Therapies-A Narrative Review. Eur Urol Focus 2021;7(4):717–21.

Surgical Management of Localized Disease and Small Renal Masses

Daniel S. Carson, MD[a], Tova Weiss, MD[a],
Lisa Xinyuan Zhang, MD[a], Sarah P. Psutka, MD, MSc[b],*

KEYWORDS

- Small renal mass • Renal cell carcinoma • Partial nephrectomy
- Radical nephrectomy

KEY POINTS

- The incidence of renal masses has increased without an increase in mortality over the past several decades.
- Earlier detection of localized disease is associated with favorable 5-year survival rates.
- Management of small renal masses includes nonsurgical and surgical approaches.
- Surgical intervention remains the gold standard. Both open and minimally invasive surgical approaches with nephron sparing or radical excision can be offered depending on individual evaluation.
- Shared decision-making is mandatory when determining the correct surgical treatment option for a patient with a localized renal tumor. This should follow elicitation of patient priorities, taking into account baseline renal function, competing comorbidities, body habitus, and prior surgery, tumor characteristics and oncologic risk, and a balanced discussion of surgical risks and expectations for recovery.

INTRODUCTION
Localized Disease

Renal cancer is the seventh most common neoplasm globally with increasing incidence rates attributed to the ubiquity of cross-sectional imaging.[1,2] However, renal cancer associated mortality is declining,[3,4] likely due to both stage migration toward earlier stage disease[4–6] and advances in management of advanced disease with novel immunotherapies and targeted agents.[2,7,8]

[a] Department of Urology, University of Washington, Seattle, WA, USA; [b] Department of Urology, University of Washington, Fred Hutchinson Cancer Center, Harborview Medical Center, 1959 NE Pacific Street, Box 356510, Seattle, WA 98195, USA
* Corresponding author.
E-mail address: spsutka@uw.edu

Hematol Oncol Clin N Am 37 (2023) 877–892
https://doi.org/10.1016/j.hoc.2023.05.003
0889-8588/23/© 2023 Elsevier Inc. All rights reserved.

Localized disease is defined as tumor confined within the kidney capsule without evidence of nodal or distant metastases, including both solid and complex cystic masses. Localized disease comprises clinical stage 1 and 2 tumors classified based by size as follows: Stage 1a: less than 4 cm, which comprise small renal masses (SRMs), Stage1b: 4 to 7 cm, Stage 2a: 7 to 10 cm, and Stage 2b: 10 cm or larger, without extension into the pararenal or renal sinus fat, the renal vasculature, or the urinary collecting system.[9] The objective of this narrative review will be to detail the contemporary approach to the surgical management of the nonmetastatic SRMs and localized disease.

Epidemiology of Small Renal Masses and Localized Renal Cell Carcinoma

The incidence of renal mass detection has increased over the past 30 years, with approximately 73,000 new cases detected in the United States in 2020 and more than 300,000 worldwide.[4] The incidence of renal tumors is higher in men than women with a ratio of 1.5:1 and the rate of diagnosis peaks in the seventh decade. Most SRMs and localized disease are incidentally diagnosed on cross-sectional imaging.[10] Symptomatic presentation including flank pain, hematuria, or palpable mass are suggestive of locally advanced or metastatic disease and rarely observed in patients with SRMs. Risk factors associated with malignant renal masses include smoking, hypertension, chronic kidney disease, sedentary lifestyle, diabetes, diet, and obesity, and environmental exposures to perfluorinated chemicals and aristolochic acid.[1,2]

Differential Diagnosis

Renal masses include benign and malignant tumors with variable oncologic potential dependent on histologic subtype and grade. More than 90% of *malignant* renal masses are renal cell carcinoma (RCC)[4,5,11]; however, the true incidence of benign versus malignant masses remains unknown. Imaging features help in predicting malignancy as the risk of malignancy and higher histologic grade are associated with increasing tumor size.[12] Furthermore, increasing tumor size is correlated with increased likelihood of aggressive histology for malignant masses.[13] This may be helpful when considering counseling and management options for SRMs and localized disease. Contemporary American Urologic Association guidelines emphasize the importance of shared decision-making with patients when electing treatment for renal masses, and especially SRMs, and endorse percutaneous renal mass biopsy (RMB) to facilitate histologic diagnosis and risk stratification for SRMs to guide treatment election.[3]

Natural History of Small Renal Masses

The increasing incidence of renal tumors resulted in greater numbers of patients undergoing treatment, however, Smaldone and colleagues posited that earlier detection may not change the absolute numbers of aggressive tumors detected, ultimately leading to overtreatment of predominantly indolent, or, in some cases, benign masses.[14] The natural history of SRMs demonstrates low rates of metastasis in tumors growing between 1 and 3 mm/y, with metastases typically occurring in larger (>3 cm) and faster growing tumors.[15,16] *Active surveillance* (AS) involves observing SRMs with imaging at 3 to 6 month intervals, with the goal of proceeding to intervention only in those patients who demonstrate concerning growth kinetics or for patient preference. Multiple international guidelines now endorse AS for select patients with SRMs less than 2 cm in size to reduce the risk of overtreatment.[3]

PREOPERATIVE EVALUATION AND RISK STRATIFICATION

When evaluating a patient with localized renal masses, obtaining a detailed medical history including a careful assessment of competing comorbidities, baseline renal disease is essential as are assessing frailty and estimating life expectancy using validated tools such as the Lee Schonberg Index.[17–21] Past surgical history, especially history of abdominal surgeries is essential to guide decisions regarding surgical approaches. Genetic counseling should also be considered for patients with renal malignancy, and high-risk factors, including young age (<46 year old), multifocal or bilateral renal masses, personal or family history, suggest a familial renal neoplastic syndrome such as von Hippel–Lindau disease or first- or second-degree relatives with a history of renal malignancy.[3]

After radiographic diagnosis, RMB can help guide treatment decisions and is important in establishing histology in cases of metastatic disease where a tissue diagnosis is needed. Per the National Comprehensive Cancer Network (NCCN) guidelines, RMB can also be considered when initiating AS or at follow-up interval if not done previously and is recommended before thermal ablation to confirm malignancy.[22] Ultimately, like other diagnostic or treatment paradigms, the decision to pursue RMB is shared between physician, patient, and family. In a recent study by Kurtzman and colleagues, 86% of patients that underwent RMB stated that the results facilitated decision-making, with 92% rating the RMB as useful. Importantly, 86% of patients reporting lack of certainty regarding treatment choice pre-biopsy, reported feeling sure of their treatment decision after undergoing RMB[23]

RMB are safe, with a risk of major complications including procedure-related hemorrhage, arteriovenous fistula, infection, and pneumothorax occurring in less than 1%.[24,25] Nondiagnostic biopsies can occur in up to 14% of cases with increased risks in very small and cystic renal masses, in patients with skin-to-mass distances greater than 10 cm, and when aspirates are used rather than core biopsies.[26] In contemporary series, RMB diagnosis of malignant disease and histology are concordant with final histologic pathology with high rates of accuracy (up to 98%).[27] Current guidelines endorse RMB to provide histologic diagnosis in patients considering surveillance versus definitive treatment and before ablative procedures.[3,4]

NONSURGICAL MANAGEMENT OPTIONS

Patients with SRMs (<3 cm) may undergo AS with serial imaging to monitor for tumor growth, biopsy, symptoms, or patient preference triggering definitive treatment. Imaging and clinical evaluations are performed at regular intervals, with thoracic imaging obtained at baseline and then followed annually. The risk of metastatic progression on AS is low, with a CSM risk of 0.6%. Patients with high surgical risk may be offered ablative techniques such as cryoablation, radiofrequency ablation (RFA), or microwave ablation, which have similar outcomes to partial nephrectomy (PN), but inferior overall survival (OS) is likely due to selection bias. Delayed treatment is pursued by 34% of patients on AS, with tumor growth and patient/physician preference being the most common reasons for treatment.

Patients with SRM less than 3 cm in size may undergo AS with serial imaging to monitor tumor growth, and definitive treatment is triggered by robust growth kinetics, biopsy, symptoms, or for patient preference.[3,4] Imaging with abdominal computed tomography (CT) or MRI with contrast within 6 months of initiation of AS and then with follow-up CT, MRI, or ultrasound (US) at 3 to 6 month intervals to monitor for tumor progression. In patients with stable tumor size, interval imaging may be extended to annually.[3,4,28] Follow-up also includes annual clinical evaluations and renal function monitoring with thoracic imaging at baseline and then for symptoms, restaging in case of progression, or for follow-up of an identified abnormality thereafter.

A recent meta-analysis reported that 34% of patients on AS pursued delayed treatment after an average of 27.8 ± 10.6 months on AS citing tumor growth (41%), patient- or physician-preference (52%) or symptom management (7%) as the triggers for intervention.[29] Across meta-analyses, the risk of metastatic progression on AS seems to be less than 2%, with a cancer specific mortality (CSM) risk of 0.6%.[8,29–31]

In patients with SRM desiring definitive treatment but with high surgical risk, ablative techniques, such as cryoablation, RFA, or microwave ablation represent definitive treatment options with equivalent oncologic outcomes to PN in clinical Stage T1a (cT1a) renal masses if secondary or repeated treatments are included.[3,4,11] The available literature demonstrates an association between inferior OS and ablative approaches; however, this likely is related to the high burden of comorbidity in many of the available ablation cohorts.[11]

SURGICAL MANAGEMENT
The Evolving Role of Partial Nephrectomy

Surgical intervention remains the standard of care for management of localized renal tumors, and PN is the favored surgical option when feasible to mitigate the downstream complication of renal insufficiency.[32] Per multiple international current guideline statements, PN is appropriate and favored for patients with unilateral tumors that are stage 1–3a (involvement of the renal sinus fat or perinephric fat) and technically feasible for partial resection[3,4,22,33] and PN is preferred surgical option of choice for many clinical settings including solitary kidney, multifocal or bilateral masses, familial renal tumors, and young patients or those with comorbidities which may impact renal function (Table 1). Various scoring systems have been developed to characterize tumor complexity and to determine candidacy for PN incorporating tumor size, location, adjacency to hilum, endo/exophytic extension, renal vascular anatomy, renal pelvic anatomy, and degree of perinephric fat.[34]

The role of PN in larger and centrally located renal tumors (eg, cT1b and above) remains controversial. Results from a recent SEER database-based study demonstrated equivalent local control following PN versus radical nephrectomy (RN) for T1b tumors.[35] Similarly, other reports have observed no significant difference in CSM with PN versus RN for carefully selected pT2 tumors.[36] In the EORTC 30904 trial, patients receiving PN suffered less postoperative renal function decline, whereas RN was associated with improvements in OS[37] (Table 2). However, critiques of this trial include a high degree of cross-over between arms, under accrual, over 10% of

Table 1 Decision-making for nephron sparing versus radical nephrectomy[14]	
Partial Nephrectomy and Nephron-Sparing Approach[14]	**Radical Nephrectomy**
cT1a	When all of the following are met:
Anatomical or functional solitary kidney	High tumor complexity that would be challenging even in experienced hands
Bilateral tumor	Normal contralateral kidney
Known familial RCC	New eGFR likely be > 45
Preexisting chronic kidney disease (CKD) or proteinuria	No preexisting CKD/proteinuria

Table 2
Pathologic, functional, and oncologic outcomes in partial nephrectomy for cT1 RCC

Study	Type	Number of Patients	Age (Years)	Tumor Size (cm)	ccRCC	PSM	Follow-Up (Months)	CKD Upstaging	DFS	MFS	CSS	OS
Carbonara et al,[74] 2021	RAPN	85	58	3.0	76.5%	8.2%	88	20.1%	91.7%		97.7%	91.7%
Bertolo,[84] 2019	RAPN	278	60	3.2	65.5%	4.3%	46	8.3% at 1 y	96.4% at 5 y	96.7% at 5 y	98.2% at 5 y	91.7% at 5 y
Chang,[89] 2018	OPN	122	54	2.5	61.1%	2.5%	64	20%		98.4%	90.2% at 5 y	
	LPN	122	53	2.7	66.4%	4.1%	60	3%		99.2%	86.9% at 5 y	
	RAPN	122	53	2.8	70.5%	2.5%	60	33.6%		98.4%	88.2% at 5 y	
Van Poppel et al,[37] 2011 IOI	OPN	268	62	3.0	84.7%	1.1%	111		93.9%		97%	75%

Abbreviations: CSS, cancer-specific survival; DFS, disease-free survival; LPN, laparoscopic partial nephrectomy; MFS, metastasis-free survival; OPN, open partial nephrectomy; OS, overall survival; PSM, positive surgical margin; RAPN, robotic-assisted partial nephrectomy.

patients with non-RCC at the time of surgery. A recent large systematic review of 21 case-control studies including 11,204 patients concluded that PN is a viable treatment option for larger renal tumors due to acceptable surgical morbidity, equivalent cancer control, and superior preservation of renal function, with even the potential for better long-term survival.[36]

Cost-effectiveness must also be taken into account in surgical decision-making. In older studies, open surgeries were determined to be more cost-effective than laparoscopic or robotic surgeries due to the high cost of equipment in the operating room, whereas recent studies suggest parity between approaches; operating room costs are still higher in minimally invasive surgery (MIS) surgeries, they are counteracted by decreased length of stay.[38,39] An ongoing large-scale research study funded by the National Institutes of Health (NIH) was initiated in July 2022 to examine the cost-effectiveness of PN versus RN, for which results are eagerly anticipated.

Overview of Nephron-Sparing Surgical Options

Open partial nephrectomy

Minimally invasive approaches to PN have gained popularity, largely related to dissemination of robotic-assisted techniques and expertise; however, the open approach is still preferred in certain situations. Tumor complexity, for example, as described by the RENAL nephrometry score, reflecting size, and location with respect to the hilar vasculature and collecting system are the key factors that may influence the decision regarding approach.[40] Other factors that may influence the decision for open approach include patient body habitus, history of prior abdominal surgery, anticipated prolonged clamp time, and solitary kidney status[21] as well as surgeon experience and training. For example, in patients with posterior tumors, a surgeon's comfort with laparoscopically approaching the retroperitoneum may lead to favoring a flank approach.

Adequate visualization is essential for open PN including exposure of the renal hilum. The most common approach for an open PN is retroperitoneal via a flank incision through 10th or 11th intercostal spaces. Alternative access options include transperitoneal approaches via subcostal flank, midline, or thoraco-abdominal incisions **(Fig. 1)**.

Minimally invasive partial nephrectomy

Laparoscopic PN was the first minimally invasive technique reported for management of SRMs.[41] With increasing experience with laparoscopic techniques and evolution of

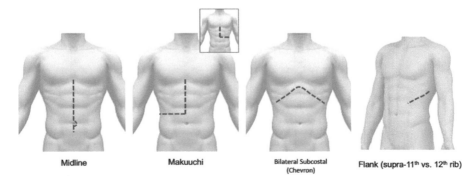

Midline   Makuuchi   Bilateral Subcostal   Flank (supra-11th vs. 12th rib)
                                    (Chevron)

Fig. 1. Diagram of incisions for open RN or PN.

the approach, they were applied to larger and more complex tumors. With the widespread adoption of robotic-assisted laparoscopic surgery, there has been a shift away from the pure laparoscopic approach due to improved dexterity, enhancements of intracorporeal visualization, enhanced retraction, and a shorter learning curve.[42] Nevertheless, laparoscopic PN remains a viable nephron-sparing minimally invasive option in experienced hands.

For a laparoscopic three-port transperitoneal PN, patients are positioned in a modified flank position with the operating room table in flexion to expand the space between iliac crest and inferior costal margin. The primary camera port is placed at the level of umbilicus. A subcostal port is placed inferior to costochondral angle and lateral to rectus and an additional working port is placed in the mid-clavicular line lateral to camera port resulting in triangulation of the target anatomy. When performing right-sided surgery, an additional 5 mm subxiphoid port can be placed for liver retraction (Fig. 2).

Although the transperitoneal approach is most common, for posteriorly located tumors, and in patients with concern for extensive intraperitoneal adhesions, robotic-assisted retroperitoneal PN is increasingly used to facilitate treatment for posteriorly located tumors and in patients with concern for extensive intraperitoneal adhesions. More recently, the single-port approach has been described as well.[43] Port placement for standard transperitoneal four-arm approach using the Da-Vinci Xi and the retroperitoneal approach are presented in Fig. 2.[44] Experiences with single-port access have recently been described in which access is obtained through a single 2.5 cm periumbilical incision. After entry into the peritoneum is established a multichannel gel port is placed.[45]

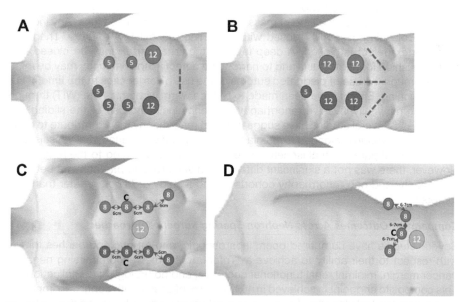

Fig. 2. Port placement for minimally invasive approaches to surgery for small renal masses (c = camera port). (A) Laparoscopic port sites with Pfannenstiel extraction site. (B) Hand-assisted laparoscopic port sites (low midline vs Gibson hand-port sites). (C) Robotic-assisted laparoscopic transperitoneal port sites (Da Vinci Xi). (D) Robotic-assisted laparoscopic retroperitoneal port sites (left) (Da Vinci Xi).

Surgical approach

During open or minimally invasive *transperitoneal* cases, exposure of the kidney is achieved by medialization of the ipsilateral colon, kocherization of the duodenum and elevation of the liver on the right, and cranial retraction of the spleen and pancreas on the left, to expose the anterior surface of the kidney and renal hilum. To minimize bleeding during tumor excision, the renal hilum is isolated to permit vascular clamping of the renal artery. However, this practice may result in renal injury due to ischemia with the potential for subsequent renal function decline with no consensus regarding the minimum warm ischemic period that will result in permanent renal dysfunction. Thus, it is recommended to minimize clamp time as much as is safe and feasible,[46] with a general recommendation to limit warm ischemia to 25 to 30 minutes or less. Limiting ischemic time is particularly pertinent in patients with baseline chronic kidney disease, who may be at higher risk for declines in renal function after nephron sparing.[47] One option to reduce ischemia-related renal function decline includes cold ischemia, which is generally used during the open approaches by packing the mobilized kidney in ice.[48,49] Alternative approaches include early unclamping, selective clamping, super-selective clamping, and off-clamp techniques.[50–53] In patients with baseline renal insufficiency, particularly for small, exophytic, peripherally located tumors, off-clamp PN may be attempted in experienced hands, albeit with increased risk of perioperative blood loss.[53,54]

Intraoperative ultrasound is frequently used to provide detailed, real-time anatomic information regarding tumor localization, characteristics, border delineation and can be especially helpful in cases of partially or completely endophytic tumors.[55–59] Then, tumor excision is generally undertaken sharply. In some cases, the tumor may be enucleated along the pseudocapsule, maximizing preservation of normal renal parenchyma, whereas others advocate for excision of a margin of normal parenchyma to minimize the risk of a positive surgical margin.[60,61] Small perforating vessels may be clipped or oversewn at the time of mass excision to minimize blood loss. Any incision into the collecting system is closed with a running monofilament suture. Then, the renal cortex defect is closed. A deep layer of the renal cortex may be closed in a running fashion for hemostasis and to narrow the defect. Capsular injury may be minimized through the use of pledgeted sutures or the use of larger clips at the time of suture tensioning. Efforts have been made to reduce warm ischemia time (WIT) through improving minimally invasive renorrhaphy efficiency including use of the sliding clip technique.[62] Several studies have suggested that renorrhaphy may contribute to renal dysfunction through prolonged ischemia time, disruption of parenchymal vessels, and collateral renal parenchymal ischemia due to compression related to the repair.[63–65] However, there was not a significant difference in vascularized parenchyma between renorrhaphy and non-renorrhaphy cohorts during a study of PN on greater than T1b tumors.[64]

Comparative Outcomes Across Nephron-Sparing Surgery Approaches

Several studies have compared open, laparoscopic, and robotic approaches for PN with respect to their ability to achieve a "Trifecta outcome" encompassing negative cancer margin, minimal renal functional decrease, and no urological complications.[66] This composite endpoint is achieved in 40% to 85% of cases, with continued improvements over the last decade, despite increased complexity of tumor anatomy.[66–68] A meta-analysis of 60,808 patients demonstrated that the widespread adoption of the robotic-assisted approach is associated with lower blood loss and resultant rates of transfusion, and reduced risk of postoperative complications, lower readmission rate, shorter length of stay, and less estimated glomerular filtration rate (eGFR) decline compared with the open approach.[69] However, when adjusting for tumor complexity, rates of intraoperative and short-term complications and changes in renal function are comparable between the open and minimally invasive approaches,[69–71] whereas the robotic approach is associated with similar or longer operative and WIT times compared with the open approach.[68] Compared with pure laparoscopic approaches, especially for complex renal masses, the robotic approach is associated with favorable perioperative outcomes, including lower rates of conversion to radical surgery, shorter WIT, shorter length of stay (LOS), and less eGFR decline.[72] Robotic approaches have been applied for increasingly complex renal masses, such as completely endophytic or hilar tumors, and several studies have shown that open and robotic approaches offer comparable perioperative outcomes even in these highly complexes cases.[73–75]

In terms of oncologic outcomes, the positive surgical margin rate following PN is low, regardless of surgical approaches, ranging from 1% to 4.5%.[70,74,76,77] Factors associated with positive margins after PN include solitary kidney, bilateral disease, multiple tumors, higher nephrometry score, and pathologic stage.[78–82] Cancer-specific survival (CSS) at 5 years is 90% to 96%, and OS at 5 years is 93% to 98% following PN for SRMs.[79,83,84] As such, PN via open or minimally invasive approaches are considered the standard of care for the definitive management of SRMs and are generally associated with excellent surgical safety and long-term oncologic benefit.

Radical Nephrectomy

RN involves the removal of the entire kidney and perirenal fat contained within Gerota's fascia. It can be performed via open, laparoscopic, or robotic approaches. When choosing an approach, surgical history, body habitus, tumor size and location, and complexity of vasculature are considered. For large tumors with concern for invasion of surrounding structures or tumor thrombus, an open approach is often preferred via flank (retroperitoneal) or anterior (transperitoneal) approaches.

For the flank approach, patients are positioned in the lateral decubitus flexed position. Supracostal flank incisions are generally performed superior to the ipsilateral 11th or 12th ribs from the posterior axillary line to the linea semilunaris. The intercostal muscle is divided, permitting entry into the retroperitoneum, which is mobilized from the pleural attachments and peritoneum and undersurface of the rib, avoiding the intercostal neurovascular bundle and diaphragm. The extraperitoneal approach via the flank reduces the risk of bowel injury, postoperative ileus, negates the need for lysis of adhesions in cases with multiple prior abdominal surgeries, and is favored for posteriorly located tumors undergoing open PN.

Midline, subcostal, or chevron incisions can be used for an anterior transperitoneal approach (see **Fig. 1**). A midline incision is performed from below the xiphoid to just below the umbilicus and is favored for cases of inferior vena cava (IVC) thrombus, bilateral disease, or when a nephroureterectomy is pursued. A modified or full Makuuchi incision may be used for large lateral tumors or IVC thrombi. The subcostal approach offers excellent renal exposure and can be converted into a chevron incision (bilateral subcostal) in cases of bilateral tumors, for the management of IVC thrombus or locally advanced tumors. Midline and subcostal approaches are limited with respect to access to a posterior SRM for PN. Paramedian incisions are rarely performed but can be used in special circumstances, such as to avoid an existing colostomy.[85]

Laparoscopic and robotic approaches are generally favored in smaller tumors without tumor thrombi and without local invasion although, with rapid adoption of robotic techniques, are being increasingly used for complex tumors as well. The advantages of a minimally invasive approach include decreased blood loss, shorter length of stay, less risk of postoperative ileus, and increased cosmesis. The decision of location of port placement should emphasize ease of renal access and access to the hilum.

Postoperative Complications

When choosing between PN and RN for localized renal tumors, a comprehensive discussion of the risks and expected recovery and outcomes associated with each approach is necessary for shared decision. Although infectious risks are equivalent, PN carries and increased risk of blood loss and need for transfusion.[11,36,37,86]

PN also is associated with the unique risks of pseudoaneurysms and urinary fistulae. Pseudoaneurysm describes a form of vascular malformation associated with significant delayed bleeding that occurs after approximately 2% of PNs.[87] Selective arterial embolization may be required to control bleeding but can compromise subsequent renal function. Urine leak after PN occur in less than 3% of cases and may results in urinoma, infection/abscesses, and increased risk of postoperative ileus, metabolic derangement, and acute kidney injury. In severe cases, urine leak may necessitate follow-up procedures such as ureteral stent or percutaneous nephrostomy to decompress the upper tract, divert the urinary stream, and facilitate healing or placement of additional percutaneous drains to drain a urinoma. With appropriate management, urinary fistulae will resolve in approximately 98% of cases within a median of 11 days.[88] While rare, pseudoaneurysms and urine leaks are more common following PN for endophytic, central/interpolar, and larger masses that abut the collecting system and central renal vasculature as well as following surgeries with higher blood loss and failure to use a sliding-clip or bolstered nephrorrhaphy technique.[87]

SUMMARY

The incidence of SRMs and localized RCC has increased; however, the indolent nature of these tumors has generated a focus on careful risk stratification and risk-adapted treatment, with a prioritization of sparing functional renal parenchyma while appropriately managing the mass from an oncologic perspective. The ultimate goal is to optimize oncologic outcomes while minimizing overtreatment, and associated risks of potential risk of perioperative decline in renal function and quality of life, as well as increased surgical morbidity, mortality, and cost. Following comprehensive evaluation, patients may be offered a variety of management strategies including AS, percutaneous treatment, and surgical intervention. Five-year survival rates remain relatively high for localized disease and SRMs. However, further work is warranted to refine predicative models to further improve patient-specific outcomes in management of SRMs and localized disease.

CLINICS CARE POINTS

- The incidence of renal masses has increased without an increase in mortality over the past several decades.
- Earlier detection of localized disease is associated with favorable 5-year survival rates.
- Management of small renal masses includes nonsurgical and surgical approaches.
- Surgical intervention remains the gold standard. Both open and minimally invasive surgical approaches with nephron sparing or radical excision can be offered depending on individual

evaluation with a priority placed on performing nephron-sparing surgery (in the form of a PN) when feasible.

- Shared decision-making is mandatory when determining the correct surgical treatment option for a patient with a localized renal tumor. This should follow elicitization of patient priorities, taking into account baseline renal function, competing comorbidities, body habitus, and prior surgery, tumor characteristics and oncologic risk, and a balanced discussion of surgical risks and expectations for recovery.

FINANCIAL DISCLOSURES/CONFLICTS OF INTEREST

None.

REFERENCES

1. Capitanio U, Montorsi F. Renal cancer. Lancet 2016;387(10021):894–906.
2. Bukavina L, Bensalah K, Bray F, et al. Epidemiology of Renal Cell Carcinoma: 2022 Update. Eur Urol 2022;82(5):529–42.
3. Campbell SC, Clark PE, Chang SS, et al. Renal Mass and Localized Renal Cancer: Evaluation, Management, and Follow-Up: AUA Guideline: Part I. J Urol 2021; 206(2):199–208.
4. Campbell SC, Uzzo RG, Karam JA, et al. Renal Mass and Localized Renal Cancer: Evaluation, Management, and Follow-up: AUA Guideline: Part II. J Urol 2021; 206(2):209–18.
5. Campbell S, Uzzo RG, Allaf ME, et al. Renal Mass and Localized Renal Cancer: AUA Guideline. J Urol 2017;198(3):520–9.
6. Kane CJ, Mallin K, Ritchey J, et al. Renal Cell Cancer Stage Migration Analysis of the National Cancer Data Base. Cancer 2018;113(1):78–83.
7. Motzer RJ, Hutson TE, Tomczak P, et al. Sunitinib versus interferon alfa in metastatic renal-cell carcinoma. N Engl J Med 2007;356(2):115–24.
8. Sung WW, Ko PY, Chen WJ, et al. Trends in the kidney cancer mortality-to-incidence ratios according to health care expenditures of 56 countries. Sci Rep 2021;11(1):1479.
9. Ward RD, Tanaka H, Campbell SC, et al. 2017 AUA Renal Mass and Localized Renal Cancer Guidelines: Imaging Implications. Radiographics 2018;38(7): 2021–33.
10. Kane CJ, Mallin K, Ritchey J, et al. Renal cell cancer stage migration: analysis of the National Cancer Data Base. Cancer 2008;113(1):78–83.
11. Pierorazio PM, Johnson MH, Patel HD, et al. Management of Renal Masses and Localized Renal Cancer: Systematic Review and Meta-Analysis. J Urol 2016; 196(4):989–99.
12. Frank I, Blute ML, Cheville JC, et al. Solid renal tumors: An analysis of pathological features related to tumor size. J Urol 2003;170(6 I):2217–20.
13. Bhindi B, Thompson RH, Lohse CM, et al. The Probability of Aggressive Versus Indolent Histology Based on Renal Tumor Size: Implications for Surveillance and Treatment. Eur Urol 2018;74(4):489–97.
14. Smaldone MC, Smaldone MC, Corcoran AT, et al. Active surveillance of small renal masses. Net Rev Urol 2013;10:266–74.
15. Smaldone MC, Kutikov A, Egleston BL, et al. Small renal masses progressing to metastases under active surveillance: a systematic review and pooled analysis. Cancer 2012;118(4):997–1006.

16. Thompson RH, Hill JR, Babayev Y, et al. Metastatic renal cell carcinoma risk according to tumor size. J Urol 2009;182(1):41–5.

17. Lee SJ, Boscardin WJ, Kirby KA, et al. Individualizing life expectancy estimates for older adults using the Gompertz Law of Human Mortality. PLoS One 2014;9(9): e108540.

18. Lee SJ, Lindquist K, Segal MR, et al. Development and validation of a prognostic index for 4-year mortality in older adults. JAMA 2006;295(7):801–8.

19. Schonberg MA, Davis RB, McCarthy EP, et al. Index to predict 5-year mortality of community-dwelling adults aged 65 and older using data from the National Health Interview Survey. J Gen Intern Med 2009;24(10):1115–22.

20. Campi R, Berni A, Amparore D, et al. Impact of frailty on perioperative and oncologic outcomes in patients undergoing surgery or ablation for renal cancer: a systematic review. Minerva Urol Nephrol 2022;74(2):146–60.

21. Chandrasekar T, Boorjian SA, Capitanio U, et al. Collaborative Review: Factors Influencing Treatment Decisions for Patients with a Localized Solid Renal Mass. Eur Urol 2021;80(5):575–88.

22. Network NCC. Kidney Cancer (Version 3.2023). https://www.nccn.org/professionals/physician_gls/pdf/kidney.pdf. Published 2022. Accessed 12/01/2022.

23. Kurtzman J, Wang C, Martina LP, Chung R, Anderson C. MP28-14 UTILITY OF RENAL MASS BIOPSY IN SHARED DECISION MAKING FOR RENAL MASS TREATMENT. *Journal of Urology.* 2022;207(Supplement 5):e466.

24. Blute ML Jr, Drewry A, Abel EJ. Percutaneous biopsy for risk stratification of renal masses. Ther Adv Urol 2015;7(5):265–74.

25. Volpe A, Kachura JR, Geddie WR, et al. Techniques, safety and accuracy of sampling of renal tumors by fine needle aspiration and core biopsy. J Urol 2007; 178(2):379–86.

26. Patel HD, Johnson MH, Pierorazio PM, et al. Diagnostic Accuracy and Risks of Biopsy in the Diagnosis of a Renal Mass Suspicious for Localized Renal Cell Carcinoma: Systematic Review of the Literature. J Urol 2016;195(5):1340–7.

27. Shannon BA, Cohen RJ, de Bruto H, et al. The value of preoperative needle core biopsy for diagnosing benign lesions among small, incidentally detected renal masses. J Urol 2008;180(4):1257–61 [discussion: 1261.

28. Pierorazio PM, Johnson MH, Ball MW, et al. Five-year analysis of a multi-institutional prospective clinical trial of delayed intervention and surveillance for small renal masses: the DISSRM registry. Eur Urol 2015;68(3):408–15.

29. Gupta M, Alam R, Patel HD, et al. Use of delayed intervention for small renal masses initially managed with active surveillance. Urol Oncol 2019;37(1):18–25.

30. Cheaib* J, Alam R, Kassiri B, et al. PD45-10 active surveillance for small renal masses is safe and non-inferior: 10-year update from the DISSRM registry. J Urol 2020;203(Supplement 4):e917.

31. Klatte T, Berni A, Serni S, et al. Intermediate- and long-term oncological outcomes of active surveillance for localized renal masses: a systematic review and quantitative analysis. BJU Int 2021;128(2):131–43.

32. Boorjian SA, Uzzo RG. The evolving management of small renal masses. Curr Oncol Rep 2009;11(3):211–7.

33. Ljungberg B, Albiges L, Abu-Ghanem Y, et al. European Association of Urology Guidelines on Renal Cell Carcinoma: The 2022 Update. Eur Urol 2022;82(4): 399–410.

34. Hou W, Yan W, Ji Z. Anatomic features involved in technical complexity of partial nephrectomy. Urology 2015;85(1):1–7.

35. Liu X, Huang X, Zhao P, et al. Survival benefit of nephron-sparing surgery for patients with pT1b renal cell carcinoma: A population-based study. Oncol Lett 2020; 19(1):498–504.
36. Mir MC, Derweesh I, Porpiglia F, et al. Partial Nephrectomy Versus Radical Nephrectomy for Clinical T1b and T2 Renal Tumors: A Systematic Review and Meta-analysis of Comparative Studies. Eur Urol 2017;71(4):606–17.
37. Van Poppel H, Da Pozzo L, Albrecht W, et al. A prospective, randomised EORTC intergroup phase 3 study comparing the oncologic outcome of elective nephron-sparing surgery and radical nephrectomy for low-stage renal cell carcinoma. Eur Urol 2011;59(4):543–52.
38. Golombos DM, Chughtai B, Trinh QD, et al. Minimally invasive vs open nephrectomy in the modern era: does approach matter? World J Urol 2017;35(10): 1557–68.
39. Klinghoffer Z, Tarride J-E, Novara G, et al. Cost-utility analysis of radical nephrectomy versus partial nephrectomy in the management of small renal masses: adjusting for the burden of ensuing chronic kidney disease. Canadian Urological Association Journal 2013;7(3–4):108–13.
40. Canter D, Kutikov A, Manley B, et al. Utility of the R.E.N.A.L. Nephrometry Scoring System in Objectifying Treatment Decision-making of the Enhancing Renal Mass. Urology 2011;78(5):1089–94.
41. Winfield HN, Donovan JF, Godet AS, et al. Laparoscopic partial nephrectomy: initial case report for benign disease. J Endourol 1993;7(6):521–6.
42. Choi JE, You JH, Kim DK, et al. Comparison of perioperative outcomes between robotic and laparoscopic partial nephrectomy: a systematic review and meta-analysis. Eur Urol 2015;67(5):891–901.
43. Palacios AR, Morgantini L, Trippel R, et al. Comparison of Perioperative Outcomes Between Retroperitoneal Single-Port and Multiport Robot-Assisted Partial Nephrectomies. J Endourol 2022;36(12):1545–50.
44. Ghani KR, Porter J, Menon M, et al. Robotic retroperitoneal partial nephrectomy: a step-by-step guide. BJU Int 2014;114(2):311–3.
45. Kaouk J, Garisto J, Eltemamy M, et al. Pure Single Site Robot-Assisted Partial Nephrectomy Using the SP Surgical System: Initial Clinical Experience. Urology 2019;124:282–5.
46. Klatte T, Ficarra V, Gratzke C, et al. A Literature Review of Renal Surgical Anatomy and Surgical Strategies for Partial Nephrectomy. Eur Urol 2015;68(6):980–92.
47. Lane BR, Campbell SC, Demirjian S, et al. Surgically Induced Chronic Kidney Disease May be Associated with a Lower Risk of Progression and Mortality than Medical Chronic Kidney Disease. J Urol 2013;189(5):1649–55.
48. Rogers CG, Ghani KR, Kumar RK, et al. Robotic Partial Nephrectomy with Cold Ischemia and On-clamp Tumor Extraction: Recapitulating the Open Approach. Eur Urol 2013;63(3):573–8.
49. Lane BR, Russo P, Uzzo RG, et al. Comparison of Cold and Warm Ischemia During Partial Nephrectomy in 660 Solitary Kidneys Reveals Predominant Role of Nonmodifiable Factors in Determining Ultimate Renal Function. J Urol 2011; 185(2):421–7.
50. Nguyen MM, Gill IS. Halving Ischemia Time During Laparoscopic Partial Nephrectomy. J Urol 2008;179(2):627–32.
51. Benway BM, Baca G, Bhayani SB, et al. Selective versus nonselective arterial clamping during laparoscopic partial nephrectomy: impact upon renal function in the setting of a solitary kidney in a porcine model. J Endourol 2009;23(7): 1127–33.

52. Desai MM, de Castro Abreu AL, Leslie S, et al. Robotic Partial Nephrectomy with Superselective Versus Main Artery Clamping: A Retrospective Comparison. Eur Urol 2014;66(4):713–9.
53. Smith GL, Kenney PA, Lee Y, et al. Non-clamped partial nephrectomy: techniques and surgical outcomes. BJU Int 2011;107(7):1054–8.
54. Kaczmarek BF, Tanagho YS, Hillyer SP, et al. Off-clamp Robot-assisted Partial Nephrectomy Preserves Renal Function: A Multi-institutional Propensity Score Analysis. Eur Urol 2013;64(6):988–93.
55. Kaczmarek BF, Sukumar S, Petros F, et al. Robotic ultrasound probe for tumor identification in robotic partial nephrectomy: Initial series and outcomes. Int J Urol 2013;20(2):172–6.
56. Hughes-Hallett A, Pratt P, Mayer E, et al. Intraoperative ultrasound overlay in robot-assisted partial nephrectomy: first clinical experience. Eur Urol 2014; 65(3):671–2.
57. Simmons MN, Ching CB, Samplaski MK, et al. Kidney tumor location measurement using the C index method. J Urol 2010;183(5):1708–13.
58. Hekman MCH, Rijpkema M, Langenhuijsen JF, et al. Intraoperative Imaging Techniques to Support Complete Tumor Resection in Partial Nephrectomy. Eur Urol Focus 2018;4(6):960–8.
59. Di Cosmo G, Verzotti E, Silvestri T, et al. Intraoperative ultrasound in robot-assisted partial nephrectomy: State of the art. Arch Ital Urol Androl 2018;90(3): 195–8.
60. Minoda R, Takagi T, Yoshida K, et al. Comparison of Surgical Outcomes Between Enucleation and Standard Resection in Robot-Assisted Partial Nephrectomy for Completely Endophytic Renal Tumors Through a 1:1 Propensity Score-Matched Analysis. J Endourol 2021;35(12):1779–84.
61. Chung HC, Kang TW, Lee JY, et al. Tumor enucleation for the treatment of T1 renal tumors: A systematic review and meta-analysis. Investig Clin Urol 2022;63(2): 126–39.
62. Benway BM, Wang AJ, Cabello JM, et al. Robotic Partial Nephrectomy with Sliding-Clip Renorrhaphy: Technique and Outcomes. Eur Urol 2009;55(3):592–9.
63. Tachibana H, Takagi T, Kondo T, et al. Comparison of perioperative outcomes with or without renorrhaphy during open partial nephrectomy: A propensity score-matched analysis. Int Braz J Urol 2018;44(3):467–74.
64. Takagi T, Kondo T, Omae K, et al. Assessment of Surgical Outcomes of the Non-renorrhaphy Technique in Open Partial Nephrectomy for ≥T1b Renal Tumors. Urology 2015;86(3):529–33.
65. Shatagopam K, Bahler CD, Sundaram CP. Renorrhaphy techniques and effect on renal function with robotic partial nephrectomy. World J Urol 2020;38(5):1109–12.
66. Hung AJ, Cai J, Simmons MN, et al. "Trifecta" in partial nephrectomy. J Urol 2013; 189(1):36–42.
67. Porpiglia F, Mari A, Bertolo R, et al. Partial Nephrectomy in Clinical T1b Renal Tumors: Multicenter Comparative Study of Open, Laparoscopic and Robot-assisted Approach (the RECORd Project). Urology 2016;89:45–51.
68. Xia L, Wang X, Xu T, et al. Systematic Review and Meta-Analysis of Comparative Studies Reporting Perioperative Outcomes of Robot-Assisted Partial Nephrectomy Versus Open Partial Nephrectomy. J Endourol 2017;31(9):893–909.
69. Tsai SH, Tseng PT, Sherer BA, et al. Open versus robotic partial nephrectomy: Systematic review and meta-analysis of contemporary studies. Int J Med Robot 2019;15(1):e1963.

70. Casale P, Lughezzani G, Buffi N, et al. Evolution of Robot-assisted Partial Ne-phrectomy: Techniques and Outcomes from the Transatlantic Robotic Nephron-sparing Surgery Study Group. Eur Urol 2019;76(2):222–7.
71. Israel GM, Bosniak MA. How I do it: evaluating renal masses. Radiology 2005; 236(2):441–50.
72. Lin P, Wu M, Gu H, et al. Comparison of outcomes between laparoscopic and robot-assisted partial nephrectomy for complex renal tumors: RENAL score ≥7 or maximum tumor size >4 cm. Minerva Urol Nephrol 2021;73(2):154–64.
73. Harke NN, Mandel P, Witt JH, et al. Are there limits of robotic partial nephrec-tomy? TRIFECTA outcomes of open and robotic partial nephrectomy for completely endophytic renal tumors. J Surg Oncol 2018;118(1):206–11.
74. Carbonara U, Simone G, Minervini A, et al. Outcomes of robot-assisted partial ne-phrectomy for completely endophytic renal tumors: A multicenter analysis. Eur J Surg Oncol 2021;47(5):1179–86.
75. Khene ZE, Peyronnet B, Gasmi A, et al. Endophytic Renal Cell Carcinoma Treated with Robot-Assisted Surgery: Functional Outcomes - A Comprehensive Review of the Current Literature. Urol Int 2020;104(5–6):343–50.
76. Borghesi M, Schiavina R, Chessa F, et al. Retroperitoneal Robot-Assisted Versus Open Partial Nephrectomy for cT1 Renal Tumors: A Matched-Pair Comparison of Perioperative and Early Oncological Outcomes. Clin Genitourin Cancer 2018; 16(2):e391–6.
77. Ray S, Cheaib JG, Biles MJ, et al. Local and Regional Recurrences of Clinically Localized Renal Cell Carcinoma after Nephrectomy: A 15 Year Institutional Expe-rience with Prognostic Features and Oncologic Outcomes. Urology 2021;154: 201–7.
78. Wood EL, Adibi M, Qiao W, et al. Local Tumor Bed Recurrence Following Partial Nephrectomy in Patients with Small Renal Masses. J Urol 2018;199(2):393–400.
79. Kim H, Kim JK, Ye C, et al. Recurrence after radical and partial nephrectomy in high complex renal tumor using propensity score matched analysis. Sci Rep 2021;11(1):2919.
80. Mouracade P, Kara O, Maurice MJ, et al. Patterns and Predictors of Recurrence after Partial Nephrectomy for Kidney Tumors. J Urol 2017;197(6):1403–9.
81. Takagi T, Yoshida K, Wada A, et al. Predictive factors for recurrence after partial nephrectomy for clinical T1 renal cell carcinoma: a retrospective study of 1227 cases from a single institution. Int J Clin Oncol 2020;25(5):892–8.
82. Petros FG, Metcalfe MJ, Yu KJ, et al. Oncologic outcomes of patients with posi-tive surgical margin after partial nephrectomy: a 25-year single institution experi-ence. World J Urol 2018;36(7):1093–101.
83. Permpongkosol S, Bagga HS, Romero FR, et al. Laparoscopic versus open par-tial nephrectomy for the treatment of pathological T1N0M0 renal cell carcinoma: a 5-year survival rate. J Urol 2006;176(5):1984–8 [discussion: 1988-1989].
84. Bertolo R, Garisto J, Dagenais J, et al. Transperitoneal robot-assisted partial ne-phrectomy with minimum follow-up of 5 years: oncological and functional out-comes from a single institution. Eur Urol Oncol 2019;2(2):207–13.
85. Kalapara AA, Frydenberg M. The role of open radical nephrectomy in contempo-rary management of renal cell carcinoma. Transl Androl Urol 2020;9(6):3123–39.
86. Huang R. Partial Nephrectomy Versus Radical Nephrectomy for Clinical T2 or Higher Stage Renal Tumors%3A A Systematic Review and Meta-Analysis. Fron-tiers in oncology 2021;11.
87. Peyton CC, Hajiran A, Morgan K, et al. Urinary leak following partial nephrectomy: a contemporary review of 975 cases. Can J Urol 2020;27(1):10118–24.

88. Massouh Skorin R, Mahfouz A, Escovar la Riva P. Systematic review on active treatment for urinary fistula after partial nephrectomy. Actas Urol Esp 2022; 46(7):387–96.
89. Chang KD, Abdel Raheem A, Kim KH, et al. Functional and oncological outcomes of open, laparoscopic and robot-assisted partial nephrectomy: a multicentre comparative matched-pair analyses with a median of 5 years' follow-up. BJU Int 2018;122(4):618–26.

Role of Surgery in Metastatic Renal Cell Carcinoma

Check for updates

José Ignacio Nolazco, MD, MMSc[a,b], Steven Lee Chang, MD, MS[a,*]

KEYWORDS

- Renal cell carcinoma • Cytoreductive nephrectomy • Metastasectomy

KEY POINTS

- In 2018, the CARMENA trial, a phase III randomized controlled clinical trial established systemic therapy (sunitinib) is non-inferior to cytoreductive nephrectomy (CN) as upfront therapy (followed by sunitinib) for metastatic renal cell carcinoma (mRCC) thus concluding that CN no longer represents the sole standard of care treatment option for patients with mRCC.
- Appropriate contemporary indications for CN include the palliation of severe symptoms, the treatment of select cases of metastatic non-clear cell renal cell carcinoma, consolidative surgery following systemic therapy, as well as for patients with oligometastatic disease.
- Surgical metastasectomy has been associated with improved overall survival although these procedures commonly have high morbidity. The best outcomes are associated with a complete metastasectomy of solitary pulmonary metastases.
- Given the heterogeneous nature of mRCC, there will never be a single approach for therapy. It is increasingly important to selectively integrate surgery with systemic therapeutic options through a multidisciplinary approach with urology, medical oncology, and other health professionals. The roles of CN and metastasectomy will continue to evolve in concert with current and future systemic therapeutic strategies for mRCC.

Historically, the mainstay of treatment for all renal masses concerning for RCC has been extirpative surgery. In 1969, Dr Charles Robson of the University of Toronto reported a series of 88 patients treated with radical nephrectomy, many of them with advanced disease, and reported a five-year survival of 52%,[1] thereby establishing surgery as the cornerstone for the treatment of RCC albeit in absence of effective systemic therapy. In the setting of localized disease, a radical nephrectomy or partial nephrectomy is performed with the intention of eliminating the totality of disease (Can reference

[a] Division of Urological Surgery, Brigham and Women's Hospital, Harvard Medical School, 45 Francis Street, Boston, MA 02115, USA; [b] Servicio de Urología, Hospital Universitario Austral, Universidad Austral, Pilar, Argentina
* Corresponding author.
E-mail address: SLCHANG@bwh.harvard.edu

Hematol Oncol Clin N Am 37 (2023) 893–905
https://doi.org/10.1016/j.hoc.2023.05.004
0889-8588/23/© 2023 Elsevier Inc. All rights reserved.
hemonc.theclinics.com

Daniel S. Carson and colleagues' article, "Surgical Management of Localized Disease and Small Renal Masses," in this issue[2]). In contrast, for patients with mRCC, a cytoreductive nephrectomy (CN) involves the resection of the primary renal mass and potentially loco-regional disease in an effort to reduce of the overall burden of disease; similarly, surgical metastasectomy refers to the resection of distant sites of metastatic disease. Over the past several decades, surgery for localized disease has been advanced through the advent of minimally invasive approaches and nephron-sparing surgical strategies as well as the recognition of consequences of intervention such as post-treatment renal. In contrast, for patients with mRCC, the role of surgery has been–and will continue to be–influenced by the development of systemic therapies.

CYTOREDUCTIVE NEPHRECTOMY AND CYTOKINE THERAPIES

In the 1980s, cytokine therapy (ie, high-dose interleukin-2 [IL-2] and interferon-alpha [INFα]) was considered the standard systemic therapy for mRCC largely because of a lack of improved overall survival (OS) associated with either chemotherapy or hormonal therapy alone.[3] In the 1990s, two phase III randomized controlled trials, SWOG 8949[4] and the EORTC 3094,[5] both randomized patients to CN followed by INFα versus INFα alone (ie, no surgery). Combined, these trials demonstrated an approximately six-month OS advantage in the arm undergoing CN compared to the arm receiving INFα alone (13.6 Vs. 7.8 months, respectively); CN was associated with a 31% reduction in the risk of death (p = 0.002).[6] Proposed reasons for the improved outcomes among patients undergoing CN included the reduction in tumor volume reducing the development of aggressive biological clones to potentially metastasize, as well as the removal of the immunological sink of the primary renal mass, which could sequester immune cells from destroying cancer cells. Other investigators theorized that the primary tumor may secrete immunosuppressive cytokines thus allowing the mRCC to progress unhindered.[7] Regardless of the rationale, the level 1 evidence from SWOG 8949 and EORTC 3094 established upfront CN as the standard of care for mRCC in the early 2000s.

SURGERY AND THE EVOLVING LANDSCAPE OF SYSTEMIC THERAPIES

With the availability of systemic therapies for mRCC that were more tolerable and achieved a greater response compared to cytokine therapies, the role of cytoreductive nephrectomy was naturally questioned. In 2014, Heng and colleagues retrospectively analyzed the International Metastatic Renal Cell Carcinoma Database Consortium (IMDC) with mRCC who received targeted therapy (TT) comparing 982 patients who underwent CN with 676 patients who did not undergo CN. This study demonstrated an OS benefit associated with CN (20.6 months versus 9.5 months) equating to a 40% reduction in the risk of death (hazard ratio [HR] 0.6, 95% confidence interval [CI]: 0.52 to 0.69, p < 0.0001).[8] Similarly, Hanna and colleagues conducted a retrospective study utilizing the large National Cancer Database (NCDB); this study compared 5,374 patients who underwent CN and TT vs. 10,016 patients who received TT alone and concluded that CN was associated with a 55% reduction in the risk of death (OS: 17.1 months versus 7.7 months; HR 0.45, 95% CI: 0.40 to 0.50, p < 0.001).[9] Other retrospective studies also demonstrated a similar OS benefit associated with CN for patients with mRCC receiving IO.[10]

CARMENA and SURTIME Trials

Despite the consistency of the results from retrospective studies evaluating outcomes of CN with TT, the widely accepted optimal approach to assess the role of surgery in mRCC is through a phase III prospective randomized controlled trial to minimize bias and confounding. The CARMENA (Cancer du Rein Metastatique Nephrectomie et Antiangiogeniques, NCT00930033) trial was a non-inferiority study comparing CN followed by sunitinib versus sunitinib alone as first-line therapy for patients with mRCC, clear cell type.[11] This trial enrolled 450 patients from 79 centers from 2009 to 2017, with a median follow-up of 50.9 months. Initial trial results revealed that in terms of OS sunitinib alone was not inferior to CN followed by sunitinib (HR = 0.89, 95% CI: 0.71 to 1.10), based on a pre-determined threshold of non-inferiority at HR $\leq$ 1.20.[11] An updated analysis, following 358 OS events, reaffirmed the initial finding that sunitinib alone was non-inferior to CN followed by sunitinib (HR = 0.97, 95% CI: 0.79–1.19).[12] Despite the level 1 evidence, this trial has received criticisms which have complicated the interpretation of the results. For example, 17% of patients in the sunitinib only arm received CN while 15% of patients in the CN and sunitinib arm did not receive sunitinib. Additionally, the patient population was highly enriched for patients with poor risk (57%) disease, which is a group prior investigators reported to have little or no benefit from CN,[13,14] and a higher tumor burden compared to patients in the NCDB raising questions regarding the possibility of recruitment bias and generalizability of the findings.[15] Indeed, the updated analysis showed that for patients with intermediate-to poor-risk disease (two or more IMDC risk factors), OS was significantly longer in the sunitinib alone arm (31.2 versus 17.6 months, HR = 0.65, 95% CI: 0.44 to 0.97, p = 0.03) while those presenting with one IMDC risk factor trended to having a longer OS with CN followed by sunitinib though this did not achieve statistical significance (31.4 versus 25.2 months, HR = 1.30, 95% CI: 0.85 to 1.98, p = 0.2).[12]

The SURTIME (SURgery TIME, EORTC 30073) trial, which was phase III randomized controlled trial conducted concurrent with CARMENA, investigated the role of CN with a focus on the timing of CN with respect to systemic therapy.[16] The trial participations were randomized to two arms: immediate CN, which was upfront surgery followed by sunitinib, or deferred CN, which was three cycles of sunitinib followed by CN (in the absence of progression). The primary outcome was progression-free survival (PFS) and OS was the secondary outcome. The study was severely underpowered with only 99 participants enrolled after 5.7 years falling far short of the target accrual of 458 participants. Nevertheless, the investigators reported the intention-to-treat 28-week PFS data showing no difference (p = 0.61) between the two strategies: 42% in the immediate CN arm (n = 50) versus 43% in the deferred CN arm (n = 49). The investigators also reported the intention-to-treat OS data, which was significantly in favor of the deferred CN with a median OS of 32.4 months versus immediate CN with a median OS of 15.0 months (HR = 0.57, 95% CI: 0.34 to 0.95, p = 0.03). In post-hoc analysis, a notable finding was that patients in the immediate CN arm were less likely to receive sunitinib (80% vs 97.7%) and decreased the duration of sunitinib (median duration: 172.5 days versus 248 days).[17] These findings raise the possibility that surgical trauma may render some patients, particularly those with minimal physiological reserve, unable to receive and tolerate systemic therapy. Moreover, the results of the SURTIME trial argue that in some patients, addressing distant disease expeditiously with upfront systemic therapy may result in more profound disease control and a greater beneficial impact on overall survival compared to extirpating the original site of disease.

Taken together, the CARMENA and SURTIME clinical trials conclude CN is no longer considered the only standard of care treatment for patients with mRCC, given the recent improvement in systemic therapies and the fact that sunitinib is not a standard first line option at this time. While there are ongoing prospective clinical trials evaluating the role of surgery with the contemporary regimens of IO/IO and IO/TKI regimen (**Table 1**), the findings of these trials are many years away. In the meantime,

Table 1
Ongoing randomized clinical trials looking at CN and combination therapies of immunotherapy

Clinical Trial	Identifier Number	Intervention	Aim	Study Completion
NORDIC-SUN	NCT03977571	Nivolumab + Ipilimumab	To evaluate the effect of deferred cytoreductive nephrectomy compared with no surgery following initial nivolumab combined with ipilimumab or a TKI-combination in mRCC patients	2025
Cyto-KIK Phase II	NCT04322955	Nivolumab + Cabozantinib	To determine if the use of immunotherapy nivolumab and the targeted therapy cabozantinib prior to removal of the kidney will increase the number of subjects who are without any visible kidney cancer in their body at some point during the course of treatment.	2027
PROBE [85] Phase III	NCT04510597	Nivolumab, Pembrolizumab, Avelumab	To compare the effect of adding surgery (by randomization after 12 months of ICI systemic therapy) to a standard-of-care immunotherapy-based drug combination versus a standard-of-care immunotherapy-based drug combination alone in patients mRCC.	2033

there are many important questions regarding the integration of surgery with systemic therapy in the care of patients with mRCC. Do the current state-of-the-art systemic therapeutic regimens, which have superior outcomes compared to sunitinib, render CN completely unnecessary? If there remains a role for CN, should systemic therapies always be considered the preferred upfront strategy over CN for all patients? What is the role of metastasectomy given the changing and expanding landscape of treatments for mRCC?

CONTEMPORARY ROLE OF SURGERY FOR METASTATIC RENAL CELL CARCINOMA
Cytoreductive Nephrectomy for Palliation

Classically, RCC is associated with gross hematuria, abdominal mass, and abdominal pain. Advanced stages can also be characterized by paraneoplastic syndrome attributed to cytokine release, immune dysregulation, and the production of proteins and other substances that affect normal physiology. Larcher and colleagues[18] reported overt symptoms in two out of every three patients with mRCC. Metastatic RCC may be associated with polycythemia in up to 8% due to erythropoietin production, hypercalcemia may be present in as many as 20% due to elevated levels of parathyroid hormone-related peptide, hypertension in up to 40% increased release of renin, and constitutional symptoms in up to a third of patients.[19] A relatively unique clinical scenario associated with advanced RCC is Stauffer syndrome, an IL-6 driven transaminitis which traditionally managed effectively with nephrectomy.[20]

An upfront palliative CN may be the most expeditious and effective approach to provide relief from the symptoms associated with the primary tumor to achieve an improvement in quality of life. A focus on optimizing quality of life remains appropriate because mRCC unfortunately remains a lethal disease for the majority of patients despite the current pharmacotherapies. Therefore, the presence of intractable symptoms, which are difficult to manage conservatively and certainly those which fail supportive care measure, is an appropriate indication for CN.

Cytoreductive Nephrectomy for Metastatic Non-Clear Cell Renal Cell Carcinoma

The advancements in the understanding and management of mRCC have been largely centered on clear cell RCC (ccRCC); CARMENA and SURTIME trials limited enrollment to patients with biopsy-proven ccRCC. Nevertheless, patients with non-clear cell RCC (nccRCC) represent approximately 20% of all RCCs[21] and up to one-third of patients in some series of patients with mRCC.[22] Unfortunately despite advances in systemic therapy for metastatic ccRCC, Motzer and colleagues[23] reported worse prognosis for patients with metastatic nccRCC. Similarly, Vera-Badillo and colleagues,[24] in a systematic review and meta-analysis including 41 studies comprising 7,771 patients, demonstrated a significantly less effective result for metastatic nccRCC, with lower response rates and worse progression-free survival and overall survival when compared to metastatic ccRCC. Kassouf and colleagues analyzed 606 patients who underwent cytoreductive nephrectomy, out of which 92 had nccRRC, and found that this subgroup of patients was younger, had a higher incidence of nodal metastasis, sarcomatoid histology, and overall a worse prognosis compared to the patients with clear cell histology. The investigators concluded that CN can be performed safely in this population.[25] For these patients with metastatic nccRCC, the options for and the magnitude of benefit from current systemic therapies are relatively limited, and thus CN may play a particularly beneficial role.

Currently, the optimal systemic therapy for nccRCC remains relatively poorly defined.[26] (reference Elizabeth Pan and colleagues' article, "Managing First-Line

Metastatic Renal-Cell Carcinoma (mRCC): Favorable-Risk Disease," in this issue[27])
A major issue is that nccRCC is that it is an umbrella term encompassing a highly
heterogeneous group of tumors with different genetic, histologic, and clinical characteristics. There is a growing body of evidence that patients with known aggressive
biology such as the ones with extensive sarcomatoid/rhabdoid features or renal
medullary cancer (RMC) should typically not get upfront CN in the setting of metastatic disease. However, until level 1 data comparing systemic therapies with and
without CN are available for metastatic nccRCC, upfront CN will remain an appropriate treatment to consider for patients with metastatic nccRCC.

Cytoreductive Nephrectomy as Consolidative Surgery

Despite the proven efficacy of current IO/IO and IO/TKI regimens, it nevertheless remains uncommon for a patient with mRCC to achieve a durable complete response
through systemic therapy alone, especially in the kidney. In cases where there is an
objective response to initial systemic therapy, CN can serve as consolidative surgery
by eliminating residual disease thus improving the likelihood of a durable remission.[28]
In some cases, paraneoplastic syndrome associated with advanced disease can
severely compromise performance status and tolerability of major surgery making systemic therapy a far more practical option. In other cases, a CN may not be a legitimate
option at the time of diagnosis because the primary tumor is deemed unresectable or the
surgical morbidity unacceptably high; these situations may be secondary to the invasion
of the primary tumor to surrounding structures such as the liver, pancreas, bowel, and
body wall or due to the extensive encasement of the disease around the renal hilar
vessels or extensive cavo-atrial thrombus. In these circumstances, initial systemic therapy may allow patients to improve health and increase the physiologic reserve necessary to tolerate surgery as well as downstage the disease to reduce surgical morbidity.

The aforementioned SURTIME trial represents the strongest argument for consolidative CN as the patients in the delayed surgery arm had a significantly increased
OS by approximately 15 months (HR: 0.57, 95% CI: 0.34 to 0.95, p = 0.032).[16] Furthermore, the authors reported that the preoperative systemic therapy did not increase the
surgical morbidity which is a concern due to possible reactive changes of the primary
tumor obliterating natural anatomic planes of dissection, which generally guide the
surgical resection. These results also support the findings of prior phase II studies
demonstrating both feasibility of a delayed surgery strategy as well as a measurable
reduction in the disease burden with CN following initial systemic therapy with sunitinib[29] and pazopanhib.[30]

Multiple questions however remain with the approach for CN as consolidative surgery. Ideally, this approach is employed once there is no longer any radiographically
visible disease beyond the primary tumor. However, recognizing that not all metastatic
disease is detectable with even state-of-the-art imaging modalities, should there be a
requisite amount of time for the primary tumor to be the sole radiographic site of disease? And, if there remains radiographically identifiable metastatic disease but
response to systemic therapy appears to have plateaued or was a mixed response,
should patients receive second/third-line systemic therapies prior to pursuing consolidative CN? Lastly, in that ideal clinical scenario where a consolidative CN results in a
state with no evidence of disease (NED), can patients shift to imaging surveillance only
or should systemic therapy resume postoperatively and for what duration? These
questions surrounding consolidative CN are currently unanswered and in the absence
of well-designed clinical trials, it is critically important for a concerted effort between
the medical oncologist and the urologist to personalize the treatment plan incorporating consolidative CN.

Oligometastatic Metastatic Renal Cell Carcinoma

Oligometastatic RCC refers to a clinical scenario in which mRCC is associated with a very limited amount of distant disease such that most of the disease is represented by the primary renal mass. The main rationale for upfront and expeditious CN in the setting of oligometastatic disease is the potential to eradicate all metastatic disease without the use of systemic therapy if the primary tumor along with the limited metastatic sites are eliminated effectively and efficiently.[31]

There are currently no level 1 data demonstrating benefit for the use of CN in patients with oligometastatic disease. This specific type of patient was not assessed in the CARMENA trial which focused on patients with a relatively higher volume of metastatic disease compared to other cohorts of patients with mRCC.[15] Observational studies report that oligometastatic RCC managed with a combination of CN and metastasectomy can be associated with prolonged survival though the biological basis is not clear.[32,33] Removing the primary tumor could eliminate the source of potential new metastases.[7] This idea is supported by the TRACERx Renal study, which compared biopsies of the primary tumor and metastatic disease and found that metastatic sites were both more homogeneous and harbored fewer driver somatic alterations compared to their matched primary tumors.[26] Additionally, there are reports of patients with oligometastatic RCC experiencing spontaneous resolution of the metastatic disease.[34–37] Although the biological mechanism of spontaneous regression is not yet completely understood, it has been proposed that the relative increase in the number of immune cells fighting the tumor (Natural Killers and CD8+ T cells), after cytoreductive surgery, leads to enhanced efficacy of the immune system.[38]

Surgical Metastasectomy

Surgical metastasectomy, the surgical removal of metastatic tumors that have spread from the primary tumor to other parts of the body, can play an important role in the management of patients with mRCC. However, the decision to perform metastasectomy in mRCC is complex and dependent on several factors including the location and extent of the metastases, the overall health and fitness of the individual patient, as well as the response to prior therapy and the expected response to future therapies.

To date, there has been no prospective randomized clinical trial evaluating the benefits of surgical metastasectomy in the management of mRCC. Retrospective studies are clearly associated with a significant potential for selection bias preferentially the best surgical candidates (ie, healthiest patients) with the most resectable and limited disease. Nevertheless, the available data suggest that surgical resection of metastases in patients with mRCC is associated with improved overall survival. Sun and colleagues[39] analyzed 6,994 patients with mRCC from the NCDB; the 1,976 patients who underwent metastasectomy had improved survival compared to patients not undergoing metastasectomy (HR: 0.83, 95% CI: 0.77–0.90, p < 0.001). Lyon and colleagues[40] revealed in a cohort of 586 patients that those 158 who underwent complete metastasectomy presented a two-year OS of 81% vs. 53% for those who had an incomplete metastasectomy or no metastasectomy (HR 0.47, 95% CI: 0.34–0.65, p < 0.001). Alt and colleagues[41] analyzed the survival of 125 patients who underwent complete metastasectomy in a cohort of 887 metastatic RCC and demonstrated that metastasectomy was associated with a significant prolongation of median cancer-specific survival (4.8 years vs. 1.3 years; P < .001). Furthermore, subgroup analysis of KEYNOTE-564, a phase III clinical trial assessing the benefit of adjuvant therapy, showed that adjuvant pembrolizumab was uniquely benefit for patients with M1 disease following complete metastasectomy (HR for disease-free survival:

0.28, 95% CI: 0.12 to 0.66).[42] Based on the available data, the most appropriate clinical scenario for metastasectomy is one in which all radiographically visible disease can be feasibly surgically resected.

Ultimately, the survival benefits of surgical metastasectomy differ based not only on the volume and number of metastatic sites, but also the location of metastases. Some examples include.

Lung metastasis

The lung is the most common site for metastasis in mRCC.[43] Hofmann and colleagues[44] investigated 64 patients with mRCC who underwent pulmonary metastasectomy and found that complete metastasectomy was associated with superior outcomes (versus incomplete metastasectomy, the 5-year survival was 39.9% vs 0% and the median survival was 46.6 months versus 13.3 months). A retrospective review of patients with mRCC in the NCDB, pulmonary metastasectomy was associated with improved survival (HR: 0.83, 95% CI: 0.77 to 0.90, p < 0.001).[39] The ideal clinical scenario that appear to benefit the most from metastasectomy is patients with resectable solitary and pulmonary-only metastasis.[45]

Bone metastasis

Bone metastasis is found in 20% to 35% of patients with mRCC,[46,47] representing the second most common site for metastasis from RCC.[43] Individuals with single metastases without a pathological fracture often experience the greatest benefit in terms of extended prognosis following metastasectomy.[48] Resection of a bone metastasis can be curable in select patients.[49] Even when not curable, surgical intervention may be indicated in patients with intractable pain, a pathological fracture has occurred or is impending, spinal instability exists, and spinal cord compression or curative intent can be achieved.[50] As an alternative to surgery, radiotherapy plays a crucial role in the palliation of bone lesions.[51]

Liver metastasis

Liver metastasis is present in approximately 20% of metastatic renal cancers.[43] Surgical excision of liver metastases from renal cancer may be a viable treatment option for select individuals.[52] The most crucial factor in choosing candidates for liver resection is achieving a margin-negative resection.[53] An alternative treatment is transarterial chemoembolization which has also been shown to have benefit in addressing liver metastases.[54]

Surgical metastasectomy is not equally beneficial for all patients with mRCC. One of the largest studies available analyzed 2,911 patients with mRCC who previously underwent CN from the Surveillance, Epidemiology, and End Results Program (SEER) registry and found that metastasectomy was associated with improved OS (HR: 0.875, 95% CI: 0.773 to 0.991, p = 0.015).[55] Importantly, this study resulted in a nomogram stratifying patients into low-, intermediate-, and high-risk groups based on tumor grade, T stage, N stage, the location of the metastases; low-risk was characterized by low stage, low grade, node negative for the primary tumor, and solitary pulmonary metastasis. Based on these categories, surgical metastasectomy was only associated with a reduction in cancer-specific mortality in the low-risk group (12.8% reduction in the risk for 3-year cancer-specific mortality [HR: 0.689, 95% CI: 0.507 to 0.938, p = 0.008]) while those in the intermediate- and high-risk groups saw no benefit. While this nomogram has not yet been validated, it highlights that patient selection remains extremely important and the decision for metastasectomy should be made on an individualized basis.

The decision to pursue surgical metastasectomy must be carefully weighed again the potential for surgical morbidity and mortality. Meyer and colleagues assessed the National Inpatient Sample from 2000 to 2011 and identified 1,102 patients with mRCC who underwent metastasectomy. In the cohort, nearly half (45.7%) experienced an in-hospital complication, and over one-quarter (27.5%) developed a major complication (Clavien III-V complication); the in-hospital mortality rate was 2.4%.[56] In particular, resection of liver metastases was associated with the highest risk for a complication (OR: 2.59, 95% CI: 1.84 to 3.62, p < 0.001). Even though pulmonary metastases are typically considered a "favorable" site of metastatic disease from an oncologic perspective, pulmonary metastasectomy is nevertheless associated with a range of complications including pneumonia, supraventricular tachyarrhythmia, nerve palsy, chylothorax, and upper gastrointestinal bleeding.[57] Metastasectomy represents among the most complex and challenging of procedures even if minimally invasive surgeries are employed.[58] Fortunately, systemic therapy utilization in a preoperative context does not appear to significantly increase the risk of perioperative complications for surgical metastasectomy.[59]

SUMMARY

The management of mRCC is continually evolving. While surgery was arguably the only effective treatment in the past, the changing landscape of systemic therapies over the past two decades has served to improved quality and quantity of life for patients with mRCC but at the same time created new challenges in formulating treatment plans by healthcare professionals. Until non-surgical therapies reliably achieve a durable complete response for patients with mRCC, surgery will remain a cornerstone of treatment. At this time, CN may be indicated as upfront therapy for patients with intractable symptoms, in those with nccRCC histology, and for cases of oligometastatic mRCC. However, the most common forms of surgery for patients with mRCC may be a consolidative CN and metastasectomy since upfront systemic therapy is now widely adopted. Following an approach favoring "personalization over protocolization," the treatment plan for each patient should be tailored through a multidisciplinary approach and established through shared decision making with patients and their families.

Moving forward, more well-designed clinical trials are necessary to evaluate novel treatment options developed from the growing understanding of the molecular and immunological characteristics of mRCC. There are multiple ongoing clinical trials (see **Table 1**) aim to assess the benefit of CN in comparison to current treatment regimen comprised of IO and TKI agents. Interestingly, future advancements in immunotherapy, such as vaccines, may potentially increase the role of upfront surgery because a surgical specimen may be necessary to generate highly personalized treatments which are both effective and minimally toxic. Overall, the role of surgery will continue to change in concert with developments in systemic therapy and other non-surgical treatments.

CLINICS CARE POINTS

- Systemic therapy is non-inferior to cytoreductive nephrectomy in the management of metastatic renal cell carcinoma based on recent phase III randomized clinical trials (CARMENA, SURTIME).

- While no longer considered the standard of care, cytoreductive nephrectomy continues to remain a cornerstone of management for patients with metastatic renal cell carcinoma. It is now commonly employed as consolidative therapy following systemic therapy. Additionally, cytoreductive nephrectomy is appropriately considered for the palliation of symptoms, for patients with non-clear cell histology, and for oligometastatic disease.

- Surgical metastasectomy may improve overall survival and the best outcomes are associated with a complete metastasectomy which achieves a no evidence of disease state.
- For patients with metastatic renal cell carcinoma, both cytoreductive nephrectomy and metastasectomy are associated with significant morbidity and mortality. Thus, the decision for surgery must be weighed against the potential for substantial surgical trauma especially if it would impact the timely use of systemic therapy.

FUNDING

None.

DISCLOSURE

There are no disclosures.

REFERENCES

1. Robson CJ, Churchill BM, Anderson W. The results of radical nephrectomy for renal cell carcinoma. 1969. J Urol 2002;167(2 Pt 2):873–5 [discussion: 876-877].
2. Psutka SP. Surgical management of localized disease and small renal masses. Hematol Oncol 2023;37(5). In Press.
3. Amato RJ. Chemotherapy for renal cell carcinoma. Semin Oncol 2000;27(2): 177–86.
4. Flanigan RC, Salmon SE, Blumenstein BA, et al. Nephrectomy followed by interferon alfa-2b compared with interferon alfa-2b alone for metastatic renal-cell cancer. N Engl J Med 2001;345(23):1655–9.
5. Mickisch GH, Garin A, van Poppel H, et al. Radical nephrectomy plus interferon-alfa-based immunotherapy compared with interferon alfa alone in metastatic renal-cell carcinoma: a randomised trial. Lancet Lond Engl 2001;358(9286): 966–70.
6. Flanigan RC, Mickisch G, Sylvester R, et al. Cytoreductive nephrectomy in patients with metastatic renal cancer: a combined analysis. J Urol 2004;171(3):1071–6.
7. Flanigan RC. Debulking nephrectomy in metastatic renal cancer. Clin Cancer Res 2004;10(18 Pt 2). 6335S-41S.
8. Heng DYC, Wells JC, Rini BI, et al. Cytoreductive nephrectomy in patients with synchronous metastases from renal cell carcinoma: results from the International Metastatic Renal Cell Carcinoma Database Consortium. Eur Urol 2014;66(4): 704–10.
9. Hanna N, Sun M, Meyer CP, et al. Survival analyses of patients with metastatic renal cancer treated with targeted therapy with or without cytoreductive nephrectomy: a national cancer data base study. J Clin Oncol 2016;34(27):3267–75.
10. Bakouny Z, El Zarif T, Dudani S, et al. Upfront cytoreductive nephrectomy for metastatic renal cell carcinoma treated with immune checkpoint inhibitors or targeted therapy: an observational study from the international metastatic renal cell carcinoma database Consortium. Eur Urol 2023;83(2):145–51.
11. Méjean A, Ravaud A, Thezenas S, et al. Sunitinib alone or after nephrectomy in metastatic renal-cell carcinoma. N Engl J Med 2018;379(5):417–27.
12. Méjean A, Ravaud A, Thezenas S, et al. Sunitinib alone or after nephrectomy for patients with metastatic renal cell carcinoma: is there still a role for cytoreductive nephrectomy? Eur Urol 2021;80(4):417–24.

13. Manley BJ, Tennenbaum DM, Vertosick EA, et al. The difficulty in selecting patients for cytoreductive nephrectomy: an evaluation of previously described predictive models. Urol Oncol 2017;35(1):35.e1–5.
14. Powles T, Blank C, Chowdhury S, et al. The outcome of patients treated with sunitinib prior to planned nephrectomy in metastatic clear cell renal cancer. Eur Urol 2011;60(3):448–54.
15. Arora S, Sood A, Dalela D, et al. Cytoreductive nephrectomy: assessing the generalizability of the CARMENA trial to real-world national cancer data base cases. Eur Urol 2019;75(2):352–3.
16. Bex A, Mulders P, Jewett M, et al. Comparison of immediate vs deferred cytoreductive nephrectomy in patients with synchronous metastatic renal cell carcinoma receiving sunitinib: the SURTIME randomized clinical trial. JAMA Oncol 2019;5(2):164–70.
17. Abu-Ghanem Y, van Thienen JV, Blank C, et al. Cytoreductive nephrectomy and exposure to sunitinib - a post hoc analysis of the immediate surgery or surgery after sunitinib malate in treating patients with metastatic kidney cancer (SURTIME) trial. BJU Int 2022;130(1):68–75.
18. Larcher A, Fallara G, Rosiello G, et al. Cytoreductive nephrectomy in metastatic patients with signs or symptoms: implications for renal cell carcinoma guidelines. Eur Urol 2020;78(3):321–6.
19. Palapattu GS, Kristo B, Rajfer J. Paraneoplastic syndromes in urologic malignancy: the many faces of renal cell carcinoma. Rev Urol 2002;4(4):163–70.
20. Blay JY, Rossi JF, Wijdenes J, et al. Role of interleukin-6 in the paraneoplastic inflammatory syndrome associated with renal-cell carcinoma. Int J Cancer 1997; 72(3):424–30.
21. Valenca LB, Hirsch MS, Choueiri TK, et al. Non-clear cell renal cell carcinoma, part 1: histology. Clin Adv Hematol Oncol HO 2015;13(5):308–13.
22. Renshaw AA, Richie JP. Subtypes of renal cell carcinoma. Different onset and sites of metastatic disease. Am J Clin Pathol 1999;111(4):539–43.
23. Motzer RJ, Bacik J, Mariani T, et al. Treatment outcome and survival associated with metastatic renal cell carcinoma of non-clear-cell histology. J Clin Oncol 2002;20(9):2376 81.
24. Vera-Badillo FE, Templeton AJ, Duran I, et al. Systemic therapy for non-clear cell renal cell carcinomas: a systematic review and meta-analysis. Eur Urol 2015; 67(4):740–9.
25. Kassouf W, Sanchez-Ortiz R, Tamboli P, et al. Cytoreductive nephrectomy for metastatic renal cell carcinoma with nonclear cell histology. J Urol 2007;178(5): 1896–900.
26. Turajlic S, Xu H, Litchfield K, et al. Tracking cancer evolution reveals constrained routes to metastases: TRACERx renal. Cell 2018;173(3):581–94.e12.
27. McKay R, Pan E. Managing first-line metastatic renal-cell carcinoma (mRCC): favorable-risk disease. Hematol Oncol 2023;37(5). In Press.
28. Thomas AA, Campbell SC. Consolidative surgery after targeted therapy for renal cell carcinoma. Urol Oncol 2013;31(6):914–9.
29. Powles T, Kayani I, Blank C, et al. The safety and efficacy of sunitinib before planned nephrectomy in metastatic clear cell renal cancer. Ann Oncol 2011; 22(5):1041–7.
30. Powles T, Sarwar N, Stockdale A, et al. Safety and efficacy of pazopanib therapy prior to planned nephrectomy in metastatic clear cell renal cancer. JAMA Oncol 2016;2(10):1303–9.
31. Hellman S, Weichselbaum RR. Oligometastases. J Clin Oncol 1995;13(1):8–10.

32. Ishihara H, Takagi T, Kondo T, et al. Prognostic impact of metastasectomy in renal cell carcinoma in the postcytokine therapy era. Urol Oncol 2021;39(1):77.e17–25.

33. Yu X, Wang B, Li X, et al. The significance of metastasectomy in patients with metastatic renal cell carcinoma in the era of targeted therapy. BioMed Res Int 2015; 2015:176373.

34. Okazaki A, Kijima T, Schiller P, et al. Spontaneous regression of multiple pulmonary metastases accompanied by normalization of serum immune markers following cytoreductive nephrectomy in a patient with clear-cell renal cell carcinoma. IJU Case Rep 2021;4(2):95–9.

35. Ueda K, Suekane S, Mitani T, et al. Spontaneous regression of multiple pulmonary nodules in a patient with unclassified renal cell carcinoma following laparoscopic partial nephrectomy: a case report. Mol Clin Oncol 2016;5(1):49–52.

36. Chan BPH, Booth CM, Manduch M, et al. Spontaneous regression of metastatic pulmonary renal cell carcinoma in the setting of sarcomatoid differentiation of the primary tumour. Can Urol Assoc J J Assoc Urol Can 2013;7(9–10):E587–9.

37. Lekanidi K, Vlachou PA, Morgan B, et al. Spontaneous regression of metastatic renal cell carcinoma: case report. J Med Case Reports 2007;1(1):89.

38. Ricci SB, Cerchiari U. Spontaneous regression of malignant tumors: Importance of the immune system and other factors (Review). Oncol Lett 2010;1(6):941–5.

39. Sun M, Meyer CP, Karam JA, et al. Predictors, utilization patterns, and overall survival of patients undergoing metastasectomy for metastatic renal cell carcinoma in the era of targeted therapy. Eur J Surg Oncol J Eur Soc Surg Oncol Br Assoc Surg Oncol 2018;44(9):1439–45.

40. Lyon TD, Thompson RH, Shah PH, et al. Complete surgical metastasectomy of renal cell carcinoma in the post-cytokine era. J Urol 2020;203(2):275–82.

41. Alt AL, Boorjian SA, Lohse CM, et al. Survival after complete surgical resection of multiple metastases from renal cell carcinoma. Cancer 2011;117(13):2873–82.

42. Choueiri TK, Tomczak P, Park SH, et al. Pembrolizumab as post nephrectomy adjuvant therapy for patients with renal cell carcinoma: Results from 30-month follow-up of KEYNOTE-564. J Clin Oncol 2022;40(6_suppl):290.

43. Bianchi M, Sun M, Jeldres C, et al. Distribution of metastatic sites in renal cell carcinoma: a population-based analysis. Ann Oncol 2012;23(4):973–80.

44. Hofmann H-S, Neef H, Krohe K, et al. Prognostic factors and survival after pulmonary resection of metastatic renal cell carcinoma. Eur Urol 2005;48(1):77–81 [discussion: 81-82].

45. Kavolius JP, Mastorakos DP, Pavlovich C, et al. Resection of metastatic renal cell carcinoma. J Clin Oncol 1998;16(6):2261–6.

46. Woodward E, Jagdev S, McParland L, et al. Skeletal complications and survival in renal cancer patients with bone metastases. Bone 2011;48(1):160–6.

47. Lipton A, Colombo-Berra A, Bukowski RM, et al. Skeletal complications in patients with bone metastases from renal cell carcinoma and therapeutic benefits of zoledronic acid. Clin Cancer Res 2004;10(18 Pt 2). 6397S-403S.

48. Fottner A, Szalantzy M, Wirthmann L, et al. Bone metastases from renal cell carcinoma: patient survival after surgical treatment. BMC Musculoskelet Disord 2010;11:145.

49. Grünwald V, Eberhardt B, Bex A, et al. An interdisciplinary consensus on the management of bone metastases from renal cell carcinoma. Nat Rev Urol 2018;15(8): 511–21.

50. Wood SL, Brown JE. Skeletal metastasis in renal cell carcinoma: current and future management options. Cancer Treat Rev 2012;38(4):284–91.

51. McDonald R, Ding K, Brundage M, et al. Effect of radiotherapy on painful bone metastases: a secondary analysis of the NCIC clinical trials group symptom control trial SC.23. JAMA Oncol 2017;3(7):953–9.
52. Pinotti E, Montuori M, Giani A, et al. Surgical treatment of liver metastases from kidney cancer: a systematic review. ANZ J Surg 2019;89(1–2):32–7.
53. Thelen A, Jonas S, Benckert C, et al. Liver resection for metastases from renal cell carcinoma. World J Surg 2007;31(4):802–7.
54. Matsuda H, Tamada S, Kato M, et al. Transarterial chemoembolization of liver metastasis from renal cell carcinoma. Urol Case Rep 2018;17:79–81.
55. Wu K, Liu Z, Shao Y, et al. Nomogram predicting survival to assist decision-making of metastasectomy in patients with metastatic renal cell carcinoma. Front Oncol 2020;10:592243.
56. Meyer CP, Sun M, Karam JA, et al. Complications after metastasectomy for renal cell carcinoma—a population-based assessment. Eur Urol 2017;72(2):171–4.
57. Kudelin N, Bölükbas S, Eberlein M, et al. Metastasectomy with standardized lymph node dissection for metastatic renal cell carcinoma: an 11-year single-center experience. Ann Thorac Surg 2013;96(1):265–71.
58. Becher E, Jericevic D, Huang WC. Minimally invasive surgery for patients with locally advanced and/or metastatic renal cell carcinoma. Urol Clin North Am 2020;47(3):389–97.
59. McCormick B, Meissner MA, Karam JA, et al. Surgical complications of presurgical systemic therapy for renal cell carcinoma: a systematic review. Kidney Cancer Clifton Va 2017;1(2):115–21.

Adjuvant and Neoadjuvant Therapy in Renal Cell Carcinoma

Teele Kuusk, MD, PhD[a,b,c], Axel Bex, MD, PhD[b,c,d],*

KEYWORDS

- Renal cell carcinoma • Neoadjuvant • Adjuvant • Nephrectomy
- Perioperative therapy • Immune checkpoint inhibitors

KEY POINTS

- Results of the vascular endothelial growth factor receptor-tyrosine kinase inhibitor (TKI) trials have been largely inconsistent.
- Of tested immune checkpoint inhibitors in the adjuvant setting only pembrolizumab for 1 year improved disease-free survival in patients with clear-cell renal cell carcinoma (ccRCC) at intermediate-high and high risk of recurrence.
- Single-arm neoadjuvant trials with immunotherapy have generated data on safety, efficacy, and immune infiltrates.

INTRODUCTION AND RATIONALE

Surgical complete resection is standard of care for patients with locally advanced or limited metastatic renal cell carcinoma (RCC). Unfortunately, these patients have a high risk to develop locally recurrent disease and systemic progression. Based on validated risk scores, high-risk patients have a 2-year local or systemic recurrence rate of more than 50%, and only one-third of patients are metastasis-free at 3 years.[1] High-risk patients with no evidence of disease following complete resection may benefit from adjuvant and neo-adjuvant systemic treatment strategies that primarily aim to prolong disease-free survival (DFS) and ultimately overall survival (OS). Based on the efficacy of vascular endothelial growth factor receptor (VEGFR)-targeted therapy (TT) in advanced disease, several phase 3 randomized controlled trials (RCTs) investigated adjuvant therapy targeting VEGFR after resection of high-risk nonmetastatic

[a] Homerton University Hospital, London, UK; [b] Specialist Centre for Kidney Cancer, Royal Free London NHS Foundation Trust, Pond Street, London NW3 2QG, UK; [c] Department of Urology, The Netherlands Cancer Institute, Plesmanlaan 121, Amsterdam 1066 CX, The Netherlands; [d] Division of Surgery and Interventional Science, University College London, Pond Street, London NW3 2QG, UK
* Corresponding author.
E-mail address: a.bex@ucl.ac.uk

Hematol Oncol Clin N Am 37 (2023) 907–920
https://doi.org/10.1016/j.hoc.2023.05.020
0889-8588/23/© 2023 Elsevier Inc. All rights reserved.

RCC. The results did not show an OS benefit with conflicting DFS benefit, and all except one trial did not show a DFS advantage.[2,3]

Subsequently, the efficacy of immune checkpoint inhibitors (ICIs) in metastatic RCC[4] has generated enthusiasm for their potential use in the perioperative space. This narrative review gives an overview of the current status of perioperative systemic therapies for patients with locally advanced RCC. In general, immunotherapy with ICI augments an existing adaptive immune response.[5] The rationale for perioperative immunotherapy is that it may eradicate residual tumor cells and maintain surveillance against micrometastases even after treatment discontinuation.[6,7]

ADJUVANT THERAPY
Adjuvant Trials with Targeted Therapy

Before the introduction of ICI therapy into the treatment paradigm, 6 adjuvant phase 3 RCTs had been performed in the era of TT (ASSURE,[8] S-TRAC,[2] PROTECT,[9] ATLAS,[10] SORCE,[3] and EVEREST[11]; **Table 1**). Following VEGFR-tyrosine kinase inhibitor (TKI) trials with sunitinib, sorafenib, pazopanib, and axitinib, the Food and Drug Administration (FDA) approved only sunitinib for the adjuvant treatment of patients with RCC at high risk of recurrence following nephrectomy.[12] This approval was based on S-TRAC, a multicenter double-blind placebo-controlled trial of 615 patients at high risk for recurrent RCC following nephrectomy, which led to a statistically significant improvement of DFS with sunitinib compared with placebo.[2] Because the other trials failed to detect a statistically significant benefit for adjuvant VEGFR-TKI therapy, it has been argued that the inclusion of a well-defined high-risk group on full-dose sunitinib might have led the S-TRAC trial to demonstrate a significant DFS benefit.[13] However, a subset analysis from the ASSURE trial (which also explored adjuvant sunitinib) that included the highest-risk patients and those starting with full dose sunitinib did not show any DFS or OS benefit.[14]

The EVEREST trial compared everolimus 10 mg orally daily for 54 weeks versus placebo within 12 weeks following radical or partial nephrectomy for intermediate-high (pT1 G3-4 N0 to pT3a G1-2 N0) or very high-risk (pT3a G3-4 to pT4 G-any or N+) clear cell and non–clear-cell RCC. Results were reported after a median follow-up of 76 months, 4 prespecified interim analyses, and after 556 DFS events occurred among 1499 eligible patients by the time of final study analysis in February 2022. The primary endpoint, recurrence-free survival (RFS), had a hazard ratio (HR) of 0.85 (95% CI 0.72–1.00; $P = .0246$) in favor of everolimus but narrowly missed the prespecified, one-sided significance level of 0.022. Despite selection for higher risk patients, the trial struggled with the required events for final analysis, which is reflected in the long 6-year RFS estimate of 64% for everolimus and 61% for placebo. In a subgroup analysis, a 21% RFS improvement was observed in the very high-risk group (HR 0.79, 95% CI 0.65–0.97) in favor of everolimus. Grade 3 to 4 adverse events (AEs) occurred in 46% of patients who received everolimus and 11% of those in the placebo arm.[11] Results are hypothesis generating, suggesting a subgroup of patients may derive benefit from mammalian target of rapamycin (mTOR) inhibition, although toxicities must be considered as well.

ADJUVANT TRIALS WITH IMMUNE CHECKPOINT INHIBITOR

Six phase 3 RCTs with ICI therapy as adjuvant either as monotherapy or combination in patients with high-risk RCC were designed: IMmotion 010 (NCT03024996 studying atezolizumab vs placebo),[15] CheckMate 914 (NCT03138512 studying nivolumab and ipilimumab or nivolumab vs placebo),[16] Keynote-564 (NCT03142334 studying

Table 1
Completed trials with targeted therapy in the adjuvant setting

Trial	N	Patient Characteristics	Treatment Arms	Treatment Duration	Primary End Point
S-TRAC: Sunitinib Trial in Adjuvant Renal Cancer Treatment[6] NCT00375674	615	High risk per modified UISS criteria Clear-cell RCC	Sunitinib vs Placebo	1 y	DFS ITT 0.76; 95% CI, 0.59–0.98; P = .03
ASSURE: Adjuvant Sorafenib or Sunitinib for Unfavorable RCC[19] NCT00326898	1943	Intermediate-high: pT1b G3/4, pT2 G_{any} pT3a G1/2 Very-high: pT3a G3-4, pT3-4 G_{any} N1 Clear-cell RCC	Sunitinib vs Sorafenib vs Placebo	1 y	DFS ITT SUN: 1.02; 97·5% CI 0.85–1.23, P = .8038 SOR: 0.97; 97·5% CI 0.80–1.17, P = 0·7184
SORCE: Sorafenib in Patients with Resected Primary RCC at High/ Intermediate Risk of Relapse[7] NCT00492258	1711	Intermediate- and high risk per Leibovich score (3–5 and 6–11) Clear-cell/non-cc RCC	3y Sorafenib vs 1y Sorafenib vs Placebo	1 and 3 y	DFS ITT 3y SOR: 1.01; 95% CI, 0.82–1.23; P = .946 1y SOR: 0.94; 95% CI, 0.77–1.14; P = .509
EVEREST: Everolimus for Renal Cancer Ensuing Surgical Therapy[9] NCT01120249	1545	Intermediate-high: pT1b G3/4, pT2 G_{any} pT3a G1/2 Very-high: pT3a G3-4, pT3-4 G_{any} N1 Clear-cell/non-cc RCC	Everolimus vs Placebo	54 wk	RFS ITT 0.85; 95% CI, 0.72–1.00; P = .051
PROTECT: Pazopanib as an Adjuvant Treatment for Localized RCC[16] NCT01235962	1538	pT2 G3/4, pT3-4 G_{any} N1 clear-cell RCC	Pazopanib vs Placebo	1 y	DFS ITT 0.86; 95% CI, 0.70–1.06; P = .165
ATLAS: Adjuvant Axitinib Therapy of Renal Cell Cancer in High Risk Patients[17] NCT01599754	724	≥pT2 and/or N+, any Fuhrman grade	Axitinib vs Placebo	1–3 y	DFS ITT 0.87; 95% CI, 0.66–1.147; P = .3211

Abbreviations: DFS, disease free survival; RFS, relapse free survival; ITT, intention to treat.

pembrolizumab vs placebo),[17] LITESPARK-022 (NCT05239728 studying pembrolizumab with or without belzutifan),[18] RAMPART (NCT03288532 studying durvalumab and tremelmiumab or durvalumab vs placebo),[19] and PROSPER RCC (NCT03055013 studying perioperative nivolumab vs surgery alone).[20] All but LITESPARK and RAMPART have reported results (**Table 2**). IMmotion 010 and Keynote-564 enrolled high-risk patients (which resulted in a higher event rate compared with other studies) as well as patients after complete metastasectomy; the PROSPER trial was later amended to include this population too. Notably, while Keynote-564 enrolled patients with metachronous metastatic disease or those rendered surgically no evidence of disease (NED) within 1 year of nephrectomy, IMmotion 010 enrolled patients who were rendered surgically NED greater than 1 year after nephrectomy. RAMPART and PROSPER are the only trials that included RCC of variant histologies. Length of treatment was predominantly 1 year, apart from Checkmate-914, which used only 6 months of therapy. Across the studies, patients were ineligible if they received earlier treatment with drugs specifically targeting T-cell costimulation or immune checkpoint pathways; any earlier systemic anticancer treatment of RCC; or a live or attenuated vaccine in the 30 days before study treatment. The trials were designed with different ICIs including programmed cell death protein-1 (PD-1) and programmed cell death protein-ligand-1 (PD-L1) inhibitors, as well as their combination with anti-cytotoxic T lymphocyte associated protein-4 (CTLA4) or a hypoxia inducible factor-2 alpha (HIF-2α) inhibitor, and are each reviewed in detail.

ADJUVANT TREATMENT WITH PD-1 INHIBITION

Keynote-564 reported in 2021 and was the first and only adjuvant ICI phase III trial with positive DFS data, the primary endpoint of the study.[17] In this trial, pembrolizumab given for 17 cycles at 3-week intervals was evaluated versus placebo. A total of 994 patients with intermediate (pT2, grade 4 or sarcomatoid, N0 M0; or pT3, any grade, N0, M0) or high risk (pT4, any grade, N0 M0; or pT any stage, and grade, or N+, M0), or M1 NED after primary tumor plus soft tissue metastases completely resected 1 year or lesser from nephrectomy, were included. At initial presentation, the median follow-up was 24.1 months. DFS was significantly improved in the pembrolizumab group versus placebo (HR 0.68, 95% CI: 0.53–0.87, P = .001). The estimated 24-month DFS rate was 77% versus 68% for pembrolizumab and placebo, respectively. Benefit occurred across several subgroups of patients including those with M1 NED postsurgery (n = 58, 6%). At 24.1 months follow-up, OS showed a statistically insignificant trend toward a benefit in the pembrolizumab arm (HR 0.54, 95% CI 0.30–0.96, P = .0164). At this time, only a few OS events have occurred, with 2-year OS rates of 97% for pembrolizumab versus 94% for placebo. An update at a median follow-up of 30 months[21] confirmed the positive DFS results (HR 0.63, 95% CI 0.50–0.80) while OS data remained immature (HR 0.52, 95% CI 0.31–0.86; P = .0048). Grade 3 to 5 all-cause AEs were noted in 32.2% versus 17.7% of patients for pembrolizumab and placebo, respectively. Quality of life assessment by functional kidney symptom inde- disease-related symptoms (FKSI-DRS) and core quality of life questionnaire (QLQ30) did not show a statistically significant or clinically meaningful deterioration in health-related QoL or symptom scores for either adjuvant pembrolizumab or placebo. DFS data for the CheckMate 914 monotherapy (arm B are eagerly awaited),[16,22] as discussed in detail below.

Adjuvant Treatment with PD-L1 Inhibition

The IMmotion 010 phase III trial investigated a PD-L1 inhibitor with a primary endpoint of DFS.[15] Patients received atezolizumab 1200 mg IV (16 cycles of therapy every

Table 2
Completed trials with immunotherapy in the perioperative setting

Study	N	Intervention	Primary Endpoint	Risk Assessment and Subtype	DFS (mo) Median (95% CI) HR	OS (mo) Median (95% CI) HR
Keynote-564 NCT03142334 Median follow-up of 30.1 mo[26]	994	Pembro 200 mg IV Q3W (17 cycles) vs Placebo	DFS in the ITT by IR	pTNM pT2 grade 4 or sarcomatoid; pT3 any grade pT4 any grade, pN1; M1 NED <12 mo after nephrectomy clear-cell	PEMBRO: NR (NE) PLACEBO: NR (NE) HR: 0.63 (95% CI: 0.50–0.80) P < .002 DFS at 24 mo: PEMBRO: 78.3% PLACEBO: 67.3%	PEMBRO: NR (NE) PLACEBO: NR (NE) HR: 0.52 (95% CI: 0.31–0.86) not significant alive at 30 mo: PEMBRO: 95.7% PLACEBO: 91.4%
IMmotion 010 NCT03024996 Median follow-up of 44.7 mo[27]	778	Atezo 1200 mg IV Q3W (16 cycles or 1 y) vs placebo	DFS in the ITT by IR	pTNM: pT2 grade 4 or sarcomatoid; pT3 a grade 3–4; pT3b/cT4 any grade, pN1 M1 NED synchronous or ≥12 mo after nephrectomy Clear-cell component	ATEZO: 57.2 (44.6-NE) PLACEBO: 49.5 (47.4-NE) HR: 0.93 (95% CI: 0.75–1.15) P = .4950 DFS at 24 mo: NR	ATEZO: NE (59.8-NE) PLACEBO: NE (NE-NE) HR: 0.97 (95% CI: 0.67–1.42) alive at 24 mo: NR
CheckMate 214 Arm A NCT03138512 Median follow-up of 37.0 mo[21]	816	Nivo 240 mg IV Q2W (× 12 cycles) + Ipi 1 mg/kg IV Q6W (× 4 cycles) vs placebo	DFS in the ITT by BICR	By TNM: pT2a grade 3–4; pT2b/T3/T4 any grade, pN1 clear-cell component	NIVO + IPI: NR (NE) PLACEBO: 50.7 (48.1-NE) HR: 0.92 (95% CI: 0.71–1.19) P = .5347 DFS at 24 mo: NIVO + IPI: 76.4% PLACEBO: 74.0%	NIVO + IPI:NR (NE) PLACEBO: NR (NE) HR: NR NIVO + IPI: 33/405 events PLACEBO: 28/411 events
PROSPER NCT03055013 Median follow up not reported[24]	779	One dose preoperative nivolumab 480 mg IV followed by adjuvant nivolumab 480 mg IV for 9 doses vs Surgery alone	RFS in the ITT by IR	cTNM: ≥cT2 (7 cm) or cTany cN1 clear-cell and non-cc	NIVO: NR (NE) Observation: NR (NE) HR: 0.97 (95% CI: 0.74–1.28) P = .43	NIVO: NR (NE) Observation: NR (NE) HR: 1.48 (95% CI: 0.89–2.48) P = .93

Abbreviations: Atezo, atezolizumab; DFS, disease free survival; Ipi, Ipilimumab; ITT, intention to treat; NE, Not evaluable; Nivo, nivolumab; NR, Not reached; Pembro, pembrolizumab; RFS, relapse free survival.

3 weeks up to 1 year) or placebo as adjuvant therapy. A total of 778 patients with an increased risk of recurrence defined as pT2, grade 4 or sarcomatoid, N0 M0; or pT3, grade 3 to 4, N0, M0; pT3b/c/T4, any grade, N0 M0; or pT any stage or grade, pN1, M0, or M1 NED after primary tumor plus soft tissue metastases completely resected either synchronous or if metachronous, 12 months or greater from nephrectomy were enrolled. The minimum follow-up was 38.6 months. DFS per investigator assessment was not met in the atezolizumab group versus placebo (HR 0.93, 95% CI 0.75–1.15, $P = .4950$). None of the exploratory subgroups suggested a DFS benefit with atezolizumab; the M1 NED subgroup (n = 108), the sarcomatoid subgroup, and the subgroup expressing 1% or greater PD-L1 had HRs of 0.93 (0.58–1.49), 0.77 (0.44–1.36), and 0.83 (0.63–1.10), respectively. There was also no improvement in OS. Grade 3 or 4 all-cause and treatment AEs occurred in 27.2% and 14.1% versus 21.1% and 4.7% of patients for atezolizumab and placebo, respectively. There were no treatment-related grade 5 AEs.

Adjuvant Treatment with Immune Checkpoint Inhibitor Combination Therapy

CheckMate 914 was the first trial to report on adjuvant ICI combination therapy. Part A compared nivolumab plus ipilimumab with placebo, whereas Part B compared nivolumab monotherapy with both placebo and the nivolumab/ipilimumab combination.[22] In both parts of the trial, treatment continued until completion of 12 cycles, unacceptable toxicity, disease recurrence, week 36, or withdrawal of consent, whichever occurred first. The data published to date concern part A, which evaluated nivolumab 240 mg Q2W for 12 cycles with ipilimumab 1 mg/kg Q6W for 4 cycles versus placebo as adjuvant for a total of 816 patients. Enrolled patients had pT2a, grade 3 or 4, N0 M0; pT2b/T3/T4, any grade, N0 M0; or pT any stage, any grade, pN1, M0. With a median follow-up of 37 months,[16] the primary endpoint of DFS per investigator assessment was not met in the nivolumab plus ipilimumab group versus placebo (HR 0.92, 95% CI 0.71–1.19; $P = .5347$).

All-cause AEs of any grade led to discontinuation of nivolumab plus ipilimumab in 129 (32%) of patients in the experimental arm. Treatment-related grade 3 or greater AEs were observed in 28% in the nivolumab plus ipilimumab arm and 2% in the placebo arm, with 4 deaths considered related to combination therapy.

Perioperative and Neoadjuvant Therapy

Neoadjuvant therapy seeks to exploit the presence of tumor neoantigens in situ before surgical removal. A higher disease burden may aid in stimulating an immune response and may result in better response to therapy.[23] With primary in place, there is an abundance of tumor antigen for cross-priming a robust antitumor CD8+ T-cell response.[24] Randomized data do not exist in RCC but studies in melanoma support that neoadjuvant ICI therapy may generate a stronger immune response from the activation of tumor-infiltrating lymphocytes (TILs) against tumor neoantigens compared with adjuvant therapy.[25] In the SWOG S1801 trial of resected stage III/IV melanoma, neoadjuvant pembrolizumab significantly improved event-free survival versus adjuvant therapy (HR 0.59, 95% CI 0.40–0.86; $P = .0015$).

Perioperative Trials

The only phase 3 trial in the perioperative space is PROSPER, which compared nivolumab with observation in localized RCC undergoing nephrectomy.[20] Patients were randomized to 1 cycle of nivolumab followed by radical or partial nephrectomy, and then adjuvant nivolumab (480 mg IV every 4 weeks) for 9 doses versus surgery alone. Patients with either high risk or oligometastatic clinical stage T2Nx or greater or

$T_{any}N$ + RCC of any histology were included. Oligometastatic ($\leq$3 metastases) patients were eligible only if they underwent local therapy for metastatic sites. In total, 819 patients with clear cell (87%) and non–clear RCC were included. The primary endpoint of RFS was similar between the arms (HR 0.97, 95% CI 0.74–1.28; P = .43) and the trial was stopped early by the data safety monitoring committee, with median follow-up of 16 months. Although immature, OS was not statistically different (HR: 1.48, 95% CI 0.89–2.48; P = .93). Grade 3 to 4 treatment-related AEs occurred in 15% of patients in the nivolumab arm and 4% in the control arm. Trial design issues, such as mixed subtypes, different definitions for recurrence, short pretreatment with nivolumab and follow-up, and heavy censoring all may have contributed to the negative results from PROSPER.

Neoadjuvant Therapy

Currently, neoadjuvant therapy for locally advanced RCC is not standard of care. In the era of VEGFR-TT, single-arm phase II trials primarily aimed at downsizing of the primary tumor to exploit changes in size for nephron sparing strategies or to facilitate tumor thrombectomy. Two prospective phase 2 trials were conducted with neoadjuvant axitinib, demonstrating a median reduction of tumor size by 17% to 28% as well as improvement of RENAL nephrometry score complexity and downstaging.[26,27] In another single-arm phase 2 trial designed to reduce venous tumor thrombus (VTT), 20 patients with resectable clear-cell RCC and VTT received up to 2 months of axitinib before resection. Of patients enrolled, 37.5% (6/16) with inferior vena cava VTT and 25% (1/4) with renal vein thrombus had a reduction in VTT level, leading to less invasive surgery than originally planned in 41.2% (7/17) of patients.[28]

Due to their properties that differ from VEGFR-TT, neoadjuvant ICI strategies may be beneficial in eradicating disease beyond the rationale of reducing tumor size. Neoadjuvant anti-PD-1 therapy could potentially induce tumor-specific CD8+ T cell expansion and improve response and survival.[29] Preclinical and early clinical research suggests that for patients with high-risk nonmetastatic RCC, a significantly greater therapeutic efficacy may be gained by neoadjuvant immune therapies instead of an adjuvant approach to eradicate distant micrometastases following primary tumor resection.[23] This hypothesis requires testing in a randomized trial beyond PROSPER. In metastatic clear-cell renal cell carcinoma (ccRCC), translational data from the ADAPTeR trial (NCT02446860, a phase 2 trial of nivolumab before resection) suggest that in patients with clinical response, neoadjuvant anti-PD-1 therapy maintains and boosts a preexisting intratumoral clonal T-cell response likely recognizing the same antigens.[30] The quest to understand response and resistance to ICI therapy has resulted in several neoadjuvant phase I/II studies that either have reported or are currently ongoing **(Table 3)**.

Phase 1b and 2 Neoadjuvant Immune Checkpoint Inhibitor Studies

Single-arm safety and efficacy studies investigated neoadjuvant nivolumab in the nonmetastatic setting.[31,32] These trials are characterized by small patient numbers, and they failed to demonstrate a response in the primary tumor. Additionally, pathological responses with nivolumab monotherapy have not been well described. Another perioperative phase 1b study tested safety and efficacy of durvalumab plus tremelimumab in advanced RCC[33] but had to be stopped due to toxicity. Previous translational research suggests a modulatory effect of VEGFR-TKI on TILs, which could be harnessed in synergy with anti-PD-1 ICI.[34] NEOAVAX, a single-arm neoadjuvant combination trial of avelumab (a PD-L1 inhibitor) and axitinib enrolled patients with a hybrid high-risk of recurrence, defined as clinical advanced stage in combination with biopsy

Table 3
Response and surgical safety in neoadjuvant therapy in RCC

Publication	Number of patients	Response to Therapy in primary Tumor	Change in Surgical Approach
Bex et al,[24] 2022 Neoadjuvant axitinib (TKI) and avelumab (PD-L1 inhibitor)[a]	34 pt	30% PR	NA
Stewart et al,[30] 2022 Neoadjuvant axitinib (TKI)	17 pt	16.7% PR 72.2% SD 11.1% PD	29.4% improvement in the "level of control" of IVC/ renal vein 41.1% less extensive surgery performed than was planned before axitinib treatment
Wood et al,[40] 2020 Neoadjuvant pazopanib[b]	21 pt	38% PR	Unchanged
Carlo et al,[34] 2022 Neoadjuvant nivolumab	18 pt	100% SD	No nivolumab related complications
Gorin et al,[35] 2022 Neoadjuvant nivolumab	17 pt	100% SD	No Clavien grade ≥ III postoperative complications Quality of life remained stable
Ornstein et al,[36] 2020 Neoadjuvant durvalumab ± tremelimumab	29 pt	NA	No treatment-related delays to nephrectomy or surgical complications
Margulis et al,[41] 2021 Neoadjuvant SBRT[c]	6 pt	NA	No 90 d grade 4–5 AEs were observed

IVC, inferior vena cava.
[a] Bex A, et al. Efficacy, safety, and biomarker analysis of neoadjuvant avelumab/axitinib in patients (pts) with localized renal cell carcinoma (RCC) who are at high risk of relapse after nephrectomy (NeoAvAx). Journal of Clinical Oncology 40, no. 6_suppl 2022: 289-289.
[b] Wood CG, et al. Neoadjuvant pazopanib and molecular analysis of tissue response in renal cell carcinoma. JCI Insight. 2020 19;5(22):e132852.
[c] Margulis V, et al. Neoadjuvant SABR for Renal Cell Carcinoma Inferior Vena Cava Tumor Thrombus-Safety Lead-in Results of a Phase 2 Trial. Int J Radiat Oncol Biol Phys. 2021 Jul 15;110(4):1135-1142.

grades.[24] Primary endpoint was RECIST partial response (PR) in the primary tumor, which was met at 30%. PR in the primary tumor was associated with a trend toward improved DFS. Preliminary IHC analysis of the immune infiltrate in resected tumors demonstrated a significant increase in CD8+ densities in patients without a recurrence, suggesting expansion of a preexisting immune response.[24]

Ongoing Trials

Presently, several phase 2 trials with ICI combination therapy in the neoadjuvant setting are ongoing,[35,36] including lenvatinib and pembrolizumab, a combination that has demonstrated high-response rates in the metastatic setting[4] (**Table 4**). The NESCIO trial is unique because it is the only study randomizing between nivolumab and combinations of this drug with either relatlimab (a LAG-3 inhibitor) or ipilimumab.[37] Safety and efficacy are the primary endpoints. However, at present neoadjuvant ICI therapy for patients with RCC at high risk of recurrence is not investigated in randomized trials against placebo or adjuvant therapy.

In the adjuvant space, 2 RCTs investigate ICI combinations. RAMPART, a phase 3 multiarm RCT design, assesses durvalumab alone or in combination with tremelimumab every 4 weeks for 13 cycles versus observation.[19] RAMPART includes intermediate and high-risk patients by Leibovich risk assessment (Leibovich score 3–11) and is one of the 2 trials including non–clear-cell RCC in addition to ccRCC. Primary endpoints are DFS and OS. This trial may require a change in trial design following the approval of adjuvant pembrolizumab as an option for patients with locally advanced intermediate-to-high risk RCC.[38] Building on the success of Keynote-564, LITESPARK-022 (NCT05239728) recently opened for accrual.[18] Patients are randomized 1:1 to receive belzutifan, a HIF-2α inhibitor, 120 mg orally once daily plus pembrolizumab 400 mg IV every 6 weeks (Q6W) or oral placebo plus pembrolizumab 400 mg IV Q6W. Pembrolizumab treatment will be administered for up to 9 doses (~1 year); belzutifan and placebo may be continued for a maximum of 54 weeks. Eligibility follows the criteria of the Keynote-564 trial with the exception that patients are included with metastasectomy to NED in the first 2 years after nephrectomy with curative intent, as well as those with microscopic positive surgical margins, a novelty in adjuvant trial designs. The primary endpoint is investigator-assessed DFS, with OS as a key secondary endpoint. The trial aims to enroll 1600 patients and plans to report in 2030. There are other ongoing concepts in development within the National Cancer Institute cooperative groups.

DISCUSSION AND RECOMMENDATIONS

Perioperative treatment in the era of ICI therapy is a rapidly evolving field. Keynote-564 remains the only trial to demonstrate an improved DFS in the adjuvant setting but mature OS data and biomarkers predictive of outcome and AEs are currently unavailable. Although the results of IMmotion 010 may reflect the poor efficacy and OS results seen in the metastatic setting with PD-L1 inhibitors in the IMmotion 151 and Javelin 100 trials, the results of CheckMate 914 and PROSPER require different explanations. Nivolumab and ipilimumab leads to durable remission and long-term OS in metastatic disease, and nivolumab and pembrolizumab are both anti PD-1. The high treatment discontinuation rate of 33% in CheckMate 914 is of concern and may have had an impact on the trial outcomes. Ultimately, patient selection is critical. Although tumour, node, metastasis (TNM) risk is prognostic for recurrence, it may not be predictive of response to immunotherapy, and novel biomarkers are needed. Translational work suggests that patients with certain tumor gene expression profiles benefit most from ICI combination therapy.[39] In nonmetastatic disease, however, it

Table 4
Ongoing neoadjuvant phase II immune checkpoint inhibitor combination trials

Trial	n	Intervention	Endpoint
NCT04118855 China (J Huang)	N = 30	Toripalimab (PD-1) + axitinib 12 wk	Safety + efficacy
NCT03680521 MDACC	N = 25	Nivolumab (PD-1) + sitravatinib (TKI inhibiting TAM family receptors (TYRO3, AXL, MERTK) 6–8 wk	Safety + efficacy
NCT05319015 UT Southwestern (V Margulis)	N = 30 IVC II-IV	Pembrolizumab (PD-1) 200 mg Q3 × 4 + lenvatinib 20 mg pold for 12 wk + adjuvant pembrolizumab 200 mg Q3 × 13	Safety + efficacy
NCT04393350 Emory (M Bilen)	N = 22	Pembrolizumab 200 mg Q3 × 4 + lenvatinib 20 mg pold for 21 d to be repeated × 4	Safety + efficacy (suspended for safety reasons)
NCT05172440 China, Jiangsu (H Guo)	N = 20	Tislelizumab (PD-1) 200 mg week 1, 4,7 and 10 + axitinib 5 mg pold 12 wk	Safety + efficacy (not recruiting)
NCT04995016 China, Tianjin (B Huo)	N = 18	Pembrolizumab 200 mg Q3 × 4 + axitinib 5 mg POl BID for 12 wk	Safety + efficacy (not yet recruiting)
NCT04028245 Columbia	N = 14	Spartalizumab (PD-1) 400 mg + canakinumab 300 mg (monoclonal antibody targeting IL-1β Q4 × 2	Safety (Percentage proceeding to nephrectomy)
NCT05148546 NKI	N = 66	Nivolumab Q3 × 2 vs nivolumab Q3 × 2 + ipilimumab 1 mg/kg × 2 vs nivolumab Q3 × 2 + relatlimab 360 mg × 2	Safety + efficacy based on pathological response

remains to be determined if there is an association between higher pTNM stages and immune responsive gene expression profiles. The HR in an exploratory subgroup analysis of CheckMate 914 favoring nivolumab plus ipilimumab in tumors with sarcomatoid features suggests the presence of subgroups with immune-responsive tumors. The inability to control for the inclusion of immune-responsive tumor profiles in conjunction with TNM risk may explain the differences observed in DFS between Keynote-564 and CheckMate 914.

The uncertainty of adjuvant strategies raises opportunities to explore biomarker driven perioperative therapy for select patient subgroups. Recent translational data from neoadjuvant and presurgical phase 1b and 2 trials enhance our understanding of the tumor-immune microenvironment and its dynamic changes. In contrast to adjuvant studies, neoadjuvant trials allow collection of pretreatment and posttreatment tissue to investigate on-treatment differences in the tumor microenvironment and immune infiltrate, as well as in the peripheral blood, which may help to predict response to treatment.

CLINICS CARE POINTS

- Adjuvant sunitinib is approved by the FDA but not in Europe and is not widely used.

- Adjuvant pembrolizumab is a valid option for patients after resection of intermediate (pT2, grade 4 or sarcomatoid, N0 M0; or pT3, any grade, N0, M0) or high risk (pT4, any grade, N0 M0; or pT any stage and grade, N+, M0) primary tumors, or M1 resected to NED within 1 year from nephrectomy. This is FDA and The European Medicines Agency (EMA) approved.

- Patients should be informed that mature OS data and biomarkers predictive for outcome and AEs of adjuvant pembrolizumab are presently unavailable.

- Neoadjuvant therapy is not standard of care and should not be given outside clinical trials.

FINANCIAL SUPPORT AND SPONSORSHIP

None.

DISCLOSURE

A. Bex has received honoraria from BMS, MSD, and Ipsen and is currently receiving an educational grant from Pfizer for a neoadjuvant study with avelumab and axitinib in high-risk renal cancer. T. Kuusk has no conflicts of interest.

ACKNOWLEDGMENTS

None.

REFERENCES

1. Sun M, Shariat SF, Cheng C, et al. Prognostic factors and predictive models in renal cell carcinoma: a contemporary review. Eur Urol 2011;60(4):644–61.
2. Ravaud A, Motzer RJ, Pandha HS, et al. Adjuvant Sunitinib in High-Risk Renal-Cell Carcinoma after Nephrectomy. N Engl J Med 2016;375(23):2246–54.
3. Eisen T, Frangou E, Oza B, et al. Adjuvant Sorafenib for Renal Cell Carcinoma at Intermediate or High Risk of Relapse: Results From the SORCE Randomized Phase III Intergroup Trial. J Clin Oncol 2020;38(34):4064–75.

4. Bedke J, Albiges L, Capitanio U, et al. The 2021 Updated European Association of Urology Guidelines on Renal Cell Carcinoma: Immune Checkpoint Inhibitor-based Combination Therapies for Treatment-naive Metastatic Clear-cell Renal Cell Carcinoma Are Standard of Care. Eur Urol 2021. https://doi.org/10.1016/j.eururo.2021.04.042.

5. van der Leun AM, Thommen DS, Schumacher TN. CD8(+) T cell states in human cancer: insights from single-cell analysis. Nat Rev Cancer 2020;20(4):218–32.

6. Leow JJ, Ray S, Dason S, et al. The Promise of Neoadjuvant and Adjuvant Therapies for Renal Cancer. Urol Clin North Am 2023;50(2):285–303.

7. Lindner AK, Martowicz A, Untergasser G, et al. CXCR3 Expression Is Associated with Advanced Tumor Stage and Grade Influencing Survival after Surgery of Localised Renal Cell Carcinoma. Cancers 2023;15(4). https://doi.org/10.3390/cancers15041001.

8. Haas NB, Manola J, Uzzo RG, et al. Adjuvant sunitinib or sorafenib for high-risk, non-metastatic renal-cell carcinoma (ECOG-ACRIN E2805): a double-blind, placebo-controlled, randomised, phase 3 trial. Lancet 2016;387(10032):2008–16.

9. Motzer RJ, Haas NB, Donskov F, et al. Randomized Phase III Trial of Adjuvant Pazopanib Versus Placebo After Nephrectomy in Patients With Localized or Locally Advanced Renal Cell Carcinoma. J Clin Oncol 2017;35(35):3916–23.

10. Gross-Goupil M, Kwon TG, Eto M, et al. Axitinib versus placebo as an adjuvant treatment of renal cell carcinoma: results from the phase III, randomized ATLAS trial. Ann Oncol 2018;29(12):2371–8.

11. Ryan CW, Tangen C, Heath EI, et al. EVEREST: Everolimus for renal cancer ensuing surgical therapy—A phase III study (SWOG S0931, NCT01120249). J Clin Oncol 2022;40(17_suppl):LBA4500.

12. Bex A, Albiges L, Ljungberg B, et al. Updated European Association of Urology Guidelines Regarding Adjuvant Therapy for Renal Cell Carcinoma. Eur Urol 2017;71(5):719–22.

13. Sun M, Marconi L, Eisen T, et al. Adjuvant Vascular Endothelial Growth Factor-targeted Therapy in Renal Cell Carcinoma: A Systematic Review and Pooled Analysis. Eur Urol 2018;74(5):611–20.

14. Haas NB, Manola J, Dutcher JP, et al. Adjuvant Treatment for High-Risk Clear Cell Renal Cancer: Updated Results of a High-Risk Subset of the ASSURE Randomized Trial. JAMA Oncol 2017;3(9):1249–52.

15. Pal SK, Uzzo R, Karam JA, et al. Adjuvant atezolizumab versus placebo for patients with renal cell carcinoma at increased risk of recurrence following resection (IMmotion010): a multicentre, randomised, double-blind, phase 3 trial. Lancet 2022. https://doi.org/10.1016/s0140-6736(22)01658-0.

16. Motzer RJ, Russo P, Grünwald V, et al. Adjuvant nivolumab plus ipilimumab versus placebo for localised renal cell carcinoma after nephrectomy (CheckMate 914): a double-blind, randomised, phase 3 trial. Lancet 2023;401(10379):821–32.

17. Choueiri TK, Tomczak P, Park SH, et al. Adjuvant Pembrolizumab after Nephrectomy in Renal-Cell Carcinoma. N Engl J Med 2021;385(8):683–94.

18. Choueiri TK, Bedke J, Karam JA, et al. LITESPARK-022: A phase 3 study of pembrolizumab + belzutifan as adjuvant treatment of clear cell renal cell carcinoma (ccRCC). J Clin Oncol 2022;40(16_suppl):TPS4602.

19. Oza B, Frangou E, Smith B, et al. RAMPART: A phase III multi-arm multi-stage trial of adjuvant checkpoint inhibitors in patients with resected primary renal cell carcinoma (RCC) at high or intermediate risk of relapse. Contemp Clin Trials 2021;108:106482.

20. Allaf M, Kim SE, Harshman LC, et al. LBA67 Phase III randomized study comparing perioperative nivolumab (nivo) versus observation in patients (Pts) with renal cell carcinoma (RCC) undergoing nephrectomy (PROSPER, ECOG-ACRIN EA8143), a National Clinical Trials Network trial. Ann Oncol 2022;33: S1432–3.

21. Powles T, Tomczak P, Park SH, et al. Pembrolizumab versus placebo as post-nephrectomy adjuvant therapy for clear cell renal cell carcinoma (KEYNOTE-564): 30-month follow-up analysis of a multicentre, randomised, double-blind, placebo-controlled, phase 3 trial. Lancet Oncol 2022;23(9):1133–44.

22. Bex A, Russo P, Tomita Y, et al. A phase III, randomized, placebo-controlled trial of nivolumab or nivolumab plus ipilimumab in patients with localized renal cell carcinoma at high-risk of relapse after radical or partial nephrectomy (CheckMate 914). J Clin Oncol 2020;38(15_suppl):TPS5099.

23. Drake CG, Stein MN. The Immunobiology of Kidney Cancer. J Clin Oncol 2018. https://doi.org/10.1200/jco.2018.79.2648. Jco2018792648.

24. Bex A, Abu-Ghanem Y, Van Thienen JV, et al. Efficacy, safety, and biomarker analysis of neoadjuvant avelumab/axitinib in patients (pts) with localized renal cell carcinoma (RCC) who are at high risk of relapse after nephrectomy (NeoAvAx). J Clin Oncol 2022;40(6_suppl):289.

25. Patel S, Othus M, Prieto V, et al. LBA6 Neoadjvuant versus adjuvant pembrolizumab for resected stage III-IV melanoma (SWOG S1801). Ann Oncol 2022;33: S1408.

26. Lebacle C, Bensalah K, Bernhard JC, et al. Evaluation of axitinib to downstage cT2a renal tumours and allow partial nephrectomy: a phase II study. BJU Int 2019;123(5):804–10.

27. Karam JA, Devine CE, Urbauer DL, et al. Phase 2 trial of neoadjuvant axitinib in patients with locally advanced nonmetastatic clear cell renal cell carcinoma. Eur Urol 2014;66(5):874–80.

28. Stewart GD, Welsh SJ, Ursprung S, et al. A Phase II study of neoadjuvant axitinib for reducing the extent of venous tumour thrombus in clear cell renal cell cancer with venous invasion (NAXIVA). Br J Cancer 2022;127(6):1051–60.

29. Patel HD, Puligandla M, Shuch BM, et al. The future of perioperative therapy in advanced renal cell carcinoma: how can we PROSPER? Future Oncol 2019; 15(15):1683–95.

30. Au L, Hatipoglu E, Robert de Massy M, et al. Determinants of anti-PD-1 response and resistance in clear cell renal cell carcinoma. Cancer Cell 2021;39(11): 1497–518.e11.

31. Carlo MI, Attalla K, Mazaheri Y, et al. Phase II Study of Neoadjuvant Nivolumab in Patients with Locally Advanced Clear Cell Renal Cell Carcinoma Undergoing Nephrectomy. Eur Urol 2022;81(6):570–3.

32. Gorin MA, Patel HD, Rowe SP, et al. Neoadjuvant Nivolumab in Patients with High-risk Nonmetastatic Renal Cell Carcinoma. Eur Urol Oncol. Feb 2022;5(1):113–7.

33. Ornstein MC, Zabell J, Wood LS, et al. A phase Ib trial of neoadjuvant/adjuvant durvalumab +/- tremelimumab in locally advanced renal cell carcinoma (RCC). J Clin Oncol 2020;38(15_suppl):5021.

34. Guislain A, Gadiot J, Kaiser A, et al. Sunitinib pretreatment improves tumor-infiltrating lymphocyte expansion by reduction in intratumoral content of myeloid-derived suppressor cells in human renal cell carcinoma. Cancer Immunol Immunother 2015. https://doi.org/10.1007/s00262-015-1735-z.

35. Dallos M, Aggen DH, Ager C, et al. The SPARC-1 trial: A phase I study of neoadjuvant combination interleukin-1 beta and PD-1 blockade in localized clear cell renal cell carcinoma. J Clin Oncol 2021;39(6_suppl):TPS373.

36. Karam JA, Msaouel P, Matin SF, et al. A phase II study of sitravatinib (Sitra) in combination with nivolumab (Nivo) in patients (Pts) undergoing nephrectomy for locally-advanced clear cell renal cell carcinoma (accRCC). J Clin Oncol 2021;39(6_suppl):312.

37. Burgers FH, Graafland NM, Lagerveld BW, et al. 1481TiP A prospective, randomized phase II trial of neoadjuvant immunotherapy in primary clear cell renal cancer at risk for recurrence or distant metastases: The NESCIO trial. Ann Oncol 2022;33:S1224.

38. Bedke J, Albiges L, Capitanio U, et al. The 2022 Updated European Association of Urology Guidelines on the Use of Adjuvant Immune Checkpoint Inhibitor Therapy for Renal Cell Carcinoma. Eur Urol 2023;83(1):10–4.

39. Motzer RJ, Banchereau R, Hamidi H, et al. Molecular Subsets in Renal Cancer Determine Outcome to Checkpoint and Angiogenesis Blockade. Cancer Cell 2020. https://doi.org/10.1016/j.ccell.2020.10.011.

40. Wood CG, Ferguson JE 3rd, Parker JS, et al. Neoadjuvant pazopanib and molecular analysis of tissue response in renal cell carcinoma. JCI Insight 2020;5(22): e132852.

41. Margulis V, Freifeld Y, Pop LM, et al. Neoadjuvant SABR for Renal Cell Carcinoma Inferior Vena Cava Tumor Thrombus-Safety Lead-in Results of a Phase 2 Trial. Int J Radiat Oncol Biol Phys 2021;110(4):1135–42.

Role of Radiation in Treatment of Renal Cell Carcinoma

Jonathan E. Leeman, MD

KEYWORDS

- Renal cell carcinoma • Radiotherapy • Immunotherapy
- Stereotactic body radiation therapy • Radiosensitivity • Oligometastatic

KEY POINTS

- For patients with localized renal cell carcinoma (RCC) who are not surgical candidates, stereotactic body radiotherapy (SBRT) can be an effective option with favorable oncologic outcomes and a limited toxicity profile.
- Current evidence suggests an important role for SBRT in the management of oligometastatic or oligorecurrent RCC.
- Radiotherapy, in particular with SBRT, is emerging as an important tool in the multidisciplinary management of localized or metastatic RCC.

BACKGROUND AND HISTORICAL CONTEXT OF RADIOTHERAPY FOR RENAL CELL CARCINOMA

Renal cell carcinoma (RCC) has previously been considered a radioresistant histology with little role for inclusion of radiotherapy in management. Preclinical studies initially demonstrated RCC cell lines to be among the most resistant to conventionally fractionated radiation *in vitro*.[1] Early clinical trials failed to show an advantage in overall survival when delivering radiotherapy in the neoadjuvant setting prior to radical nephrectomy or adjuvantly following surgery.[2–4] A meta-analysis of clinical trials performed from 1975 to 1999 found an improvement in locoregional control with adjuvant radiotherapy but no impact on survival and, for these reasons, the role of radiotherapy in the overall management of RCC was considered limited.[5]

Importantly, these early studies typically utilized larger parallel opposed fields with doses in the range of 50 to 60 Gy delivered with conventionally fractionated treatment. Technological advances in the precision of radiotherapy delivery such as the

J.E. Leeman reports research funding from ViewRay, United States and NH, France Theraguix and speaker's honoraria from Viewray.
Department of Radiation Oncology, Dana Farber Cancer Institute/ Brigham and Women's Hospital, Boston, MA 02115, USA
E-mail address: JONATHANE_LEEMAN@dfci.harvard.edu

Hematol Oncol Clin N Am 37 (2023) 921–924
https://doi.org/10.1016/j.hoc.2023.04.015
0889-8588/23/© 2023 Elsevier Inc. All rights reserved.

development of intensity modulated radiotherapy and image guidance have led to the advent of stereotactic body radiotherapy (SBRT) and allowed for higher dose treatments that can be delivered safely in fewer fractions. The capability to deliver more effective doses of radiation more precisely has helped to overcome the perceived radioresistance of RCC. Furthermore, with high dose per fraction treatment, cell death may occur through effects on tumor vasculature and endothelium which may be particularly efficacious in the context of highly vascularized RCC tumors. An increasing body of work has also shed light on the immunomodulatory effects of radiotherapy and has provided the basis for rational combination of SBRT with immunotherapies that are active in RCC.[6–11]

RADIOTHERAPY FOR EARLY STAGE RENAL CELL CARCINOMA

Surgical resection is the standard approach for the management of localized RCC. For patients who are not appropriate candidates for surgery due to comorbidity, risks associated with nephrectomy or partial nephrectomy or extent of disease, SBRT delivered in 1 to 5 fractions has been shown to result in excellent local control rates. The largest study to date evaluating kidney SBRT is an individual patient meta-analysis from the International Radiosurgery and Oncology Consortium for Kidney (IROCK). This study evaluated a cohort of 190 patients treated with kidney SBRT with a median follow-up of 5 years.[12] The median maximum tumor dimension was 4.0 cm (range 2.8–4.9). The cumulative incidence of local failure at 5 years was 5.5%. Five-year freedom from distant failure was 87.3%, and 5-year progression-free survival was 63.6%. Risk of high-grade toxicity (grade 3+) was low (<1%). In aggregate, studies of kidney SBRT have been associated with small decreases in renal function (typically a decrease in eGFR of 0–15 mL/min/1.73 m^2 over 1–5 years).

SBRT bears certain advantages in comparison to interventional radiology-based techniques such as cryoablation and radiofrequency ablation. SBRT can be applied effectively to large tumors and tumors near vasculature or the renal pelvis and collecting system. A retrospective study of patients with larger tumors (median diameter 9.5 cm, range 7.5–24.4) found acceptable toxicity rates and a high rate of local control with only 1 patient of 11 who developed progressive disease.[13] In addition, as a noninvasive modality, SBRT may be a favorable approach for anticoagulated patients.

MR-Linacs (MRI-guided linear accelerators) offer technological advantages in the management of renal tumors. Specifically, they allow for contouring utilizing real-time higher quality MR images as opposed to CT, allow for daily adaptive planning to account for anatomical changes that occur between fractions with regard to the tumor or organs at risk (particularly bowel), and they provide real-time MR-based tracking of the targeted lesion during radiation beam delivery. Additionally, fiducial marker placement is not needed for MR-guided treatment which is particularly favorable for anticoagulated patients.[14,15]

For these reasons, the role of SBRT in the management of localized RCC is expanding and radiation oncology is increasingly participating in the multidisciplinary management of patients with kidney cancer.

RADIOTHERAPY FOR METASTATIC RENAL CELL CARCINOMA

Increasing evidence points to a role for radiotherapy in the management of metastatic RCC beyond the traditional goals of providing palliation. The landmark randomized phase II SABR-COMET trial demonstrated in improvement in 5-year overall survival (42.3% vs. 17.7%) for patients with oligometastatic solid tumors of varying histologies who were treated with standard of care therapy plus SBRT to sites of metastatic disease versus standard of care alone.[16]

In the context of oligometastatic or oligorecurrent RCC, SBRT can be employed with the goal of providing a treatment break or delaying progression or the need to switch systemic therapies. As the efficacy of systemic therapies for RCC has improved in recent years, there is an increasing place for radiotherapy to address nonresponsive sites of disease and allow patients to continue on active immunotherapy and targeted therapy regimens. A single-arm phase II study of 30 patients with metastatic RCC who received SBRT delivered to sites of oligometastatic disease found a favorable median progression free survival of 22.7 months.[17] Randomized trials are needed to better define the benefits associated with SBRT in the setting of metastatic RCC as well as potential synergistic effects between radiotherapy and immunotherapies and ongoing studies will provide valuable data in this regard (CYTO-SHRINK NCT04090710, SAMURAI NCT05327686).

Metastatic deposits from RCC can develop intraabdominally in sensitive and difficult to treat locations such as abdominal lymph nodes, nephrectomy bed recurrences, or pancreatic lesions. In such cases, MRI-guided adaptive radiotherapy should be considered when available to maximize precision of SBRT and minimize risks, particularly to adjacent radiosensitive luminal gastrointestinal organs.

CLINICS CARE POINTS

- Renal SBRT has been shown to result in high rates of long-term local control (~95%) for early-stage RCC with acceptable toxicity and relatively minor impact on renal function in the long term. SBRT should be considered as a treatment option for patients where risks of surgery are high.

- In the setting of metastatic RCC, metastasis-directed SBRT should be considered in cases of oligorecurrence with the goal of delaying progression and/or continuing active systemic therapy regimens.

- MR-guided SBRT should be considered when available due to the improved visualization and precision of radiotherapy that is provided, particularly for abdominal or pelvic lesions in challenging locations.

REFERENCES

1. Deschavanne PJ, Fertil B. A review of human cell radiosensitivity in vitro. Int J Radiat Oncol Biol Phys 1996;34(1):251–66.
2. Finney R. The value of radiotherapy in the treatment of hypernephroma-a clinical trial. Br J Urol 1973;45(3):258–69.
3. Kjaer M, Iversen P, Hvidt V, et al. A randomized trial of postoperative radiotherapy versus observation in stage II and III renal adenocarcinoma: a study by the copenhagen renal cancer study group. Scand J Urol Nephrol 1987;21(4):285–9.
4. van der Werf-Messing B. Carcinoma of the kidney. Cancer 1973;32(5):1056–61.
5. Tunio MA, Hashmi A, Rafi M. Need for a new trial to evaluate postoperative radiotherapy in renal cell carcinoma: a meta-analysis of randomized controlled trials. Ann Oncol 2010;21(9):1839–45.
6. Garnett CT, Palena C, Chakarborty M, et al. Sublethal irradiation of human tumor cells modulates phenotype resulting in enhanced killing by cytotoxic T lymphocytes. Cancer Res 2004;64(21):7985–94.

7. Kachikwu EL, Iwamoto KS, Liao YP, et al. Radiation enhances regulatory T cell representation. Int J Radiat Oncol Biol Phys 2011;81(4):1128–35.

8. Teitz-Tennenbaum S, Li Q, Okuyama R, et al. Mechanisms involved in radiation enhancement of intratumoral dendritic cell therapy. J Immunother 2008;31(4): 345–58.

9. Wersäll PJ, Blomgren H, Pisa P, et al. Regression of non-irradiated metastases after extracranial stereotactic radiotherapy in metastatic renal cell carcinoma. Acta Oncologica 2006;45(4):493–7.

10. Deng L, Liang H, Burnette B, et al. Irradiation and anti-PD-L1 treatment synergistically promote antitumor immunity in mice. J Clin Invest 2014;124(2):687–95.

11. Park SS, Dong H, Liu X, et al. PD-1 restrains radiotherapy-induced abscopal effect. Cancer Immunology Research 2015;3(6):610–9.

12. Siva S, Ali M, Correa RJM, et al. 5-year outcomes after stereotactic ablative body radiotherapy for primary renal cell carcinoma: an individual patient data meta-analysis from IROCK (the International Radiosurgery Consortium of the Kidney). Lancet Oncol 2022;23(12):1508–16.

13. Correa RJM, Rodrigues GB, Chen H, et al. Stereotactic ablative radiotherapy (SABR) for large renal tumors: a retrospective case series evaluating clinical outcomes, toxicity, and technical considerations. Am J Clin Oncol 2018;41(6): 568–75.

14. Yim K, Cagney DN, Mak RH, et al. Safety and efficacy of stereotactic mri-guided adaptive radiation therapy for localized kidney cancer. Int J Radiat Oncol Biol Phys 2022;114(3):e207.

15. Tetar SU, Bohoudi O, Senan S, et al. The role of daily adaptive stereotactic mr-guided radiotherapy for renal cell cancer. Cancers 2020;12(10):E2763.

16. Palma DA, Olson R, Harrow S, et al. Stereotactic ablative radiotherapy for the comprehensive treatment of oligometastatic cancers: long-term results of the SABR-COMET phase II randomized trial. J Clin Orthod 2020;38(25):2830–8.

17. Tang C, Msaouel P, Hara K, et al. Definitive radiotherapy in lieu of systemic therapy for oligometastatic renal cell carcinoma: a single-arm, single-centre, feasibility, phase 2 trial. Lancet Oncol 2021;22(12):1732–9.

Prognostic Models in Metastatic Renal Cell Carcinoma

Audreylie Lemelin, MD, Kosuke Takemura, MD, MPH, PhD,
Daniel Y.C. Heng, MD, MPH, FRCPC*, Matthew S. Ernst, MD, FRCPC

KEYWORDS

- Kidney neoplasms • Renal cell carcinoma • Prognosis • Risk stratification

KEY POINTS

- Metastatic renal cell carcinoma (mRCC) is a heterogeneous disease in biology and clinical outcomes, for which many prognostic risk stratification models incorporating patient factors, markers of disease burden, and treatment-related factors have been developed to guide clinicians and researchers in their decisions.
- Although the Memorial Sloan Kettering Cancer Center (MSKCC) model and French Model were developed when cytokine-based therapy was the standard of care for mRCC, the Cleveland Clinic Foundation, International Metastatic Renal Cell Carcinoma Database Consortium (IMDC) and International Kidney Cancer Working Group models were developed in the vascular endothelial growth factor targeted therapy era.
- IMDC and MSKCC models have been used to risk stratify patients in the contemporary immuno-oncology combination therapies.

INTRODUCTION

In the past decades, there have been important changes in the treatment landscape for metastatic renal cell carcinoma (mRCC). With this evolution in therapies, the overall survival (OS) of these patients has improved from a little over 1 year in the cytokine therapy era, to approximately 2 years in the era of vascular endothelial growth factor (VEGF) tyrosine kinase inhibitors, and to between 4 to 5 years with combination immunotherapy treatments.[1,2] However, it is generally recognized that the disease course and biology of mRCC can vary widely among patients and many studies have sought to identify disease and patient characteristics that can predict prognosis. As first and subsequent line treatment options are expanding, it remains a challenge to identify the preferred treatment for each patient population. Many risk stratification models that

Department of Oncology, Tom Baker Cancer Centre, University of Calgary, cc 110, 1331 - 29th Street Southwest, Calgary, Alberta T2N 4N2, Canada
* Corresponding author.
E-mail address: Daniel.Heng@albertahealthservices.ca

Hematol Oncol Clin N Am 37 (2023) 925–935
https://doi.org/10.1016/j.hoc.2023.04.016
0889-8588/23/© 2023 Elsevier Inc. All rights reserved.
hemonc.theclinics.com

incorporate patient factors, markers of disease burden, inflammation, and treatment-related factors have been developed over the years to meet that need and to allow a personalized treatment approach (**Table 1**). The following discussion will present available evidence on the prognostic models reported to date and the context of the treatment landscape in which they were validated.

DISCUSSION
Models Developed in the Cytokine-Based Therapy Era

One of the first widely adopted prognostic models developed for patients with mRCC is the Memorial Sloan-Kettering Cancer Center (MSKCC) model, published in 1999, when the available therapies were cytokine-based. It evaluated the relationship between pretreatment clinical and laboratory features and survival in 670 patients with advanced RCC.[3] Univariate analyses showed that five pretreatment characteristics were independently associated with a worse OS: Karnofsky Performance Status (KPS) < 80%, serum lactate dehydrogenase (LDH) > 1.5 times upper limit of normal (ULN), hemoglobin below the lower limit of normal (LLN), corrected serum calcium >10 mg/dL and absence of prior nephrectomy. The last factor was replaced with the time from diagnosis to treatment under 1 year. A validation study was conducted with this modified model in 463 patients with advanced RCC treated with first-line interferon-alfa.[4] Patients were stratified into a favorable, intermediate, and poor risk group based on the presence of 0, 1 to 2, and 3 or more factors, and the associated median OS was 30, 14, and 5 months, respectively. A similar study was also conducted by the Cleveland Clinic in 353 patients treated in majority with interleukin-2 or interferon-alpha with consistent results.[5]

Another prognostic model (the French model) was validated by the Groupe Français d'Immunothérapie in 782 patients treated with cytokine-based therapies.[6] The French model identified nine independent factors predictive of worse OS: the presence of biological signs of inflammation (erythrocyte sedimentation rate ≥ 100 mm/h or C-reactive protein ≥ 50 mg/L), interval from renal tumor to metastasis of less than 1 year, elevated neutrophil count (>ULN), liver metastases, bone metastases, performance status (Eastern Cooperative Oncology Group (ECOG) performance status (PS) > 0), the number of metastatic sites, elevated alkaline phosphatase and decreased hemoglobin level (<LLN). Four factors were predictive of rapid progression on cytokine-based therapy, defined as progression within 3 months of initiation, including the interval between renal cancer diagnosis and metastatic disease of less than 1 year, the presence of hepatic metastases, more than one metastatic site and elevated neutrophil count. Patients who presented with 3 or more of these characteristics had more than 80% probability of early treatment failure with cytokine-based therapy.

Models Developed in the Vascular Endothelial Growth Factor-Targeted Therapy Era

In the early 2000s, therapies targeting VEGF were shown to improve clinical outcomes and replaced cytokine-based therapy as the standard of care treatment for mRCC, leading to the development of new risk stratification models. As such, the Cleveland Clinic Foundation (CCF) investigated various clinical features as potential factors associated with the outcomes of 120 patients with mRCC who received VEGF-targeted therapies in 9 prospective clinical trials.[7] They identified 5 independent adverse prognostic factors associated with progression-free survival (PFS): Time from diagnosis to current treatment less than 2 years, baseline platelet count above 300 K/μL, baseline neutrophil count above 4.5 K/μL, baseline corrected serum calcium

Table 1
Factors included in validated prognostic models for metastatic renal cell carcinoma

	MSKCC[3,4]	French Model[6]	CCF[7]	IMDC[8]	IKCWG[10]
Patient function					
Performance status	√	√	√	√	√
Paraneoplastic syndromes					
Serum calcium	√		√	√	√
Inflammation					
Hemoglobin	√	√		√	
WBC					√
ANC		√	√	√	
Platelet			√	√	
ALP		√			√
ESR or CRP		√			
Rate of tumor growth/recurrence					
Time from dx to tx	√		√	√	√
Time from dx to met		√			
Tumor burden					
Number of met sites		√			√
LDH	√				√
Liver met		√			
Bone met		√			
Prior tx					√
Prior RT					√

Abbreviations: ALP, alkaline phosphatase; ANC, absolute neutrophil count; CCF, Cleveland Clinic Foundation; CRP, C-reactive protein; Dx, diagnosis; ESR, erythrocyte sedimentation rate; IKCWG, International Kidney Cancer Working Group; IMDC, International Metastatic Renal Cell Carcinoma Database Consortium; LDH, lactate dehydrogenase; Met, metastasis; mRCC, advanced or metastatic renal cell carcinoma; MSKCC, Memorial Sloan-Kettering Cancer Center; RT, radiation therapy; Tx, treatment; WBC, white blood cell count.

less than 8.5 mg/dL or above 10.0 mg/dL, and ECOG status above 0. Patients were stratified into 3 prognostic groups based on whether zero or 1 (favorable), 2 (intermediate), or 3 or more (poor) factors were present. The associated median PFS was 20.1, 13, and 3.9 months, respectively.

The International Metastatic Renal Cell Carcinoma Database Consortium (IMDC) compared the characteristics of 645 patients treated with first-line or second-line anti-VEGF therapy following cytokine-based therapy.[8] Six factors were associated with shorter median OS, including 4 of the 5 factors identified in the MSKCC, and 2 factors identified in the CCF model: hemoglobin < LLN, corrected calcium > ULN, KPS < 80%, time from diagnosis to treatment < 1 year, neutrophils > ULN, and platelets > ULN. The IMDC stratified patients into 3 risk groups based on the presence of zero (favorable), 1 or 2 (intermediate), or 3 or more (poor risk) factors and was associated with median OS not reached, 27 months, and 8.8 months, respectively. A subsequent external validation cohort of 1028 patients with mRCC who were treated with first-line VEGF-targeted treatment at 13 centers within the IMDC database demonstrated that the same 6 factors remained independent predictors of poor OS: the median OS was 43.2 months in the favorable risk group, 22.5 months in the intermediate risk group, and 7.8 months in the poor risk group.[9] As this external validation study was done in a real-world population, generalizability was considered a strength of the IMDC model compared to other models. An IMDC risk calculator can be found at IMDConline.com with instructions on how to use the model.

With the aim of developing a single validated model for survival in mRCC using a comprehensive international database, the International Kidney Cancer Working Group (IKCWG) used pooled data from 3748 patients treated with cytokine-based therapy.[10] The model was validated using independent data of 645 patients treated with tyrosine kinase therapy from the IMDC database, and 3 risk groups were defined using the 25th and 75th percentiles of the distribution in the validation cohort. Factors identified as prognostic included treatment, performance status, number of metastatic sites, time from diagnosis to treatment, pretreatment hemoglobin, white blood cell count, LDH, alkaline phosphatase, and serum calcium. Median OS in the favorable, intermediate, and poor risk groups was 26.9, 11.5, and 4.2 months, respectively.

To compare the 5 existing models, Heng and colleagues[9] used concordance indices in 672 patients. The concordance index was 0.657 (0.632–0.682) for the MSKCC model, 0.640 (0.614–0.665) for the French model, 0.662 (0.636–0.687) for the CCF model, 0.664 (0.639–0.689) for the IMDC model, and 0.668 (0.645–0.692) for the IKCWG model. Only the French model had a statistically lower concordance index, whereas the remaining models possessed similar prognostic ability. The IMDC model outperformed the MSKCC and French models by net reclassification index but there was no significant improvement compared to the CCF and IKCWG models. An important observation from this comparison was that more complex models such as the IKCWG did not yield significantly better results.

In an effort to identify a subset of patients for which deintensification of therapy could be considered, Schmidt and colleagues[11] have described a "very favorable risk" subgroup among 1638 patients with IMDC favorable risk disease. Three variables were identified as significant predictors of improved OS: time from diagnosis to systemic therapy $\geq$ 3 years, KPS >80, and absence of brain, liver, or bone metastases. Patients were classified into very favorable (0 factors) or favorable risk (1–3 factors), associated with a median OS of 64.8 months (58.8–70.8) and 45.6 months (42.0–50.4), respectively. An external validation study was performed by the Turkish Oncology Group Kidney Cancer Consortium in 112 favorable IMDC risk patients.[12]

The median OS was 55.8 months for very favorable risk patients and 34.2 months for favorable risk patients (P = 0.025).

In a study by Kroeger and colleagues[13], the IMDC model was also applied to 252 patients with non-clear cell RCC. The median OS for the favorable, intermediate, and poor risk groups was 31.4, 16.1 and 5.1 months, respectively (P < 0.0001), confirming that the IMDC model remains of prognostic value in patients with non-clear cell RCC.

Role of Existing Models in Immuno-Oncology Era

The treatment landscape of mRCC was again revolutionized in recent years with the emergence of checkpoint inhibitor combination therapies. The IMDC and MSKCC models have been used to risk stratify patients in the landmark clinical trials evaluating the efficacy of modern first line immuno-oncology (IO) combinations and continue to separate patients into distinct prognostic groups (**Table 2**).

In the CHECKMATE-214 trial, the combination of ipilimumab and nivolumab was compared to sunitinib[14] and the IMDC criteria were used to stratify patients. Long-term data from this trial shows a median OS of 47.0 months (95% CI 35.4–57.4, P < 0.001) in the ipilimumab and nivolumab arm versus 26.6 months (95% CI 22.1–33.5) in the sunitinib arm in the intermediate to poor-risk subgroup.[15] However, no OS benefit was shown in the favorable-risk subgroup, with PFS and overall response rate favoring sunitinib. To further characterize the association between outcomes and the IMDC prognostic group, Escudier and colleagues[16] performed a post-hoc analysis of the efficacy outcomes by the number of IMDC risk factors in 1051 patients included in CHECKMATE-214. They confirmed the benefit of the combination of nivolumab and ipilimumab for all patients with intermediate to poor-risk group, regardless of the number of IMDC factors. They also showed that while the overall response rate with nivolumab and ipilimumab was consistent across IMDC factors, it decreased as the number of factors increased in the sunitinib arm. An extended analysis of CHECKMATE-214 also studied the performance of the IMDC and MSKCC models and which factors were independent predictors of OS.[17] In the nivolumab plus ipilimumab arm, KPS <80%, corrected calcium > ULN, hemoglobin < LLN, neutrophils > ULN, and LDH >1.5 ULN retained prognostic value; however, time from diagnosis to treatment < 1 year and platelets > ULN did not. The c-indices for the IMDC and MSKCC models in the nivolumab plus ipilimumab cohort were 0.63 and 0.61, respectively.

The KEYNOTE-426[18,19] and the CHECKMATE-9ER[20,21] trials studied combinations of checkpoint inhibitors with VEGF targeted therapies, respectively, pembrolizumab with axitinib and nivolumab with cabozantinib, in the first-line setting for mRCC. Both trials used the IMDC model in subgroup analyses. A benefit of combination therapy remained in all IMDC risk groups, although the absolute differences in outcomes between the arms decreased in patients with favorable risk. Similarly, in the JAVELIN Renal 101 trial comparing avelumab plus axitinib with sunitinib, a decrease in PFS and overall response rates was observed in both arms as the number of IMDC risk factors increased.[22,23]

The last published pivotal trial using first-line combination therapy to date is the CLEAR trial, which studied lenvatinib with pembrolizumab or everolimus in comparison with sunitinib.[24,25] The MSKCC prognostic risk groups were used to stratify patients for randomization, but both the MSKCC and IMDC models were used in subgroup analyses for the efficacy outcomes. Again, the trend toward improved OS with combination therapy remained in all risk groups, but the magnitude of the difference between the arms was reduced in the favorable risk group.

Table 2
Summary of median overall survival (in months) for metastatic renal cell carcinoma prognostic models by clinical context

Line	Therapy	Prognostic Group	MSKCC[3,6]	IKCWG[11]	IMDC[9]
1st	IPI NIVO[14,26]	All			55.7
		Favorable[a]			74.1
		Int/poor			47.0
		Favorable[a]			*90% (18-mo survival)*
		Intermediate			*78% (18-mo survival)*
		Poor			*50% (18-mo survival)*
	PEMBRO AXI[19]	All			45.7
		Favorable			72.3% (42-mo survival)
		Int/poor			50.6% (42-mo survival)
	NIVO CABO[21]	All			37.7
		Favorable			NR
		Intermediate			37.6
		Poor			32.5
	AVEL AXI[23]	Favorable			NR
		Intermediate			42.2
		Poor			21.3
	PEMBRO LEN[25]	All	NR		NR
		Favorable	NR		NR
		Intermediate	43.0		43.0
		Poor	33.0		36.9
	IO-VEGF[26]	Favorable			*93% (18-mo survival)*
		Intermediate			*83% (18-mo survival)*
		Poor			*74% (18-mo survival)*
	VEGF-TT[9,10]	Favorable		26.9	43.2
		Intermediate		11.5	22.5
		Poor		4.2	7.8
	VEGF-TT nccRCC[13]	Favorable			*31.4*
		Intermediate			*16.1*
		Poor			*5.1*
	Cytokine-therapy[4]	Favorable	*30*		
		Intermediate	*14*		
		Poor	*5*		
2nd	Nivolumab[29,34]	All			25
		Favorable			32.8
		Intermediate			25.0
		Poor			10.4
	VEGF-TT post-cytokine therapy[27]	Favorable	*22.1[b]*		
		Intermediate	*11.9[b]*		
		Poor	*5.4[b]*		
	VEGF-TT[35]	Favorable			*35.8*
		Intermediate			*16.6*
		Poor			*5.4*
3rd	VEGF-TT[36]	Favorable			*29.9*
		Intermediate			*15.5*
		Poor			*5.5*

Abbreviations: AVEL AXI, avelumab plus axitinib; IKCWG, International Kidney Cancer Working Group; IMDC, International Metastatic Renal Cell Carcinoma Database Consortium; int/poor, pooled intermediate and poor risk groups; IO-VEGF, immuno-oncology agent plus vascular endothelial growth factor receptor targeted therapy; IPI NIVO, ipilimumab plus nivolumab; italics, based on retrospective real-world evidence; mRCC, advanced or metastatic renal cell carcinoma; MSKCC, Memorial Sloan Kettering Cancer Center; nccRCC, non-clear cell renal cell carcinoma; NIVO CABO, nivolumab plus cabozantinib; non-italics, based on prospective clinical trials; NR,

not yet reached; PEMBRO AXI, pembrolizumab plus axitinib; PEMBRO LEN, pembrolizumab plus lenvatinib; VEGF-TT, vascular endothelial growth factor receptor targeted therapy.
    [a] IPI NIVO is not indicated in IMDC favorable risk disease and must be interpreted with caution.
    [b] Based on 3 MSKCC criteria only (KPS <80%, hemoglobin < LLN, and corrected serum calcium > ULN).

Further, a retrospective study conducted by the IMDC has demonstrated that the IMDC prognostic model continues to stratify patients treated in the first-line setting with either ipilimumab plus nivolumab or immunotherapy plus VEGF targeted therapy into statistically distinct prognostic groups by OS in a real-world setting.[26] Among 728 patients treated with ipilimumab plus nivolumab, OS at 18 months was 90%, 78%, and 50% for favorable, intermediate, and poor risk, respectively. Among 282 patients treated with immunotherapy plus VEGF targeted therapy, OS at 18 months was 93%, 83%, and 74% for favorable, intermediate, and poor risk, respectively.

Both prospective phase III clinical trials and real-world studies inform us of the continued value of existing IMDC and MSKCC models to inform clinicians and patients on prognosis in the modern IO combination therapy era.

Role of Existing Models in Subsequent Lines of Therapy

Although the prognostic models previously discussed are often used in practice and clinical trials in subsequent line settings, limited data are available for their validation outside of the first-line setting.

The MSKCC has been investigated in the second-line setting after progression on cytokine-based therapy and 3 of the 5 original factors were found to be independent predictors of OS in a cohort of 251 patients.[27] Therefore, a modified MSKCC model consisting of KPS <80%, hemoglobin < LLN, and corrected serum calcium > ULN stratified patients into favorable, intermediate, or poor risk based on the presence of zero, 1, or 2 to 3 criteria. Median OS was 22.1, 11.9, and 5.4 months for favorable, intermediate, and poor risk, respectively.

The IMDC investigators studied 321 patients who experienced failure with initial VEGF targeted therapy and were subsequently treated with a second-line targeted agent.[28] The IMDC model was applied to this population and found to be prognostic in the second-line setting. Patients with favorable, intermediate, or poor risk disease achieved a median OS of not reached, 14.3, and 9.9 months, respectively. The association between median OS and the duration of treatment with first-line targeted therapy was also investigated in this study and identified as an important prognostic factor in the second-line setting. Patients who were on first-line therapy for less than 8 months had worse outcomes, with a median OS from the initiation of second-line therapy of 9.9 months versus 14.3 months for patients who were on first-line therapy for more than 8 months.

The IMDC model has been applied in the context of second-line immunotherapy following first-line targeted therapy. In the phase III CHECKMATE-025 trial, nivolumab was compared with everolimus in 821 mRCC patients previously treated with 1 or 2 antiangiogenic therapy.[29] In the whole population, there was a statistically significant benefit in OS in the nivolumab arm, with a hazard ratio of 0.73 (95% CI 0.57–0.93, $P = 0.002$). In subgroup analyses, the MSKCC model was used to compare the outcomes between the treatment arms with hazard ratios of 0.89 (95% CI 0.59–1.32) for favorable, 0.76 (95% CI 0.58–0.99) for intermediate, and 0.47 (95% CI 0.30–0.73) for poor risk disease, respectively.

The studies presented above show that the risk groups defined by the MSKCC and IMDC models can still inform patients, clinicians, and researchers on prognosis beyond first line.

Biological Rationale

The basis of prognostic models is the incorporation of factors that are indicative of disease aggressiveness and patient factors that influence survival. The IMDC model, for example, incorporates factors that indicate systemic inflammation (anemia, neutrophilia, and thrombocytopenia), paraneoplastic syndromes or bone metastasis (elevated serum calcium), rapid tumor growth or recurrence (time from diagnosis to treatment less than 1 year) which are representative of disease aggressiveness as well as patient functional status (KPS < 80). The MSKCC model also incorporates LDH, which is indicative of tumor growth and burden of disease (see **Table 1**). Other markers of systemic inflammation have been explored as potential prognostic factors, but not incorporated into currently used models. Examples include elevated neutrophil–lymphocyte ratio and neutrophil–erythrocyte ratio, which have both previously been associated with poorer OS or cancer-specific survival.[30,31]

Future Directions

As we have highlighted throughout this discussion, changes in treatment paradigms have necessitated new prognostic risk stratification models in mRCC. Although the existing models incorporate important factors that remain of prognostic significance, further study is required to develop predictive markers that may help guide treatment selection. In recent years, research has been done on biomarkers, tumor microenvironment, as well as molecular and gene expression profiles and their impact on clinical outcomes. For example, Motzer and colleagues[32] described 7 distinct molecular subgroups based on genomics evaluation of 823 tumors from advanced RCC. They found that distinct angiogenesis, immune, cell cycle, metabolism, and stromal profiles were associated with different clinical outcomes when treated with VEGF targeted therapy and immunotherapy. The molecular characteristics from baseline tumor samples of patients enrolled in the phase 3 JAVELIN Renal 101 trial were also examined according to their MSKCC risk group classification.[33] Patients with poor risk disease had higher PD-L1 positive tumor cells ($P = 0.0159$), whereas patients with favorable risk disease showed an increased frequency of NOTCH2 mutations ($P = 0.0002$) and of FLT1 expression ($P = 0.007$), among other findings. A risk stratification model combining traditional risk factors with this emerging knowledge about heterogeneity in tumor biology could inform prognostication of mRCC and allow a personalized approach to treatment.

SUMMARY

The overall prognosis for patients with mRCC has markedly improved over time as new treatment options have become available; however, there remains heterogeneity in the clinical course of patients, and the ability to stratify patients by prognosis has value for patient counseling and treatment selection. The existing prognostic models combine clinical and biochemical factors to classify patients in different risk groups. These models were developed and validated when the first-line treatment options were either cytokine or VEGF targeted therapies. As the field has moved toward first-line immunotherapy combinations for most patients, the MSKCC and IMDC models have remained important prognostic tools in clinic and research, with clinical trials and retrospective studies validating their use. The development and incorporation of molecular biomarkers to these traditional models could lead to improved models that would allow clinicians and researchers to better tailor the therapy based on prognosis and therapeutic options.

CLINICS CARE POINTS

- Prognostic models exist to stratify the risk of patients with mRCC, incorporating patient factors, markers of disease burden, and treatment-related factors.
- The MSKCC and French Model were developed when cytokine-based therapy was the standard of care for mRCC and the CCF, IMDC, and IKCWG models were developed in the VEGF targeted therapy era.
- The IMDC and MSKCC models remain the most used in the IO combination therapy era, and prospective clinical trials and retrospective studies have confirmed their continued prognostic value.

DISCLOSURE

D.Y.C. Heng: Consultancy honoraria (to self) and research funding (to institution) from: BMS, Canada, Ipsen, France, Exelixis, United States, Novartis, Switzerland, Pfizer, United States, Merck, United States, Merck KGA, Eisai, Japan. A. Lemelin, K. Takemura, and M.S. Ernst: no disclosures.

REFERENCES

1. Motzer RJ, Tannir NM, McDermott DF, et al. Conditional survival and 5-year follow-up in CheckMate 214: First-line nivolumab + ipilimumab (N+I) versus sunitinib (S) in advanced renal cell carcinoma (aRCC). Ann Oncol 2021;32:S678.
2. Motzer RJ, Hutson TE, Tomczak P, et al. Overall survival and updated results for sunitinib compared with interferon alfa in patients with metastatic renal cell carcinoma. J Clin Oncol 2009 Aug 1;27(22):3584 90.
3. Motzer RJ, Mazumdar M, Bacik J, Amsterdam A, Ferrara J, et al. Survival and Prognostic Stratification of 670 Patients With Advanced Renal Cell Carcinoma. J Clin Oncol 1999;17(8):2530.
4. Motzer RJ, Bacik J, Murphy BA, et al. Interferon-alfa as a comparative treatment for clinical trials of new therapies against advanced renal cell carcinoma. J Clin Oncol 2002;20(1):289–96.
5. Mekhail TM, Abou-Jawde RM, Boumerhi G, et al. Validation and extension of the Memorial Sloan-Kettering prognostic factors model for survival in patients with previously untreated metastatic renal cell carcinoma. J Clin Oncol 2005 Feb 1; 23(4):832–41.
6. Négrier S, Escudier B, Gomez F, et al. Prognostic factors of survival and rapid progression in 782 patients with metastatic renal carcinomas treated by cytokines: a report from the Groupe Français d'Immunothérapie. Ann Oncol 2002; 13(9):1460.
7. Choueiri TK, Garcia JA, Elson P, et al. Clinical factors associated with outcome in patients with metastatic clear-cell renal cell carcinoma treated with vascular endothelial growth factor-targeted therapy. Cancer 2007 Aug;110(3):543–50.
8. Heng DY, Xie W, Regan MM, et al. Prognostic factors for overall survival in patients with metastatic renal cell carcinoma treated with vascular endothelial growth factor-targeted agents: results from a large, multicenter study. J Clin Oncol 2009;27(34):5794.
9. Heng DY, Xie W, Regan MM, et al. External validation and comparison with other models of the International Metastatic Renal-Cell Carcinoma Database

Consortium prognostic model: a population-based study. Lancet Oncol 2013 Feb;14(2):141–8.

10. Manola J, Royston P, Elson P, et al, International Kidney Cancer Working Group. Prognostic model for survival in patients with metastatic renal cell carcinoma: results from the international kidney cancer working group. Clin Cancer Res 2011 Aug;17(16):5443–50.

11. Schmidt AL, Xie W, Gan CL, et al. The very favorable metastatic renal cell carcinoma (mRCC) risk group: Data from the International Metastatic RCC Database Consortium (IMDC). J Clin Oncol 2021;39(6):339.

12. Yekedüz E, Karakaya S, Ertürk I, et al. External Validation of a Novel Risk Model in Patients With Favorable Risk Renal Cell Carcinoma Defined by International Metastatic Renal Cell Carcinoma Database Consortium (IMDC): Results From the Turkish Oncology Group Kidney Cancer Consortium (TKCC) Database. Clin Genitourin Cancer 2023;21(1):175–82.

13. Kroeger N, Xie W, Lee JL, et al. Metastatic non-clear cell renal cell carcinoma treated with targeted therapy agents: characterization of survival outcome and application of the International mRCC Database Consortium criteria. Cancer 2013 Aug 15;119(16):2999–3006.

14. Motzer RJ, Tannir NM, McDermott DF, et al. CheckMate-214 Investigators. Nivolumab plus ipilimumab versus sunitinib in advanced renal-cell carcinoma. N Engl J Med 2018;378(14):1277–90.

15. Motzer RJ, McDermott DF, Escudier B, et al. Conditional survival and long-term efficacy with nivolumab plus ipilimumab versus sunitinib in patients with advanced renal cell carcinoma. Cancer 2022;128(11):2085–97.

16. Escudier B, Motzer RJ, Tannir NM, et al. Efficacy of Nivolumab plus Ipilimumab According to Number of IMDC Risk Factors in CheckMate 214. Eur Urol 2020 Apr;77(4):449–53.

17. Mantia C, Jegede O, Regan MM, et al. Prognostic factors for patients with advanced renal cell carcinoma (aRCC) in the era of first-line (1L) treatment with immune checkpoint inhibitors (ICIs). J Clin Oncol 2022;40(16_suppl):4544.

18. Rini BI, Plimack ER, Stus V, et al. KEYNOTE-426 investigators. Pembrolizumab plus Axitinib versus Sunitinib for Advanced Renal-Cell Carcinoma. N Engl J Med 2019;380:1116–27.

19. Rini BI, Plimack ER, Stus V, et al. Pembrolizumab (pembro) plus axitinib (axi) versus sunitinib as first-line therapy for advanced clear cell renal cell carcinoma (ccRCC): Results from 42-month follow-up of KEYNOTE-426. J Clin Oncol 2021; 39(15_suppl):4500.

20. Choueiri TK, Powles T, Burotto M, et al. Checkmate 9ER Investigators. Nivolumab plus Cabozantinib versus Sunitinib for Advanced Renal-Cell Carcinoma. N Engl J Med 2021;384:829–41.

21. Motzer RJ, Powles T, Burotto M, et al. Nivolumab plus cabozantinib versus sunitinib in first-line treatment for advances renal cell carcinoma (CheckMate 9ER): long-term follow-up results from an open-label, randomised, phase 3 trial. Lancet Onco 2022;23:888–98.

22. Motzer RJ, Penkov K, Haanen J, et al. Avelumab plus Axitinib versus Sunitinib for Advanced Renal-Cell Carcinoma. N Engl J Med 2019;380:1103–15.

23. John BAG, Larkin James, Choueiri Toni K, et al. Efficacy of avelumab + axitinib (A + Ax) versus sunitinib (S) by IMDC risk group in advanced renal cell carcinoma (aRCC): Extended follow-up results from JAVELIN Renal 101. J Clin Oncol 2021;39(15_suppl):4574.

24. Motzer RJ, Alekseev B, Rha SY, et al. CLEAR Trial Investigators. Lenvatinib plus Pembrolizumab or Everolimus for Advanced Renal Cell Carcinoma. N Engl J Med 2021;384:1289–300.

25. Choueiri TK, Powles T, Porta C, et al. A phase 3 trial of lenvatinib plus pembrolizumab versus sunitinib as a first-line treatment for patients with advanced renal cell carcinoma: overall survival follow-up analysis (CLEAR study). Austin, TX: Presented at: 2021 International Kidney Cancer Symposium; 2021. Abstract E41.

26. Ernst MS, Navani V, Wells JC, et al. Outcomes for IMDC prognostic groups in contemporary first-line combination therapies for metastatic renal cell carcinoma (mRCC). Eur Urol 2023;83(6):e166–7.

27. Motzer RJ, Bacik J, Schwartz LH, et al. Prognostic Factors for Survival in Previously Treated Patients with Metastatic Renal Cell Carcinoma. J Clin Oncol 2004;22(3):454–63.

28. Heng DY, Xie W, Bjarnason GA, et al. A unified prognostic model for first- and second-line targeted therapy in metastatic renal cell carcinoma (mRCC): Results from a large international study. J Clin Oncol 2010;28(15_suppl):4523.

29. Motzer RJ, Escudier B, McDermott DF, et al. CheckMate 025 Investigators, Nivolumab versus Everolimus in Advanced Renal-Cell Carcinoma. N Engl J Med 2015;373:1803–13.

30. Hu K, Lou L, Ye J, et al. Prognostic role of the neutrophil-lymphocyte ratio in renal cell carcinoma: a meta-analysis. BMJ Open 2015;5(4):e006404.

31. Zapała Ł, Ślusarczyk A, Garbas K, et al. Complete blood count-derived inflammatory markers and survival in patients with localized renal cell cancer treated with partial or radical nephrectomy: a retrospective single-tertiary-center study. Front Biosci (Schol Ed) 2022;14(1):5.

32. Motzer RJ, Banchereau R, Hamidi H, et al. Molecular subsets in renal cancer determines outcome to checkpoint and angiogenesis blockade. Cancer Cell 2020; 38(6):803–17.

33. Choueiri TK, Haanen JBAG, Larkin JMG, et al. Molecular characteristics of renal cell carcinoma (RCC) risk groups from JAVELIN Renal 101. J Clin Oncol 2020; 38(6):744.

34. Albiges L, Negrier S, Dalban C, et al. Safety and efficacy of nivolumab in metastatic renal cell carcinoma (mRCC): Final analysis from the NIVOREN GETUG AFU 26 study. J Clin Oncol 2019;37(7_suppl):542.

35. Ko JJ, Xie W, Kroeger N, et al. The International Metastatic Renal Cell Carcinoma Database Consortium model as a prognostic tool in patients with metastatic renal cell carcinoma previously treated with first-line targeted therapy: a population-based study. Articles Lancet Oncol 2015;16:293–300.

36. Wells JC, Stukalin I, Norton C, et al. Platinum Priority-Kidney Cancer Third-line Targeted Therapy in Metastatic Renal Cell Carcinoma: Results from the International Metastatic Renal Cell Carcinoma Database Consortium. Eur Urol 2017; 71(2):204–9.

Emerging Biomarkers of Response to Systemic Therapies in Metastatic Clear Cell Renal Cell Carcinoma

Chris Labaki, MD[a,b,]*, Renee Maria Saliby, MD, MSc[a],
Ziad Bakouny, MD, MSc[a,c], Eddy Saad, MD, MSc[a],
Karl Semaan, MD, MSc[a], Marc Eid, MD, MSc[a],
Aly-Khan Lalani, MD, FRCPC[d,1], Toni K. Choueiri, MD[a,1],
David A. Braun, MD, PhD[e,1]

KEYWORDS

- Renal cell carcinoma • Biomarkers • Systemic therapy • Immunotherapy
- Targeted therapy

KEY POINTS

- Biomarkers of response to systemic therapies in patients with metastatic clear cell renal cell carcinoma (mccRCC) could help guide the optimal therapeutic regimen for the individual patient.
- To date, no clinical or molecular entity has been approved as a predictive biomarker for the treatment of patients with mccRCC.
- Comprehensive research efforts using various methods, including genomic and transcriptomic profiling, continue to evaluate multiple promising biomarkers of response to antiangiogenic and immunotherapeutic regimens in patients with mccRCC.

INTRODUCTION

Patients with metastatic clear cell renal cell carcinoma (mccRCC) treated with immune checkpoint inhibitors (ICIs) and/or vascular endothelial growth factor tyrosine kinase inhibitors (VEGF-TKIs) experience highly heterogeneous outcomes: although some

[a] Department of Medical Oncology, Dana-Farber Cancer Institute, Boston, MA, USA;
[b] Department of Medicine, Beth Israel Deaconess Medical Center, Boston, MA, USA;
[c] Department of Medicine, Brigham and Women's Hospital, Boston, MA, USA; [d] Juravinski Cancer Centre, McMaster University, Hamilton, ON, Canada; [e] Center of Molecular and Cellular Oncology (CMCO), Yale School of Medicine, New Haven, CT, USA
[1] Co-senior authors.
* Corresponding author.
E-mail address: chris_labaki@dfci.harvard.edu

Hematol Oncol Clin N Am 37 (2023) 937–942
https://doi.org/10.1016/j.hoc.2023.05.021
0889-8588/23/© 2023 Elsevier Inc. All rights reserved.

patients have deep and sustained responses, others experience upfront progressive disease or develop subsequent resistance.[1-3] There is an urgent and unmet need to develop reliable biomarkers to potentially tailor therapeutic plans for patients. Informative biomarkers should be able to specifically predict patients' response to one or more classes of systemic therapy.[4] This review aims to outline the most relevant efforts to identify predictive biomarkers of response to systemic therapies for patients with mccRCC.

PROGRAMMED CELL DEATH LIGAND 1 (PD-L1) EXPRESSION

Although programmed cell death ligand 1 (PD-L1) expression has shown prognostic relevance among patients with mccRCC, owing to its association with poor clinical outcomes, its role as a predictive biomarker remains limited.[5] Across landmark phase 3 trials, there was an inconsistency regarding the association of PD-L1 status with improved clinical outcomes in patients treated with immunotherapy-based regimens.[1,6] Unlike some other malignancies, PD-L1 expression in patients with mccRCC does not appear to reliably differentiate those who respond to these regimens versus those who do not.

GENOMIC BIOMARKERS

Tumor mutational burden (TMB) has been widely investigated as a potential biomarker for immunotherapy across multiple cancer types, as mutations can produce tumor neoantigens that further activate the antitumor immune response.[7] In fact, pembrolizumab has been approved for all patients with advanced solid malignancies with high TMB ($\geq$10 mutations per megabase) for whom no other therapeutic options were available.[8] As compared with other immune-responsive tumors (ie, melanoma, non–small cell lung cancer), RCC is characterized by low to moderate TMB but ranks high in tumor cytolytic activity.[9] Similar outcomes between patients with TMB-high and TMB-low disease were seen in the correlative analyses of multiple prospective trials (ie, CheckMate-214, JAVELIN Renal 101, and the combined analysis of the CheckMate-009, CheckMate-010, and CheckMate-025 trials).[10-12] Therefore, a patient's TMB status should not factor into the decision to pursue an immunotherapy-based treatment regimen.

Other genomic alterations have been explored as potential biomarkers in patients with mccRCC. *VHL* alterations represent the earliest genomic event in clear cell RCC and lead to an increase in hypoxia-inducible factor (HIF) activity and expression of downstream targets, such as VEGF. Alterations in *VHL* do not predict response to VEGF-TKIs when assessed across different studies.[13,31] Truncating mutations in *PBRM1*, a common genomic event in ccRCC, appear to be characterized by an improved response to the programmed-cell-death protein 1 (PD-1) inhibitor nivolumab, specifically in the VEGF-TKI refractory setting, whereas no significant associations were identified so far among treatment-naïve patients.[14-16]

TRANSCRIPTOMIC PROFILING

Whole-transcriptome profiling (ie, bulk RNA-sequencing [RNA-seq]) has been used as a strategy to evaluate the molecular states of not only the tumor but also the tumor microenvironment (TME) in relation to survival outcomes. In patients with mccRCC treated with first-line sunitinib, 4 molecular subgroups (ccrcc1 to 4) with differential responses to VEGF-TKI were identified using bulk RNA-seq, highlighted by significantly better outcomes in ccrcc2 and ccrcc3 tumors (v ccrcc1 and ccrcc4).[17] These findings were prospectively validated in the BIONIKK trial, which also evaluated the efficacy of immunotherapy regimens in relation to these molecular subgroups.[18]

Bulk RNA-seq analysis of landmark trials identified gene expression signatures selectively associated with improved responses to VEGF-TKIs (ie, sunitinib) or immunotherapy-based combinations. Correlative analyses of the phase 2 IMmotion150 trial evaluating atezolizumab with or without bevacizumab as compared with sunitinib in patients with untreated mccRCC identified 3 gene expression signatures with a predictive potential: the angiogenesis (Angio), T-effector (T-eff), and myeloid signatures.[19] High expression of the Angio signature was associated with better progression-free survival (PFS) with sunitinib therapy, whereas patients with a high expression of the T-eff signature appeared to derive a more pronounced benefit from the combination of atezolizumab and bevacizumab. In addition, increased expression of the myeloid signature was associated with worse PFS in patients treated with atezolizumab monotherapy or in combination with bevacizumab. Last, patients with high expression of both T-eff and myeloid signatures experienced poor outcomes with atezolizumab alone, as compared with those receiving atezolizumab and bevacizumab. Some of these associations were further validated in other studies, as shown by improved survival outcomes among patients from the COMPARZ trial who had high expression of the angiogenic signature.[20] Biomarker analysis of the JAVELIN Renal 101 trial, assessing the combination of avelumab and axitinib compared with sunitinib, similarly identified 2 molecular signatures selectively associated with differential benefit to the ICI-based (Immuno signature) and the VEGF-TKI (Angio signature) regimens.[11] However, these signatures have not been consistently validated in other trials and are not used clinically.

Transcriptomic profiling of 823 patients with mccRCC enrolled in the phase 3 IMmotion151 trial identified 7 molecular tumor subgroups (clusters) among participants, which were associated with improved therapeutic responses to sunitinib (eg, angiogenic/stromal and angiogenic clusters) or atezolizumab plus bevacizumab (eg, T-eff/proliferative, proliferative, and stromal/proliferative clusters).[21] Although these transcriptomic clusters have been validated at the molecular level in large cross-trial analyses (ie, JAVELIN Renal 101 trial), their association with clinical outcomes remains to be fully determined.[22] The phase 2 OPTIC RCC trial aims to prospectively validate the clinical utility of the previously identified signatures in helping to allocate therapeutic regimens (ie, ICI + ICI vs ICI + VEGF-TKI) among patients with treatment-naïve mccRCC.[23]

SINGLE-CELL PROFILING

Single-cell transcriptomic profiling has been leveraged as a strategy to further explore components of the TME and their relationship to clinical outcomes among patients with mccRCC.[24,25] Using single-cell RNA-seq, expression signatures of cancer cell subpopulations (eg, TP1 score) and immune programs (eg, immune checkpoint/evasion score) associated with the survival outcomes of patients with mccRCC treated with ICI-regimens have been identified and further validated in large data sets at the bulk (RNA-seq) level.[26]

GUT MICROBIOME

The composition of the gut microbiome has recently been shown to be associated with outcomes of patients treated with ICIs.[27,28] Furthermore, supplementation with live bacterial products in patients with mccRCC during treatment with ICI-based regimens has been shown to result in improved outcomes in two randomized phase 1 trials.[29,32] These data highlight the need to evaluate changes in and manipulation of the gut microbiome in prospective, randomized studies.[30]

SUMMARY

Although there are still no approved predictive biomarkers for patients with metastatic kidney cancer, the field has been rapidly evolving. Several landmark investigations have helped to better understand the potential influence of molecular elements on patient outcomes. Future efforts integrating multi-omics with clinicopathologic characteristics using machine-learning approaches will be important to achieve even more promising results.

CLINICS CARE POINTS

- From a clinical standpoint, biomarkers of response to systemic anti-neoplastic regimens help to tailor therapeutic strategies adapted for each patient.

- While many molecular entities have been shown to help predict the outcomes of patients with mccRCC treated with standard-of-care regimens, there is no biomarker with a regulatory approval to be used in this setting.

REFERENCES

1. Motzer RJ, Tannir NM, McDermott DF, et al. Nivolumab plus ipilimumab versus sunitinib in advanced renal-cell carcinoma. N Engl J Med 2018;378(14): 1277–90.
2. Choueiri TK, Eto M, Motzer R, et al. Lenvatinib plus pembrolizumab versus sunitinib as first-line treatment of patients with advanced renal cell carcinoma (CLEAR): extended follow-up from the phase 3, randomised, open-label study. Lancet Oncol 2023;24(3):228–38.
3. Motzer RJ, Powles T, Burotto M, et al. Nivolumab plus cabozantinib versus sunitinib in first-line treatment for advanced renal cell carcinoma (CheckMate 9ER): long-term follow-up results from an open-label, randomised, phase 3 trial. Lancet Oncol 2022;23(7):888–98.
4. Beckman RA, Clark J, Chen C. Integrating predictive biomarkers and classifiers into oncology clinical development programmes. Nat Rev Drug Discov 2011; 10(10):735–48.
5. Leite KRM, Reis ST, Junior JP, et al. PD-L1 expression in renal cell carcinoma clear cell type is related to unfavorable prognosis. Diagn Pathol 2015;10(1). https://doi.org/10.1186/S13000-015-0414-X.
6. Rini BI, Plimack ER, Stus V, et al. Pembrolizumab plus axitinib versus sunitinib for advanced renal-cell carcinoma. N Engl J Med 2019;380(12):1116–27.
7. Schumacher TN, Schreiber RD. Neoantigens in cancer immunotherapy. Science 2015;348(6230):69–74.
8. Marabelle A, Fakih M, Lopez J, et al. Association of tumour mutational burden with outcomes in patients with advanced solid tumours treated with pembrolizumab: prospective biomarker analysis of the multicohort, open-label, phase 2 KEYNOTE-158 study. Lancet Oncol 2020;21(10):1353–65.
9. Yarchoan M, Hopkins A, Jaffee EM. Tumor mutational burden and response rate to PD-1 inhibition. N Engl J Med 2017;377(25):2500–1.
10. Braun DA, Hou Y, Bakouny Z, et al. Interplay of somatic alterations and immune infiltration modulates response to PD-1 blockade in advanced clear cell renal cell carcinoma. Nat Med 2020;26(6):909–18.

11. Motzer RJ, Robbins PB, Powles T, et al. Avelumab plus axitinib versus sunitinib in advanced renal cell carcinoma: biomarker analysis of the phase 3 JAVELIN Renal 101 trial. Nat Med 2020;26(11):1733–41.

12. Motzer RJ, Choueiri TK, McDermott DF, et al. Biomarker analysis from CheckMate 214: nivolumab plus ipilimumab versus sunitinib in renal cell carcinoma. J Immunother Cancer 2022;10(3). https://doi.org/10.1136/JITC-2021-004316.

13. Cowey CL, Rathmell WK. VHL gene mutations in renal cell carcinoma: role as a biomarker of disease outcome and drug efficacy. Curr Oncol Rep 2009;11(2): 94–101.

14. Miao D, Margolis CA, Gao W, et al. Genomic correlates of response to immune checkpoint therapies in clear cell renal cell carcinoma. Science 2018; 359(6377):801–6.

15. Braun DA, Ishii Y, Walsh AM, et al. Clinical validation of PBRM1 alterations as a marker of immune checkpoint inhibitor response in renal cell carcinoma. JAMA Oncol 2019;5(11):1631–3.

16. Conway J, Taylor-Weiner A, Braun D, et al. PBRM1 loss-of-function mutations and response to immune checkpoint blockade in clear cell renal cell carcinoma. medRxiv 2020. https://doi.org/10.1101/2020.10.30.20222356.

17. Beuselinck B, Job S, Becht E, et al. Molecular subtypes of clear cell renal cell carcinoma are associated with sunitinib response in the metastatic setting. Clin Cancer Res 2015;21(6):1329–39.

18. Vano YA, Elaidi R, Bennamoun M, et al. Nivolumab, nivolumab-ipilimumab, and VEGFR-tyrosine kinase inhibitors as first-line treatment for metastatic clear-cell renal cell carcinoma (BIONIKK): a biomarker-driven, open-label, non-comparative, randomised, phase 2 trial. Lancet Oncol 2022;23(5):612–24.

19. McDermott DF, Huseni MA, Atkins MB, et al. Clinical activity and molecular correlates of response to atezolizumab alone or in combination with bevacizumab versus sunitinib in renal cell carcinoma. Nat Med 2018;24(6):749–57.

20. Hakimi AA, Voss MH, Kuo F, et al. Transcriptomic profiling of the tumor microenvironment reveals distinct subgroups of clear cell renal cell cancer: Data from a randomized phase III trial. Cancer Discov 2019;9(4):510–25.

21. Motzer RJ, Banchereau R, Hamidi H, et al. Molecular subsets in renal cancer determine outcome to checkpoint and angiogenesis blockade. Cancer Cell 2020;38(6):803–17.e4.

22. Saliby RM, Jammihal T, Labaki C, et al. Cross-trial validation of molecular subtypes in patients with metastatic clear cell renal cell carcinoma (RCC): The JAVELIN Renal 101 experience. J Clin Oncol 2022;40(16_suppl):4531.

23. Chen Y-W, Beckermann K, Haake SM, et al. Optimal treatment by invoking biologic clusters in renal cell carcinoma (OPTIC RCC). J Clin Oncol 2023; 41(6_suppl):TPS742.

24. Braun DA, Street K, Burke KP, et al. Progressive immune dysfunction with advancing disease stage in renal cell carcinoma. Cancer Cell 2021;0(0). https://doi.org/10.1016/j.ccell.2021.02.013.

25. Krishna C, DiNatale RG, Kuo F, et al. Single-cell sequencing links multiregional immune landscapes and tissue-resident T cells in ccRCC to tumor topology and therapy efficacy. Cancer Cell 2021;39(5):662–77.e6.

26. Bi K, He MX, Bakouny Z, et al. Tumor and immune reprogramming during immunotherapy in advanced renal cell carcinoma. Cancer Cell 2021;39(0):1–13.

27. Derosa L, Routy B, Fidelle M, et al. Gut bacteria composition drives primary resistance to cancer immunotherapy in renal cell carcinoma patients. Eur Urol 2020; 78(2):195–206.

28. Salgia NJ, Bergerot PG, Maia MC, et al. Stool microbiome profiling of patients with metastatic renal cell carcinoma receiving anti–PD-1 immune checkpoint inhibitors. Eur Urol 2020;78(4):498–502.

29. Dizman N, Meza L, Bergerot P, et al. Nivolumab plus ipilimumab with or without live bacterial supplementation in metastatic renal cell carcinoma: a randomized phase 1 trial. Nat Med 2022;28(4):704–12.

30. Lalani A-KA, Swaminath A, Pond GR, et al. Phase II trial of cytoreductive stereotactic hypofractionated radiotherapy with combination ipilimumab/nivolumab for metastatic kidney cancer (CYTOSHRINK). J Clin Oncol 2023;41(6_suppl): TPS750.

31. Choueiri TK, Vaziri SAJ, Jaeger E, et al. von Hippel-Lindau Gene Status and Response to Vascular Endothelial Growth Factor Targeted Therapy for Metastatic Clear Cell Renal Cell Carcinoma. J Urol 2008;180(3):860–6.

32. Ebrahimi H, Meza LA, Lee K, et al. Effect of CBM588 in combination with cabozantinib plus nivolumab for patients (pts) with metastatic renal cell carcinoma (mRCC): A randomized clinical trial. J Clin Oncol 2023;41(17_suppl):LBA104–LBA104.

Managing First-Line Metastatic Renal Cell Carcinoma
Favorable-Risk Disease

Elizabeth Pan, MD, Danielle Urman, BA, Carmel Malvar, BS,
Rana R. McKay, MD*

KEYWORDS

- Renal cell carcinoma • Favorable-risk • Immunotherapy • VEGF-TKI

KEY POINTS

- Risk stratification for metastatic renal cell carcinoma (mRCC) helps guide prognostication and treatment decision-making.
- Systemic therapy for mRCC has changed drastically in the last several years with immunotherapy and vascular endothelial growth factor tyrosine kinase inhibitors on the forefront for favorable-risk disease.
- Options for management of favorable-risk mRCC include active surveillance and systemic therapy.

INTRODUCTION
Defining Favorable-Risk Metastatic Renal Cell Carcinoma

This article focuses on favorable-risk metastatic renal cell carcinoma (mRCC) and its management. Risk stratification of newly diagnosed mRCC is important for prognostication and treatment decision-making. Heng D and colleagues[1] summarize two of the more widely accepted criteria to risk stratify RCC patients, which are the International Metastatic Renal Cell Carcinoma Database Consortium (IMDC) and Memorial Sloan-Kettering Cancer Center (MSKCC) scores. Favorable-risk disease tends to have indolent tumor biology and is associated with fewer clinical symptoms longer time to recurrence and more responsiveness to systemic therapy.[2] Although clinical features may not always inform disease biology, studies have demonstrated that favorable-risk RCC exhibits a higher expression of genes associated with the vascular endothelial growth factor (VEGF) pathway, a key component of the pathogenesis of

University of California San Diego, Moores Cancer Center, 3855 Health Sciences Drive, #0987, La Jolla, CA 92093-0987, USA
* Corresponding author.
E-mail address: rmckay@health.ucsd.edu

Hematol Oncol Clin N Am 37 (2023) 943–949
https://doi.org/10.1016/j.hoc.2023.04.017
0889-8588/23/© 2023 Elsevier Inc. All rights reserved.

RCC and vulnerable target for systemic therapy in patients with advanced disease. In addition, RCC molecular signatures derived from RNA sequencing as identified in the IMmotion150, Immotion151, and Javelin Renal101 trials suggest that favorable-risk RCC is enriched in angiogenic/stromal and the angiogenic gene clusters with greater than 50% of patients with either IMDC or MSKCC favorable-risk disease being categorized into one of these two clusters, which are associated with improved progression-free survival (PFS) independent of treatment.[3,4] A subset of very favorable-risk disease has also been described that is associated with improved clinical outcomes and includes characteristics of primary diagnosis to systemic therapy of $\geq$3 years, Karnofsky Performance Status of greater than 80, and lack of brain, liver, or bone metastasis.[5] The management of favorable-risk mRCC is based on what is known about the tumor biology and molecular profile and will further be discussed.

DISCUSSION
Active Surveillance for Favorable-Risk Metastatic Renal Cell Carcinoma

In a select group of patients with favorable-risk mRCC who are asymptomatic and have limited disease burden, active surveillance can be considered before starting systemic therapy. A Phase II prospective trial in highly selected patients with asymptomatic mRCC demonstrated that undergoing active surveillance with imaging and laboratories, in lieu of up-front systemic therapy, helps limit systemic therapy toxicity without compromising response to subsequent systemic therapy.[6] Eligible patients had mRCC of any histologic subtype who had not previously been treated with systemic therapy, though prior surgery or radiation therapy was permitted. In the 48 patients included in analysis, the median time from active surveillance to initiation of systemic therapy was 14.9. Although data regarding the selection criterion for active surveillance in patients with mRCC are limited, patients with favorable-risk and low-volume or oligometastatic and asymptomatic disease may benefit more from initial active surveillance over systemic therapy initiation.[7] Although mRCC prognostic scoring systems can help guide this decision, they are insufficient to use alone and further studies are needed.

Systemic Therapy for Favorable-Risk Metastatic Renal Cell Carcinoma

Immune checkpoint inhibitors (ICI) -tyrosine kinase inhibitors (TKI)
Although combination of ICI + VEGF-tyrosine kinase inhibitors (TKI) has demonstrated substantial efficacy for intermediate- and poor-risk mRCC, their role for patients with favorable-risk disease is less clear. The four landmark trials that compared ICI + VEGF-TKIs to sunitinib monotherapy are KEYNOTE-426 with pembrolizumab + axitinib,[8] Javelin Renal 101 with avelumab + axitinib,[9] CheckMate 9ER with nivolumab + cabozantinib,[10] and CLEAR with pembrolizumab + lenvatinib.[11] A summary of frontline ICI combination trials and their outcomes by favorable-risk status is provided in **Table 1**. Across the board, for patients with favorable-risk disease, generally ICI-VEGF-TKI combination has been associated with improved objective response rate (ORR), and complete response (CR). However, the data are more obscure when evaluating overall survival (OS) benefit with HR ranging from 0.94 to 1.22 with ICI-VEGF-TKI combinations. Although these subset analyses can be informative, these trials were not appropriately powered to statistically answer the question of whether ICI-VEGF-TKI improves OS compared with sunitinib in these specific groups. The question of whether a sequential approach with VEGF-TKI and ICI monotherapies is also worth exploring in the favorable-risk setting, and studies evaluating switching between VEGF-TKIs and ICI would inform on effective sequencing strategies. Before next-generation VEGF-TKIs,

Table 1
Summary of first-line ICI combination regimens by favorable risk status

	CheckMate-214 (Ipi/Nivo) (n = 550 vs n = 546)	Keynote-426 (Axi/Pembro) (n = 432 vs n = 429)	CheckMate-9ER (Cabo/Nivo) (n = 323 vs n = 328)	CLEAR (Len/Pembro) (n = 355 vs n = 357)	Javelin Renal 101 (Avelumab/Axi) (n = 442 vs n = 444)
FDA approval	2018, 1L for int/poor risk	2019, 1L	2021, 1L	2021, 1L	2019, 1L
Favorable/Intermediate/Poor percentage	23/61/17	32/55/13	23/58/19	31/58/9	22/64/12
Median follow-up, mo	67.7	42.8	32.9	33.7	42.2
OS (favorable), HR (CI)	74.1 vs 68.4 0.94 (0.65–1.37)	NR vs NR[a] 1.06 (0.60–1.86)	NR vs 47.6 1.07 (0.63–1.79)	NR vs NR 1.22 (0.66–2.26)	N/A[b]
PFS (favorable), HR (CI)	12.4 vs 28.9 1.60 (1.13–2.26)	20.7 vs 17.8 0.76 (0.56–1.03)	21.4 vs 13.9 0.75 (0.5–1.13)	28.1 vs 12.9 0.41 (0.28–0.62)	N/A 0.5 (0.26–0.97)
ORR (favorable), %	30 vs 52	69 vs 50	66 vs 44	68 vs 51	68 vs 38

Abbreviation: NR, not reached.
[a] Reported at interim analysis, minimum follow-up of 23 mo.
[b] Not available.

ICIs, and their combinations in the treatment of mRCC, Voog and colleagues[12] demonstrated that rechallenge with a second or third TKI provided clinical benefit without cumulative toxicity. However, the treatment landscape has changed drastically in the last decade, and studies evaluating sequencing monotherapies may have to evolve to include combination therapies.

In light of these limitations in evaluating outcomes of patients with favorable-risk disease across these studies, a meta-analysis sought to determine whether applying an intensified strategy to the favorable-risk cohort in these trials had meaningful benefit. Results from the meta-analysis revealed a significant prolongation of radiographic progression-free survival (rPFS) with immune checkpoint inhibitot (ICI) + VEGF-TKI compared with sunitinib with a 39% reduction of the risk of progression (HR = 0.63; $P < 0.00001$). There was also a higher ORR with combination ICI + VEGF-TKI compared with sunitinib in the favorable-risk subgroup in the KEYNOTE-426 (69.6% vs 50.4%) and Javelin Renal 101 (67% vs. 39.6%) trials. There was no observed OS advantage (hazard ratio (HR) 0.99; 95% CI 0.74–1.33; $P = 0.95$).[13] The ORR benefit may be particularly useful in the setting of favorable-risk RCC with high tumor burden or symptomatic disease where early disease control is crucial. Furthermore, CR rates are higher with the combination therapy compared with sunitinib and several studies have demonstrated that the depth of response is associated with improved long-term outcomes.[14]

ICI–ICI

Although dual ICI combinations are widely used in intermediate and poor-risk disease, there role in favorable-risk mRCC is more nuanced.[15] Landmark trials that compared dual checkpoint inhibition to sunitinib monotherapy including CheckMate-214[16] (ipilimumab + nivolumab versus sunitinib). CheckMate-214 has overall inconclusive evidence to support the use of ipilimumab + nivolumab versus sunitinib in favorable-risk disease. Although ORR and PFS favored sunitinib in intermediate- and poor-risk disease (ORR 29% with ipilimumab + nivolumab vs 52% with sunitinib; PFS 15.3 months with ipilimumab + nivolumab vs 25.1 months with sunitinib), OS was numerically longer with ipilimumab + nivolumab with an HR of 0.94 and a follow-up time of 67 months though this is not statistically significant. In addition, the CR rate was double the one with sunitinib suggesting that a subset of patients may derive long-term benefit with dual ICI. A follow-up study was reported on treatment-free survival based on 42-month results of the CheckMate 214 trial, and reported 20% of favorable-risk patients were treatment-free compared with just 9% with sunitinib.[17] Favorable-risk RCC with sarcomatoid features is another population that may benefit from dual ICI given their more inflammatory milieu.[3] The benefit of dual ICI combinations in treating favorable-risk disease is still evolving.[15] Atkins and colleagues[18] showed a potential benefit in sequential step-up ICI, in which patients with treatment-naïve favorable-risk clear cell renal cell carcinoma (ccRCC) unresponsive to nivolumab monotherapy had notable benefit with nivolumab + ipilimumab salvage (ORR 57.1%, median duration of response 27.6 months). Other studies evaluating sequential nivolumab followed by ipilimumab have not shown a benefit in ORR rates (15% in favorable-risk disease per the phase 2 OMNIVORE study[19]); however, additional studies are needed to determine the ideal subgroup of patients with favorable-risk disease that may benefit most from dual ICI.

Tyrosine kinase inhibitor

In patients with favorable-risk RCC who require systemic therapy, monotherapy with an anti-VEGF-TKI may still play a role, particularly where there is concern for toxicity from

ICI or those with very indolent disease. Although combination therapy is favored for most patients with favorable-risk disease, single-agent VEGF-TKIs can be considered in select patients accounting for performance status, comorbidities, and goals of care. There may also be a role for sequential therapy of VEGF-TKI followed by ICI on progression or vice versa.

Novel approaches. Therapies for favorable-risk RCC on the horizon include the combination of belzutifan, an Hypoxia inducible factor 2a (HIF-2α) inhibitor, plus cabozantinib. Findings from the phase 2 LITESPARK-003 trial presented at the 2022 ESMO Congress showed that this regimen demonstrated antitumor activity in patients with treatment-naïve advanced ccRCC across all IMDC risk groups. Patients with favorable-risk disease saw an ORR of 62%, with two (10%) patients having achieved a CR and 11 (52%) patients having a partial response (PR); the disease control rate was 90%. In the overall population, the median duration of response was 28.6 months.[20] These data are promising for future directions of favorable-risk RCC treatment, and additional combinations incorporating HIF-2α inhibitors, such as belzutifan plus lenvatinib, are being investigated in front-line RCC with the inclusion of favorable-risk patients.

SUMMARY

The treatment of favorable-risk RCC has been evolving in the era of ICI combination treatments. Per National Comprehensive Cancer Network guidelines, the aforementioned ICI + VEGF-TKI combinations are recommendations for first-line treatment of favorable-risk mRCC.[21] In general, there is a clinically relevant role for ICI + VEGF-TKI in favorable-risk disease despite the lack of OS advantage at the present time, and it is important to balance the risk of overtreatment with the benefit of improving clinical outcomes. For those patients who require systemic therapy, generally ICI-VEGF-TKIs are preferred given the benefit in ORR and PFS. For patients who are unfit or have low tumor burden, indolent disease pattern, or medical comorbidities that may preclude from immunotherapy, TKI monotherapy can be considered to prevent overtreatment and risk of additional treatment-related toxicity. One thing to remember is in case of favorable-risk and oligometastatic state, localized therapies with surgery, radiation or ablation should also be entertained. Ultimately, choosing between these regimens depends on several clinical factors and also the patient's goals of care. A shared decision-making process should be had with patients and their caregivers to determine the optimal treatment of any given patient. Currently, predictive biomarkers are lacking and in the absence of these, we rely on clinical factors to guide therapy selection. Despite the lack of OS benefit, dual therapy is the preferred approach for most patients who warrant treatment.

CLINICS CARE POINTS

- Favorable-risk metastatic renal-cell carcinoma (mRCC) can have an indolent tumor biology and in some selected cases can be monitored with active surveillance with deferred systemic therapy.

- Combinations of ICI and vascular endothelial growth factor tyrosine kinase inhibitors are preferred in patients with mRCC who require systemic therapy given the objective response rate and progression-free survival benefit.

- The choice of systemic therapy should be a shared decision between the physician and patient and should be based on tumor characteristics and quality of life parameters.

DISCLOSURE

R.R. McKay Advisory Board/Consultant for Aveo, AstraZeneca, Bayer, Bristol Myers Squib, Calithera, Caris, Dendreon, Exelixis, Eli Lilly, Janssen, Merck, Myovant, Novartis, Pfizer, Sanofi, Sorrento Therapeutics, Tempus, and Telix.

REFERENCES

1. Heng D, Lemelin A, Takemura K, et al. Prognostic models in metastatic RCC. Hematol Oncol Clin North Am 2023;37(5). In Press.
2. Kartolo A, Procopio G, Vera-Badillo FE. Management of favorable-risk advanced renal cell carcinoma: is dual therapy the answer? Eur Urol Open Sci 2021; 30:44–6.
3. Motzer RJ, Banchereau R, Hamidi H, et al. Molecular subsets in renal cancer determine outcome to checkpoint and angiogenesis blockade. Cancer Cell 2020;38(6):803–17.e4.
4. Saliby RM, Jammihal T, Labaki C, et al. Are the IMmotion 151-molecular signatures predictive of treatment outcomes in the JAVELIN Renal 101 trial? October 2022. Available at: https://kcrs.kidneycan.org/wp-content/uploads/2022/10/reneemaria_saliby_10.03.2022_v4-final.pdf. Kidney Cancer Research Summit 2022 PowerPoint Presentation. Accessed November 1, 2022.
5. Schmidt AL, Xie W, Gan CL, et al. The very favorable metastatic renal cell carcinoma (mRCC) risk group: data from the International Metastatic RCC Database Consortium (IMDC). J Clin Oncol 2021;39(6_suppl):339.
6. Rini B, Dorff T, Elson P, et al. Active surveillance in metastatic renal-cell carcinoma: a prospective, phase 2 trial. Lancet Oncol 2016;17(9):1317–24.
7. Harrison M, Costello B, Bhavsar N, et al. Active surveillance of metastatic renal cell carcinoma: results from a prospective observational study (MaRCC). Cancer 2021;127(13):2204–12.
8. Powles T, Plimack ER, Soulières D, et al. Pembrolizumab plus axitinib versus sunitinib monotherapy as first-line treatment of advanced renal cell carcinoma (KEYNOTE-426): extended follow-up from a randomised, open-label, phase 3 trial. Lancet Oncol 2020;21(12):1563–73.
9. Motzer RJ, Penkov K, Haanen J, et al. Avelumab plus axitinib versus sunitinib for advanced renal-cell carcinoma. N Engl J Med 2019;380(12):1103–15.
10. Choueiri TK, Powles T, Burotto M, et al. Nivolumab plus cabozantinib versus sunitinib for advanced renal-cell carcinoma. N Engl J Med 2021;384(9):829–41.
11. Motzer R, Alekseev B, Rha SY, et al. Lenvatinib plus pembrolizumab or everolimus for advanced renal cell carcinoma. N Engl J Med 2021;384(14):1289–300.
12. Voog E, Campillo-Gimenez B, Elkouri C, et al. Long survival of patients with metastatic clear cell renal cell carcinoma. Results of real life study of 344 patients. Int J Cancer 2020;146(6):1643–51.
13. Ciccarese C, Iacovelli R, Porta C, et al. Efficacy of VEGFR-TKIs plus immune checkpoint inhibitors in metastatic renal cell carcinoma patients with favorable IMDC prognosis. Cancer Treat Rev 2021;100:102295.
14. Grünwald V, McKay RR, Krajewski KM, et al. Depth of remission is a prognostic factor for survival in patients with metastatic renal cell carcinoma. Eur Urol 2015 May;67(5):952–8.
15. Manneh R, Lema M, Carril-Ajuria L, et al. Immune checkpoint inhibitor combination therapy versus sunitinib as first-line treatment for favorable-IMDC-risk advanced renal cell carcinoma patients: a meta-analysis of randomized clinical trials. Biomedicines 2022;10(3):577.

16. Motzer RJ, Tannir NM, McDermott DF, et al. Nivolumab plus ipilimumab versus sunitinib in advanced renal-cell carcinoma. N Engl J Med 2018;378(14):1277–90.

17. Regan MM, Jegede OA, Mantia CM, et al. Treatment-free survival after immune checkpoint inhibitor therapy versus targeted therapy for advanced renal cell carcinoma: 42-month results of the CheckMate 214 trial. Clin Cancer Res 2021; 27(24):6687–95.

18. Atkins MB, Jegede OA, Haas NB, et al. Phase II study of nivolumab and salvage nivolumab/ipilimumab in treatment-naive patients with advanced clear cell renal cell carcinoma (HCRN GU16-260-Cohort A). J Clin Oncol 2022 Sep 1;40(25): 2913–23.

19. McKay RR, McGregor BA, Xie W, et al. Optimized management of nivolumab and ipilimumab in advanced renal cell carcinoma: a response-based phase II study (OMNIVORE). J Clin Oncol 2020 Dec 20;38(36):4240–8.

20. Choueiri TK, Bauer T, Merchan J, et al. Phase II study of belzutifan plus cabozantinib as first-line treatment of advanced renal cell carcinoma (RCC): Cohort 1 of LITESPARK-003. Ann Oncol 2022;33(suppl 7):S660–80.

21. Motzer RJ, Jonasch E, Agarwal N, et al. NCCN Guidelines Version 2.2023 Kidney Cancer. Available at: https://www.nccn.org/professionals/physician_gls/pdf/kidney.pdf. Accessed August 27, 2022.

First-Line Treatment for Intermediate and Poor Risk Advanced or Metastatic Clear Cell Renal Cell Carcinoma

Michael T. Serzan, MD, Wenxin Xu, MD, Stephanie A. Berg, DO*

KEYWORDS

- Clear cell renal cell carcinoma • Immune checkpoint inhibitors
- Vascular endothelial growth factor receptor tyrosine kinase inhibitor
- IMDC intermediate and poor risk

KEY POINTS

- Patients with IMDC intermediate and poor risk ccRCC have been historically characterized by a disease with an aggressive clinical course and poor response to available treatments.
- Systemic therapy targeting immune checkpoints (anti-PD1) combined with either ipilimumab (anti-CTLA) or VEGFR TKI have significantly improved outcomes for patients with intermediate and poor risk ccRCC.
- Patients treated with ipilimumab and nivolumab may benefit from durable antitumor responses and treatment free intervals, while also having the risks of primary progressive disease and irAE.
- Patients treated with ICI plus VEGFR TKI may benefit from early and deep tumor shrinkage, while also having the risks of developing treatment resistance and chronic VEGFR-associated toxicities.

INTRODUCTION AND BACKGROUND

Advanced or metastatic clear cell renal cell carcinoma (ccRCC) is a heterogenous disease with diverse underlying biology, clinical presentation, and response to systemic therapies. Historically, immune-based therapy with cytokines such as interferon alpha and high-dose interleukin 2 (HD-IL2) was the standard of care centered on durable responses in a minority of patients. Targeted therapies against the vascular endothelial growth factor receptor (VEGFR) (and to a lesser extent, mammalian target of rapamycin (mTOR)) demonstrated responses in a higher proportion of patients relative to cytokine

Department of Medical Oncology, Dana-Farber Cancer Institute, 44 Binney Street D1230, Boston, MA 02115, USA
* Corresponding author.
E-mail address: stephaniea_berg@dfci.harvard.edu

Hematol Oncol Clin N Am 37 (2023) 951–964
https://doi.org/10.1016/j.hoc.2023.04.018
0889-8588/23/© 2023 Elsevier Inc. All rights reserved.

therapies. However, the duration of response and overall survival (OS) of patients treated with VEGFR tyrosine kinase inhibitors (TKI) varied widely. In efforts to estimate ccRCC prognosis and response to VEGFR TKI therapy, the International Metastatic RCC Database Consortium (IMDC) and Memorial Slone-Kettering Cancer Center (MSKCC) developed criteria to classify patients into favorable, intermediate, and poor risk groups based on pretreatment clinical (time of diagnosis to treatment, performance status) and laboratory (calcium, blood cell counts, and lactose dehydrogenase level) factors. The IMDC and MSKCC risk models identified patients at highest risk for disease progression on VEGFR TKI and served as stratification factors for clinical trials investigating combination regimens. For patients with intermediate and poor risk ccRCC, immune checkpoint inhibitors (ICI) combined with VEGFR TKIs have demonstrated significant improvements in overall response rate (ORR), progression free survival (PFS), and OS relative to monotherapy with the VEGFR TKI sunitinib. Despite these improvements, there are no validated biomarkers to guide selection of the optimal regimen for individual patients. Furthermore, many patients with intermediate and poor risk disease do not achieve durable disease remission and/or experience adverse effects from therapy. A retrospective analysis utilizing real-world evidence demonstrated that the IMDC model stratified patients treated with ICI plus ICI, ICI plus VEGFR TKI, and VEGFR plus targeted therapy into 3 distinct risk groups (favorable, intermediate, poor), which correlated with overall survival, time to next treatment and therapy duration.[1] This chapter will focus on recent studies leading to US FDA approvals and ongoing clinical trials for patients with intermediate and poor risk metastatic ccRCC.

HISTORICAL TRIALS

Immunotherapy with high-dose IL2 was initially approved by the FDA in 1992 based on durable responses in a minority of patients treated on phase II trials.[2] However, widespread implementation of HD-IL2 was limited by excessive short-term toxicity requiring management at specialized care centers. A retrospective analysis of patients treated with HD-IL2 in the PROCLAIM registry demonstrated marked differences in median OS across IMDC risk groups at 64.5, 57.6, and 14 months in favorable, intermediate, and poor risk groups, respectively.[3] Although HD-IL2 remains a National Comprehensive Cancer Network (NCCN) guideline category 2B/3 recommendation, it has fallen out of clinical use as a first-line therapy for metastatic ccRCC due to excessive toxicity, administration challenges, and newer combination therapy approvals.[4]

The phase III ARCC trial was one of the earliest studies to focus on therapy for patients with metastatic ccRCC and poor prognostic features defined with pretreatment clinical and laboratory criteria (the Hudes criteria).[5] A total of 626 patients were randomized to receive interferon alpha, temsirolimus (an mTOR inhibitor), or combination temsirolimus plus interferon alpha. The temsirolimus monotherapy arm had significantly longer OS relative to interferon alpha monotherapy [hazard ratio (HR), 0.73; 95% confidence interval (CI), 0.58–0.92, P =0.001]. Thus, temsirolimus monotherapy was FDA approved for patients with metastatic ccRCC and poor prognosis features. Temsirolimus still remains an NCCN guidelines category 2B/3 recommendation, but it too has also fallen out of clinical use.

Sunitinib and pazopanib are targeted therapies against VEGFR that have demonstrated improvements in OS compared to interferon alpha and placebo, respectively, leading to FDA approvals.[6,7] The phase IV FLIPPER trial for patients with MSKCC poor risk disease demonstrated that pazopanib had similar efficacy and toxicity relative to prior studies of patients with favorable and intermediate risk disease.[8] Cabozantinib is a multikinase inhibitor of VEGFR, MET, and AXL that was compared to sunitinib in the phase II CABOSUN trial for patients with IMDC intermediate and poor risk disease.[9,10] Patients were randomized to receive cabozantinib 60 mg daily or sunitinib 50 mg daily for 4 weeks, followed by a 2-week break. Cabozantinib was associated with significant improvements relative to sunitinib, including superior PFS (HR, 0.48; 95% CI 0.31–0.74, P = 0.0008) and ORR 20% (95% CI 12–30.8) versus 9% (95% CI 3.7–17.6), respectively.[11] Although the study was not powered to detect a survival difference, cabozantinib showed a trend toward prolonged OS (HR, 0.80; 95% CI 0.53–1.21). Cabozantinib and sunitinib treatments were associated with similar grade 3 to 4 treatment-related adverse events (TRAEs) (68% vs. 65%), dose reduction (46% vs. 35%), and discontinuation (21% vs. 22%), respectively. Based on these results, cabozantinib received FDA approval and remains a standard of care monotherapy for patients with intermediate and poor risk metastatic ccRCC who have absolute contraindications to ICI. However, combination therapies with ICI are now the preferred option for most patients with metastatic RCC.

FRONT LINE SYSTEMIC THERAPY
Immune Checkpoint Inhibitor plus Immune Checkpoint Inhibitor

Early evidence that ICIs are effective for ccRCC was demonstrated in the phase I CheckMate 016 trial of nivolumab [anti-programmed death (PD1)] plus ipilimumab (anti-cytotoxic T-lymphocyte associated antigen 4 [CTLA-4]) that demonstrated an ORR of 40.4%, with 38.1% of patients experiencing grade 3 to 4 adverse effects.[12] Subsequently, the phase III Checkmate 214 trial evaluated nivolumab plus ipilimumab versus sunitinib for patients with treatment naïve metastatic ccRCC.[13,14] A total of 1096 patients were enrolled among all IMDC risk categories: favorable (23%), intermediate (59%), and poor (18%); co-primary endpoints of the study were ORR, PFS, and OS in the intermediate and poor risk groups. Patients were randomized to receive Ipilimumab 1 mg/kg plus nivolumab 3 mg/kg every 3 weeks for 4 doses (induction phase) followed by nivolumab 3 mg/kg every 2 weeks (maintenance phase) or sunitinib 50 mg daily for 4 weeks, followed by a 2-week break. Patients who experienced TRAEs due to ipilimumab plus nivolumab were not eligible to receive maintenance nivolumab and patients who achieved benefit from maintenance nivolumab without serious toxicity were allowed to continue indefinitely. With 67.7 months median follow-up, ipilimumab plus nivolumab was superior to sunitinib among those with intermediate and poor risk disease with median OS of 47 months versus 26.6 months (HR, 0.68; 95% CI 0.58–0.81, P < 0.0001).[13] A subgroup of particular interest was patients with pathologic sarcomatoid features, which may coexist within any histologic subtype of RCC and has been associated with an aggressive clinical course and lack of response to targeted therapies.[15] An exploratory post-hoc analysis of 139 patients with intermediate and poor risk disease and sarcomatoid dedifferentiation showed that the combination of ipilimumab plus nivolumab compared to sunitinib was associated with improvements in median OS [48.6 months vs. 14.2 months (HR, 0.46; 95% CI 0.30–0.70, P = 0.0004)], mPFS [26.5 months vs. 5.1 months (HR, 0.54; 95% CI 0.30–0.90, P = 0.0093)], ORR (60.8 vs. 23.1%), and complete response (CR) rate (18.9% vs. 3.1%).[16] Lastly, another subgroup analysis investigated patients in the intention to treat (ITT) population with baseline tumor programmed death ligand 1 (PD-L1) expression ≥1% had a greater magnitude of OS benefit (HR, 0.57; 95% CI 0.40–0.80) relative to patients with PD-L1 ≤1% (HR, 0.77; 95% CI 0.64–0.93); overall, there was a benefit to the combination over sunitinib independent of PD-L1 status. Although ipilimumab plus nivolumab was associated with higher ORR and CR rates compared to sunitinib, more patients also experienced primary progressive disease (17% vs. 14%) and continued treatment beyond initial investigator-assessed, RECIST-defined progression (29% vs. 24%), as permitted by the protocol.[17]

The adverse effect profile of ipilimumab plus nivolumab is distinctive from sunitinib. Patients treated with the combination experienced less grade 3 to 4 TRAEs (48% vs 64%) with 27% experiencing grade 3 to 4 immune-mediated adverse events (irAEs) and higher rates of treatment discontinuation (23% vs. 13%). Approximately 30% of patients required high-dose corticosteroid use ($\geq$40 mg prednisone daily or equivalent) for the management of irAE. Despite the risk of early irAE associated with ipilimumab plus nivolumab, many irAEs are reversible with short-term immunosuppression without impairment to long-term anti-tumor immune activity. Regan and colleagues[18] investigated antitumor efficacy and toxicity after ICI discontinuation in the CheckMate 214 trial. This analysis described a novel endpoint of treatment free survival (TFS) which was defined as time from protocol therapy cessation to time of subsequent systemic therapy or death. After 42 months of follow-up, 52% of patients with intermediate or poor risk metastatic ccRCC initially treated with ipilimumab plus nivolumab were alive, and of those, 14% were receiving nivolumab maintenance and 31% were free of subsequent therapy. The overall 42-month restricted mean TFS was 7.8 months for ipilimumab plus nivolumab and 3.3 months for sunitinib. The mean TFS for ipilimumab plus nivolumab compared to sunitinib was over twice as long for patients with intermediate and poor risk disease (6.9 months vs. 3.1 months; 95% CI, 2.5–5.0). These TFS analyses complement existing mPFS and OS outcomes by demonstrating that patients across all IMDC risk groups experienced benefit from ICI therapy with greater TFS without toxicity relative to sunitinib.[18] Patient-reported outcomes were consistently maintained or improved with ipilimumab plus nivolumab compared to sunitinib across multiple instruments, including the FKSI-19 disease-related symptoms score, FACT-G, and EQ-5D-3 L.[17]

Immune Checkpoint Inhibitor plus Anti-vascular Endothelial Growth Factor

Several large phase III trials were initiated to evaluate the efficacy and safety of ICI (anti-PD1/L1) in combination with intravenous or oral multikinase inhibitors to VEGF or VEGFR compared to sunitinib.[19–23] The phase III IMmotion 151 trial evaluated bevacizumab, an intravenous VEGF inhibitor, in combination with the PD-L1 inhibitor atezolizumab.[20] The KEYNOTE-426 and JAVELIN Renal 101 trials evaluated axitinib, a selective VEGFR 1 to 3 inhibitor with a short half-life (t½ = 2.5–6 h) in combination with pembrolizumab (anti-PD1) or avelumab (anti-PD-L1), respectively.[19,21] The CheckMate 9ER trial evaluated cabozantinib, a broad-acting VEGFR 1 to 3, MET, and AXL inhibitor with a long half-life (t½ = 99 h), in combination with nivolumab (anti-PD1).[22] The CLEAR trial evaluated lenvatinib, a broad-acting VEGFR 1 to 3, FGF, KIT, and RET inhibitor with an intermediate half-life (t½ = 28 h) in combination with pembrolizumab.[23] Of note, the IMmotion 151 and JAVELIN Renal 101 trials allowed responding patients to continue anti-PDL1 therapy indefinitely, whereas the KEYNOTE-426, CheckMate 9ER, and CLEAR trials stopped anti-PD1 therapy after a maximum of 24 months. Plus, dosing differences with VEGFR TKI differ when combined with anti-PD1 therapy versus monotherapy. For example, in CheckMate9ER the starting dose of cabozantinib is 40 mg daily when used with nivolumab compared to the standard 60 mg daily as monotherapy and in CLEAR lenvantinib is given at 20 mg daily in combination with pembrolizumab compared to 18 mg daily when combined with everolimus.

Although these trials accrued patients with treatment naïve metastatic ccRCC across all risk groups, the relative percentage of patients in each group differed across trials (**Table 1**). Each of these trails met primary endpoints of statistically significant

Table 1
Efficacy outcomes from selected first-line clinical trials in metastatic clear cell renal cell carcinoma with intermediate and poor International Metastatic RCC Database Consortium risk

Trial Name (N, Patients Enrolled)	CABOSUN[10] (N = 157)	CheckMate 214[14] (N = 1096)	Keynote-426[19] (N = 861)	JAVELIN Renal 101[21] (N = 886)	CheckMate 9ER[22] (N = 651)	CLEAR[23] (N = 1069)	COSMIC-313[24] (N = 855)
Experimental arm	Cabozantinib	Ipilimumab Nivolumab	Axitinib Pembrolizumab	Axitinib Avelumab	Cabozantinib Nivolumab	Lenvatinib Pembrolizumab	Cabozantinib Ipilimumab Nivolumab
Control arm	Sunitinib	Sunitinib	Sunitinib	Sunitinib	Sunitinib	Sunitinib	Ipilimumab Nivolumab
F: %		F: 23	F: 31	F: 21	F: 23	F: 33	
Int: %	Int: 81	Int: 58	Int: 56	Int: 62	Int: 58	Int: 56	Int: 75
P: %	P: 19	P: 19	P: 13	P: 16	P: 19	P: 10	P: 25
Follow-up (mo)	34.5	67.7	42.8	19	44	33.7	20.2
ORR (ITT), %	20 vs. 9	39 vs. 32	60 vs. 40	52 vs. 27	55.7 vs. 28.4	71 vs. 36	43 vs. 36
CR (ITT), %	0 vs. 0	12 vs. 3	10 vs. 4	4 vs. 2	12.4 vs. 5.2	16 vs. 4	3 vs. 3
PD (ITT), %	18 vs. 29	18 vs. 14	11 vs. 17	12 vs. 19	6 vs. 14	5 vs. 14	8 vs. 20
Median PFS (ITT), mo	8.6 vs. 5.3	12.3 vs. 12.3	15.7 vs. 11.1	13.3 vs. 8	16.6 vs. 8.4	23.9 vs. 9.2	15.3 vs. 11.3
Median OS (ITT), mo	26.6 vs. 21.2	55.7 vs. 38.4	45.7 vs. 40.1	NR vs. NR	49.5 vs. 35.5	NR vs. NR	NR vs. NR
PFS Int & P, HR (95% CI)	0.48 (0.31–0.74)	0.73 (0.61–0.87)	Int: 0.72 (0.57–0.90) P: 0.54 (0.34–0.86)	Int: 0.75 (0.60–0.95) P: 0.51 (0.34–0.77)	Int: 0.61 (0.48–0.79) P: 0.38 (0.25–0.58)	Int: 0.44 (0.34–0.58) P: 0.18 (0.08–0.32)	Int: 0.68 (0.54–0.86) P: 0.93 (0.64–1.35)
OS Int & P, HR (95% CI)	0.80 (0.53–1.21)	0.68 (0.58–0.81)	Int: 0.63 (0.47–0.83) P: 0.59 (0.37–0.96)	Int: 0.86 (0.61–1.20) P: 0.57 (0.36–0.89)	Int: 0.75 (0.56–1.00) P: 0.46 (0.30–0.72)	Int: 0.72 (0.50–1.05) P: 0.30 (0.04–0.64)	Int: NA P: NA

Abbreviations: CI, confidence interval; CR, complete response; F, favorable; HR, hazard ratio; Int, intermediate; mo, months; NA, not available; NR, not reached; ORR, overall response rate; OS, overall survival; P, poor; PFS, progression free survival; TRAE, treatment related adverse event.

improvements in PFS relative to sunitinib. In addition, all these regimens showed significant improvements in OS relative to sunitinib except for axitinib plus avelumab and bevacizumab plus atezolizumab.[20,21] Each of these trials demonstrated statistically significant and clinically meaningful improvements in ORR (52%–71%), CR (4%–16%), and less primary progressive disease (5%–12%) relative to sunitinib. In subset analyses between IMDC risk groups, patients with intermediate and poor risk disease treated with combination therapy appeared to have greater PFS and OS benefits compared to sunitinib (see **Table 1**). Exploratory analyses from each of these studies classified patients into subgroups according to best overall response: 100% (CR); $\geq$80%–<100% (PR1); $\geq$60%–<80% (PR2); or $\geq$30%–<60% (PR3) relative to sunitinib.[25] Patients treated with ICI plus VEGFR TKI combinations had greater depths of response relative to sunitinib. Furthermore, depth of response was associated with prolongation of PFS and OS.[19,21–23,25]

The adverse effect profile of combination anti-PD1/L1 plus VEGFR TKI regimens was similar across trials. Patients had high rates of overall grade 3 to 4 adverse events (68%–83%) (**Table 2**). The most common adverse effects were hypertension, diarrhea, rash, elevated liver enzymes, and thyroid abnormalities, which were often attributable to VEGFR TKI. Patients who experienced adverse effects were managed with dose reductions in VEGFR TKI (20%–68%) but had low rates of discontinuation of both VEGFR and anti-PD1/L1 therapies (5%–13%).[19,21–23] Dose reductions and dose delays should be expected based on a patient's tolerability during combination treatment. Patient-reported outcome scores pertaining to disease-related symptoms were improved with cabozantinib plus nivolumab; however, similar between axitinib plus pembrolizumab and lenvatinib plus pembrolizumab compared to sunitinib. All 3 combination therapies led to improvement in patient-reported time to clinical deterioration.[26,27]

Immune Checkpoint Inhibitor plus Immune Checkpoint Inhibitor plus Vascular Endothelial Growth Factor Receptor Tyrosine Kinase Inhibitor

Although doublet therapies have consistently demonstrated superior outcomes compared to VEGFR TKI monotherapies, the role of triplet therapies in the first-line setting remained uncertain until results of the phase III COSMIC-313 trial were reported. COSMIC-313 randomized patients with treatment naïve intermediate (75%) or poor risk (25%) ccRCC to cabozantinib 40 mg daily plus nivolumab plus ipilimumab or placebo plus nivolumab and ipilimumab; patients with favorable risk disease were not eligible for this trial. Patients in both arms received induction nivolumab 3 mg/kg plus ipilimumab 1 mg/kg every 3 weeks for up to 4 doses followed by nivolumab maintenance for up to 2 years. In contrast to Checkmate 214, patients who experienced dose interruptions or adverse effects of immunotherapy during the induction phase of treatment were eligible to receive nivolumab maintenance without receiving 4 doses of ipilimumab. This trial met its primary endpoint by demonstrating superior PFS for the triplet combination (HR, 0.74; 95% CI 0.58–0.94, $P = 0.01$).[24,28] The triplet combination was associated with higher toxicity with grade 3 and 4 TRAEs occurring in 73% of patients versus 41% of patients receiving placebo plus nivolumab and ipilimumab. Rates of liver dysfunction (26% vs. 5%) and hypertension (9% vs. 6%) were higher among patients receiving triplet therapy. OS is immature at the time of this writing (most recent data cutoff 1/31/22).[24] Considering the increased toxicity associated with triplet therapy, further data and longer term follow-up from this trial are needed to determine whether this combination (cabozantinib plus nivolumab and ipilimumab) will have a role in routine clinical practice for intermediate and poor risk patients.

Table 2
Toxicity outcomes from selected first line clinical trials in metastatic clear cell renal cell carcinoma with intermediate and poor International Metastatic RCC Database Consortium risk

Trial Name (Patients Enrolled)	CABOSUN[10] (157)	CheckMate 214[14] (1096)	Keynote-426[19] (861)	JAVELIN Renal 101[21] (886)	CheckMate 9ER[22] (651)	CLEAR[23] (1069)	COSMIC-313[24] (855)
Experimental arm	Cabozantinib	Ipilimumab Nivolumab	Axitinib Pembrolizumab	Axitinib Avelumab	Cabozantinib Nivolumab	Lenvatinib Pembrolizumab	Cabozantinib Ipilimumab Nivolumab
Control arm	Sunitinib						Ipilimumab Nivolumab
Grade 3–4 TRAE, %	68 vs. 65	48 vs. 64	68 vs. 54	71 vs. 71	75 vs. 71	83 vs. 72	73 vs. 41
Dose reduction % VEGFR TKI	46 vs. 35	0 vs. 53	20 vs. 29	42 vs. 43	56 vs. 52	69 vs. 50	54 vs. 20
Discontinuation % Anti-PD1/L1		23 vs. 0	21 vs. 0	NA vs. 0	7 vs. 0	29 vs. 0	26 vs. 18
VEGFR TKI	21 vs. 22	0 vs. 13	20 vs. 12	NA vs. 13	8 vs. 17	26 vs. 14	28 vs. 14
Both			7 vs. 0	8 vs. 0	6 vs. 0	13 vs. 0	12 vs. 5

Abbreviations: NA, data not available; TRAE, treatment-related adverse event.

DISCUSSION

The success of several recent large phase III trials has dramatically improved outcomes for patients with intermediate and poor risk ccRCC. However, the selection of optimal treatment for each individual patient necessitates shared decision making incorporating the patient's goals, comorbid conditions, tumor histologic features, and adverse effect profiles of treatment regimens. For many patients with intermediate and poor risk ccRCC, treatment will consist of an anti-PD1 backbone paired with either ipilimumab or VEGFR TKI. For the minority of patients with a contraindication to ICI therapy such as active autoimmune disease, solid organ transplantation, or high-dose immunosuppressive medications, cabozantinib is a standard of care option. Because of the limited durability of response to cabozantinib for patients with intermediate and poor risk ccRCC, efforts should be made to control autoimmune disease and decrease immunosuppressive medications with the goal of utilizing ICI therapy at the time of progression.

Ipilimumab plus nivolumab is a standard of care option for patients with the goals of durable anti-tumor responses and treatment free intervals. Patients with tumors that have sarcomatoid histology should receive immunotherapy-based regimens given remarkable response to ICI therapy and reduced benefit from VEGFR TKI reported across multiple trials, with the strongest data supporting ipilimumab plus nivolumab.[16,29,30] However, with a primary PD rate approaching 20%, there is risk associated with this approach and for patients who experience primary progressive disease on ipilimumab plus nivolumab, prompt initiation of subsequent therapy with VEGFR TKI is necessary to prevent early clinical deterioration or death. In contrast, axitinib plus pembrolizumab, cabozantinib plus nivolumab, and lenvatinib plus pembrolizumab are standard of care options for patients with goals to optimize tumor shrinkage with PD rates <11%. Patients treated with ICI plus VEGFR TKI consistently demonstrated high response rates, low primary progressive disease, and prolongation of median PFS and OS relative to sunitinib. Although the maximum duration of anti-PD1 therapy was limited to 2 years in some of these trials, it remains uncertain if patients with deep response can discontinue VEGFR TKI therapy and long-term follow-up will be critical.

Because of unique composite patient populations, distinct VEGFR and anti-PD1/L1 therapies, and subtle differences in study designs, one must maintain caution against comparing outcomes across trials. Currently, there is no head-to-head data to select which ICI plus VEGFR TKI combination is optimal for individual patients; however, a recent network meta-analysis (NMA) explored the efficacy and safety of ICI-based combinations in first-line mRCC and commented on survival according to MSKCC or IMDC risk criteria.[31] As shown in **Table 1**, most patients enrolled on CheckMate 214, JAVELIN Renal 101, or CheckMate 9ER are classified as intermediate and poor risk, but CLEAR and KEYNOTE-426 had higher percentages of favorable risk patients. Although an NMA can provide insightful data utilizing indirect comparisons, it should not replace the gold standard of randomized controlled trials; head-to-head comparisons are necessary to determine the best treatment combination. Consequently, treatment decisions are often guided by slight differences in VEGFR TKI pharmacologic profiles and the clinician's prior experience in managing adverse effects.

FUTURE DIRECTIONS

Current clinical trials are utilizing the clinically based IMDC and MSKCC risk stratifications regarding patient eligibility for first-line treatments (**Table 3**). No standard prognostic biomarkers are approved for ccRCC, but many are in development and

Table 3
Ongoing phase III first-line clinical trials in metastatic clear cell renal cell carcinoma

Trial Name NCT# (Patient Total, N)	A031704/PDIGREE NCT03793166 (N = 1046)[32]	MK-6482–012 NCT04736706 (N = 1653)[33]	S1931/PROBE NCT04510597 (N = 364)[34]	RENAVIV NCT03592472 (N = 413)[35]	NORDIC-SUN NCT03977571 (N = 400)[36]	NCT04394975 (N = 380)[37]	NCT04523272 (N = 418)[38]
IMDC Patient population	Intermediate and poor	All	All	All	All	All	All
Experimental arm	Cabozantinib plus nivolumab (in patients with non-CR non-PD)[a]	Pembrolizumab plus lenvatinib plus belzutifan OR Pembrolizumab plus lenvatinib plus quavonlimab	Cytoreductive nephrectomy[b]	Pazopanib plus abexinostat[c]	Deferred nephrectomy	TQB2450 plus anlotinib	Toripalimab plus axitinib
Control arm	Nivolumab	Pembrolizumab plus lenvatinib	Systemic therapy	Pazopanib plus placebo	No surgery	Sunitinib	Sunitinib
Primary endpoint	OS	PFS, OS	OS	PFS	OS	PFS	PFS
Estimated completion year	2023	2026	2033	2023	2026	2023	2023

Abbreviations: CI, confidence interval; CR, complete response; F, favorable; HR, hazard ratio; Int, Intermediate; Mo, months; NA, not available; NR, not reached; ORR, overall response rate; OS, overall survival; P, poor; PFS, progression free survival; TRAE, treatment-related adverse event.

[a] Patients are randomized only to the experimental arm after completion of 1–4C of ipilimumab plus nivolumab and repeat imaging demonstrates stable disease or a partial response. If a complete response is demonstrated, patients receive maintenance nivolumab; if there is disease progression, patients receive cabozantinib.

[b] Patients are randomized only if non-CR non-PD after 10 to 14 weeks of initial systemic therapy: ipilimumab plus nivolumab or pembrolizumab plus nivolumab or avelumab plus axitinib.

[c] Prior immunotherapy is allowed but not required for enrollment.

described in subsequent chapters. Future risk models should incorporate molecular and genomic features that accurately predict response to therapy. Similarly, treatment of patients with metastatic ccRCC will be shaped by ongoing clinical trials in the adjuvant and first-line setting. For patients with resected high-risk localized ccRCC, adjuvant pembrolizumab prolonged disease free survival compared to placebo leading to FDA approval.[39] In contrast, adjuvant atezolizumab and adjuvant ipilimumab plus nivolumab did not prolong disease free survival.[40] Several ongoing studies are evaluating the role of adjuvant ICI therapies for high-risk resected ccRCC, which may impact selection of first-line therapy for metastatic disease if patients relapse after receiving ICI in the perioperative setting.

For patients with treatment naïve intermediate and poor risk ccRCC, the phase III CheckMate 8Y8 (NCT03873402) trial is investigating nivolumab plus ipilimumab compared to nivolumab monotherapy.[41] Although several studies have demonstrated the efficacy of the combination, this trial will be the first prospective phase III trial to evaluate whether upfront addition of anti-CTLA therapy to anti-PD-1 improves outcomes relative to anti-PD-1 monotherapy. The coprimary endpoints of this trial are PFS by blinded independent central review and ORR. Although ORR and PFS improvements are clinically relevant, these tumor shrinkage endpoints may be suboptimal to determine the benefit of dual ICI therapy, which has been demonstrated in landmarks and tails on PFS and OS curves. For patients with treatment naïve intermediate and poor risk ccRCC, Alliance A031704 (PDIGREE, NCT0379316) is a currently enrolling adaptive phase III trial.[32] After 1 to 4 cycles of nivolumab plus ipilimumab, patients with a partial response or stable disease by iRECIST are randomized to receive nivolumab alone or nivolumab plus cabozantinib; patients with a complete response receive nivolumab alone; and patients with progressive disease receive cabozantinib alone.

Patients with all risk treatment naïve metastatic ccRCC are eligible for the phase III MK6482 to 012 (NCT04736706) trial that is investigating pembrolizumab in combination with belzutifan (HIF2 inhibitor) and lenvatinib, or pembrolizumab and the CTLA-4 inhibitor quavonlimab in combination with lenvatinib, versus pembrolizumab plus lenvatinib.[33] In contrast to other studies involving CTLA-4 inhibition, quavonlimab was given for 2 years duration. Ultimately, the OS endpoint will be what determines whether these triplet combination therapies are adopted in routine practice. Additionally, 2 ongoing phase III trials based in China (NCT04523272 and NCT04394975) are testing different PD-1/PD-L1 and VEGFR TKI combination therapies versus sunitinib.[37,38]

SUMMARY

Current approved combination treatment regimens all demonstrated improved PFS and OS over VEGFR TKI monotherapy. Standard of care treatment in IMDC intermediate and poor risk disease includes PD-1 plus CTLA-4 or PD-1 plus VEGFR TKI, but no current head-to-head trials between the approved regimens are being conducted. For most patients, the choice of whether to combine PD-1 blockade with CTLA-4 blockade or a VEGFR TKI should involve shared decision making to navigate the need for a response in the short term (ICI/VEGF combinations) and potential durable response and/or treatment free survival (favoring anti-CTLA-4). Ongoing trials of novel triplet combination regimens are using modern comparator arms instead of sunitinib: for example, MK6482 to 012 with pembrolizumab plus lenvatinib, or COSMIC-313 with ipilimumab plus nivolumab. Novel combinations being studied incorporate radiation, surgery, and new therapeutic targets, which may alter our current first-line treatment paradigm. In summary, the inherent tradeoff between long-term outcomes and toxicity with ICI combinations is a shared decision when choosing among first-line therapy options. Current risk models to direct therapy are still relevant but need to be improved by incorporating prognostic genomic and molecular information.

CLINICS CARE POINTS

- Patients with IMDC intermediate and poor risk ccRCC have been historically characterized by a disease with an aggressive clinical course and poor response to available treatments.

- Systemic therapy targeting immune checkpoints (anti-PD1) combined with either ipilimumab (anti-CTLA) or VEGFR TKI have significantly improved outcomes for patients with intermediate and poor risk ccRCC.

- Patients treated with ipilimumab and nivolumab may benefit from durable antitumor responses and treatment free intervals, while also having the risks of primary progressive disease and irAE.

- Patients treated with ICI plus VEGFR TKI may benefit from early and deep tumor shrinkage, while also having the risks of developing treatment resistance and chronic VEGFR-associated toxicities

DISCLOSURE

W. Xu: consulting or advisory board: Jazz, Exelixis. M.T. Serzan: the author has nothing to disclose. S.A. Berg: consulting or advisory board: BMS, Eisai, Exelixis, Pfizer, Seattle Genetics; Honoraria: MJH Life Sciences, Aptitude Health.

REFERENCES

1. Ernst MS, Navani V, Wells JC, et al. Outcomes for International Metastatic Renal Cell Carcinoma Database Consortium Prognostic Groups in Contemporary First-line Combination Therapies for Metastatic Renal Cell Carcinoma. Eur Urol 2023. https://doi.org/10.1016/j.eururo.2023.01.001. S0302283823000015.
2. Fyfe G, Fisher RI, Rosenberg SA, et al. Results of treatment of 255 patients with metastatic renal cell carcinoma who received high-dose recombinant interleukin-2 therapy. J Clin Oncol 1995;13(3):688–96.
3. Fishman M, Dutcher JP, Clark JI, et al. Overall survival by clinical risk category for high dose interleukin-2 (HD IL-2) treated patients with metastatic renal cell cancer (mRCC): data from the PROCLAIMSM registry. j immunotherapy cancer 2019; 7(1):84.
4. National Cancer Care Network, NCCN Clinical Practice Guidelines in Oncology, *Kidney Cancer*, 2023. Version 4.2023.
5. Hudes G, Carducci M, Tomczak P, et al. Temsirolimus, Interferon Alfa, or Both for Advanced Renal-Cell Carcinoma. N Engl J Med 2007;356(22):2271–81.
6. Sternberg CN, Davis ID, Mardiak J, et al. Pazopanib in locally advanced or metastatic renal cell carcinoma: results of a randomized phase III trial. J Clin Oncol 2010;28(6):1061–8.
7. Motzer RJ, Hutson TE, Tomczak P, et al. Overall survival and updated results for sunitinib compared with interferon alfa in patients with metastatic renal cell carcinoma. J Clin Oncol 2009;27(22):3584–90.
8. Staehler M, Panic A, Goebell PJ, et al. First-line pazopanib in intermediate- and poor-risk patients with metastatic renal cell carcinoma: Final results of the FLIPPER trial. Int J Cancer 2021;148(4):950–60.

9. Choueiri TK, Halabi S, Sanford BL, et al. Cabozantinib Versus Sunitinib As Initial Targeted Therapy for Patients With Metastatic Renal Cell Carcinoma of Poor or Intermediate Risk: The Alliance A031203 CABOSUN Trial. J Clin Orthod 2017;35(6): 591–7.

10. George DJ, Hessel C, Halabi S, et al. Cabozantinib Versus Sunitinib for Untreated Patients with Advanced Renal Cell Carcinoma of Intermediate or Poor Risk: Subgroup Analysis of the Alliance A031203 CABOSUN trial. Oncol 2019;24(11): 1497–501.

11. Choueiri TK, Hessel C, Halabi S, et al. Cabozantinib versus sunitinib as initial therapy for metastatic renal cell carcinoma of intermediate or poor risk (Alliance A031203 CABOSUN randomised trial): Progression-free survival by independent review and overall survival update. European Journal of Cancer 2018;94:115–25.

12. Hammers HJ, Plimack ER, Infante JR, et al. Safety and Efficacy of Nivolumab in Combination With Ipilimumab in Metastatic Renal Cell Carcinoma: The CheckMate 016 Study. J Clin Oncol 2017;35(34):3851–8. https://doi.org/10.1200/JCO. 2016.72.1985.

13. Motzer RJ, McDermott DF, Escudier B, et al. Conditional survival and long-term efficacy with nivolumab plus ipilimumab versus sunitinib in patients with advanced renal cell carcinoma. Cancer 2022;128(11):2085–97.

14. Motzer RJ, Tannir NM, McDermott DF, et al. Nivolumab plus Ipilimumab versus Sunitinib in Advanced Renal-Cell Carcinoma. N Engl J Med 2018;378(14):1277–90.

15. Bakouny Z, Braun DA, Shukla SA, et al. Integrative molecular characterization of sarcomatoid and rhabdoid renal cell carcinoma. Nat Commun 2021;12(1):808.

16. Tannir NM, Signoretti S, Choueiri TK, et al. Efficacy and Safety of Nivolumab Plus Ipilimumab versus Sunitinib in First-line Treatment of Patients with Advanced Sarcomatoid Renal Cell Carcinoma. Clin Cancer Res 2021;27(1):78–86.

17. Cella D, Grünwald V, Escudier B, et al. Patient-reported outcomes of patients with advanced renal cell carcinoma treated with nivolumab plus ipilimumab versus sunitinib (CheckMate 214): a randomised, phase 3 trial. Lancet Oncol 2019;20(2): 297–310.

18. Regan MM, Jegede OA, Mantia CM, et al. Treatment-free Survival after Immune Checkpoint Inhibitor Therapy versus Targeted Therapy for Advanced Renal Cell Carcinoma: 42-Month Results of the CheckMate 214 Trial. Clin Cancer Res 2021; 27(24):6687–95.

19. Rini BI, Plimack ER, Stus V, et al. Pembrolizumab plus Axitinib versus Sunitinib for Advanced Renal-Cell Carcinoma. N Engl J Med 2019. https://doi.org/10.1056/ NEJMoa1816714.

20. Motzer RJ, Powles T, Atkins MB, et al. Final Overall Survival and Molecular Analysis in IMmotion151, a Phase 3 Trial Comparing Atezolizumab Plus Bevacizumab vs Sunitinib in Patients With Previously Untreated Metastatic Renal Cell Carcinoma. JAMA Oncol 2022;8(2):275.

21. Motzer RJ, Penkov K, Haanen J, et al. Avelumab plus Axitinib versus Sunitinib for Advanced Renal-Cell Carcinoma. N Engl J Med 2019. https://doi.org/10.1056/ NEJMoa1816047.

22. Choueiri TK, Powles T, Burotto M, et al. Nivolumab plus Cabozantinib versus Sunitinib for Advanced Renal-Cell Carcinoma. N Engl J Med 2021;384(9):829–41.

23. Motzer R, Alekseev B, Rha SY, et al. Lenvatinib plus Pembrolizumab or Everolimus for Advanced Renal Cell Carcinoma. N Engl J Med 2021;384(14):1289–300.

24. Powles T, Motzer RJ, Albiges L, et al. Outcomes by IMDC risk in the COSMIC-313 phase 3 trial evaluating cabozantinib (C) plus nivolumab (N) and ipilimumab (I) in

first-line advanced RCC (aRCC) of IMDC intermediate or poor risk. J Clin Oncol 2023;41(suppl 6):abstr 605.

25. Suárez C, Choueiri TK, Burotto M, et al. Association between depth of response (DepOR) and clinical outcomes: Exploratory analysis in patients with previously untreated advanced renal cell carcinoma (aRCC) in CheckMate 9ER. J Clin Orthod 2022;40(16_suppl):4501.

26. Motzer R, Porta C, Alekseev B, et al. Health-related quality-of-life outcomes in patients with advanced renal cell carcinoma treated with lenvatinib plus pembrolizumab or everolimus versus sunitinib (CLEAR): a randomised, phase 3 study. Lancet Oncol 2022;23(6):768–80.

27. Cella D, Motzer RJ, Suarez C, et al. Patient-reported outcomes with first-line nivolumab plus cabozantinib versus sunitinib in patients with advanced renal cell carcinoma treated in CheckMate 9ER: an open-label, randomised, phase 3 trial. Lancet Oncol 2022;23(2):292–303.

28. Choueiri T, Powles T, Albiges L, et al. Phase III study of cabozantinib (C) in combination with nivolumab (N) and ipilimumab (I) in previously untreated advanced renal cell carcinoma (aRCC) of IMDC intermediate or poor risk (COSMIC-313). Ann Oncol 2022;33(suppl_7):S808–69.

29. Rini BI, Plimack ER, Stus V, et al. Pembrolizumab (pembro) plus axitinib (axi) versus sunitinib as first-line therapy for metastatic renal cell carcinoma (mRCC): Outcomes in the combined IMDC intermediate/poor risk and sarcomatoid subgroups of the phase 3 KEYNOTE-426 study. J Clin Orthod 2019; 37(15_suppl):4500.

30. Choueiri TK, Larkin JMG, Pal SK, et al. Efficacy and biomarker analysis of patients (pts) with advanced renal cell carcinoma (aRCC) with sarcomatoid histology (sRCC): Subgroup analysis from the phase III JAVELIN renal 101 trial of first-line avelumab plus axitinib (A + Ax) vs sunitinib (S). Ann Oncol 2019;30:v361.

31. Bosma NA, Warkentin MT, Gan CL, et al. Efficacy and Safety of First-line Systemic Therapy for Metastatic Renal Cell Carcinoma: A Systematic Review and Network Meta-analysis. European Urology Open Science 2022;37:14–26.

32. National Cancer Institute (NCI). PD-Inhibitor (Nivolumab) and Ipilimumab Followed by Nivolumab vs. VEGF TKI Cabozantinib With Nivolumab: A Phase III Trial in Metastatic Untreated REnal Cell CancEr PDIGREE. clinicaltrials.gov; 2023. Available at: https://clinicaltrials.gov/ct2/show/NCT03793166Accessed 30 January, 2023.

33. Merck Sharp & Dohme LLC. An Open-Label, Randomized Phase 3 Study to Evaluate Efficacy and Safety of Pembrolizumab (MK-3475) in Combination With Belzutifan (MK-6482) and Lenvatinib (MK-7902), or MK-1308A in Combination With Lenvatinib, Versus Pembrolizumab and Lenvatinib, as First-Line Treatment in Participants With Advanced Clear Cell Renal Cell Carcinoma (CcRCC). clinicaltrials.gov; 2023. Available at: https://clinicaltrials.gov/ct2/show/NCT04736706. Accessed 30 January, 2023.

34. Southwest Oncology Group. Phase III Trial of Immunotherapy-Based Combination Therapy With or Without Cytoreductive Nephrectomy for Metastatic Renal Cell Carcinoma (PROBE Trial). clinicaltrials.gov; 2022. Available at: https://clinicaltrials. gov/ct2/show/NCT04510597. Accessed 30 January, 2023.

35. Xynomic Pharmaceuticals, Inc. A Randomized, Phase 3, Double-Blind, Placebo-Controlled Study of Pazopanib With or Without Abexinostat in Patients With Locally Advanced or Metastatic Renal Cell Carcinoma(RENAVIV). clinicaltrials.gov; 2022. Available at: https://clinicaltrials.gov/ct2/show/NCT03592472Accessed 30 January, 2023.

36. Fristrup N. Multicenter Randomized Trial of Deferred Cytoreductive Nephrectomy in Synchronous Metastatic Renal Cell Carcinoma Receiving Checkpoint Inhibitors: A DaRenCa and NoRenCa Trial Evaluating the Impact of Surgery or No Surgery. The NORDIC-SUN-Trial. clinicaltrials.gov; 2022. Available at: https://clinicaltrials.gov/ct2/show/NCT03977571. Accessed 30 January, 2023.

37. Chia Tai Tianqing Pharmaceutical Group Co., Ltd. A Randomized, Positive Parallel Controlled, Multicenter Phase III Study of TQB2450 Injection Combined With Anlotinib Hydrochloride Capsule Versus Sunitinib in Subjects With Advanced Renal Cancer. clinicaltrials.gov; 2020. Available at: https://clinicaltrials.gov/ct2/show/NCT04523272Accessed 30 January, 2023.

38. Shanghai Junshi Bioscience Co., Ltd. A Phase III, Randomized, Open-Label, Active Controlled, Multicenter Study on Toripalimab Combined With Axitinib Versus Sunitinib Monotheraphy as a First-Line Treatment for Unresectable or Metastatic Renal Cell Carcinoma (RCC). clinicaltrials.gov; 2021. Available at: https://clinicaltrials.gov/ct2/show/NCT04394975Accessed 30 January, 2023.

39. Choueiri TK, Tomczak P, Park SH, et al. Adjuvant Pembrolizumab after Nephrectomy in Renal-Cell Carcinoma. N Engl J Med 2021;385(8):683–94.

40. Pal SK, Uzzo R, Karam JA, et al. Adjuvant atezolizumab versus placebo for patients with renal cell carcinoma at increased risk of recurrence following resection (IMmotion010): a multicentre, randomised, double-blind, phase 3 trial. Lancet 2022;400(10358):1103–16.

41. Bristol-Myers Squibb. A Phase 3b, Randomized, Double-Blind Study of Nivolumab Combined With Ipilimumab Versus Nivolumab Monotherapy for Patients With Previously Untreated Advanced Renal Cell Carcinoma and Intermediate- or Poor-Risk Factors. clinicaltrials.gov; 2023. Available at: https://clinicaltrials.gov/ct2/show/NCT03873402Accessed 30 January, 2023.

Managing Metastatic Renal Cell Carcinoma after Progression on Immunotherapy

Regina Barragan-Carrillo, MD[a,b,1], Ameish Govindarajan, MD[a,1],
Adam Rock, MD[a], Rubens C. Sperandio, MD[c],
Sumanta K. Pal, MD[a,*]

KEYWORDS

- Renal cell carcinoma • Immunotherapy • Targeted therapy

KEY POINTS

- The standardization of treatment in the subsequent lines for patients with metastatic renal cell carcinoma treated with first-line immunotherapy remains an unmet need.
- More than 50% of patients who progress on first-line treatment with an immune checkpoint inhibitor (ICI)-based combination are eligible for second-line treatment.
- Vascular endothelial growth factor receptor-tyrosine kinase inhibitors (VEGFR-TKIs) have shown promising results after exposure to an ICI-based combination in the second-line setting. Overall treatment response is approximately 30%, with more than 75% of patients obtaining disease control.
- Rechallenge with immunotherapy alone may be safe but seems to have limited efficacy, with an overall response rate of 7% to 13%.
- Promising new regimens, including those with novel mechanisms of action, such as hypoxia-inducible factor-2α inhibition and ICI with VEGFR-TKI combinations, are currently being evaluated in phase 3 trials.

INTRODUCTION

Real-world data suggest that 35.5% of patients with renal cell carcinoma (RCC) are administered immune checkpoint inhibitor (ICI)-based regimens as their initial

[a] Department of Medical Oncology and Therapeutics Research, City of Hope Comprehensive Cancer Center, 1500 East Duarte Road, Duarte, CA 91010, USA; [b] Department of Hematology and Oncology, Instituto Nacional de Ciencias Médicas y Nutrición "Salvador Zubiran", Vasco de Quiroga 15 Tlalpan, Mexico City 14080, Mexico; [c] Centro de Oncologia e Hematologia Einstein Família Dayan-Daycoval, Hospital Israelita Albert Einstein, Av. Albert Einstein, 627/701 - Morumbi, São Paulo, 05652-900, Brasil
[1] Both authors contributed equally to this study.
* Corresponding author.
E-mail address: spal@coh.org
Twitter: @ReginaBarCar (R.B.-C.); @AGovindarajanMD (A.G.); @RCSperandio (R.C.S.); @montypal (S.K.P.)

Hematol Oncol Clin N Am 37 (2023) 965–976
https://doi.org/10.1016/j.hoc.2023.05.005
0889-8588/23/© 2023 Elsevier Inc. All rights reserved.

treatment, and this figure is projected to increase in the coming years.[1] Despite significant advances in treatment, the vast majority of patients who undergo ICI-based therapy will ultimately experience disease progression and require further systemic treatment.[2] Based on data from phase 3 clinical trials of first-line ICI combinations, roughly 50% of patients receive a second-line treatment consisting of either a VEGFR-TKI, ICI/VEGFR-TKI combination, or dual ICIs.[3–6] However, choosing second-line therapy and beyond primarily relies on clinicians' preference instead of evidence-based guidelines, with data guiding such selections predating the introduction of front-line ICIs.

Further, recommendations provided by guidelines are often based on smaller trials or retrospective cohorts, and some agents may not have an appropriate indication in this context. To address this, the current review will detail relevant studies that can help guide treatment selection among patients with metastatic renal cell carcinoma (mRCC) who experience disease progression after front-line ICIs.

RATIONALE FOR TREATMENT

Retrospective data suggest that patients who experience disease progression on first-line combination therapy with VEGFR-TKI and ICI regimens can still benefit from active treatment, assuming adequate performance status.[7] The BEYOND study examined a retrospective cohort of 42 patients with mRCC who progressed after receiving a combination of cabozantinib and nivolumab. Patients could then receive either best supportive care (BSC; 42.9%) or active treatment (57.3%).[7] Active treatment options included everolimus (28.6%), sorafenib (16.7%), sunitinib (4.8%), high-dose interleukin-2 (4.8%), or lenvatinib plus everolimus (2.4%). Patients undergoing active treatment had a median overall survival (OS) of 13 months (95% confidence interval [CI] 4–not reached [NR]) versus 3 months (95% CI 2–4) among patients receiving BSC. According to current guidelines, the available treatment options in the second-line treatment setting include VEGFR-TKIs, with or without readministration of ICI therapy.[8,9] However, there is currently no high-quality evidence supporting recommendations for either of these treatment options.

TYROSINE KINASE INHIBITORS

The majority of evidence concerning treatment after disease progression on an ICI is derived from retrospective data. Broadly speaking, VEGFR-TKIs seem to offer a disease-free survival duration ranging from 6.4 to 8.8 months, with an overall response rate of 28% to 45% as second-line treatment following ICI exposure.[10,11] In a longitudinal retrospective cohort study of patients with mRCC who experienced disease progression on monotherapy or doublet combination ICI, VEGFR-TKI was administered as the second-line therapy.[12] Treatment options included sunitinib, sorafenib, axitinib, or pazopanib. VEGFR-TKIs therapy was associated with a complete response among 1.5% of patients, a partial response among 39.7% of patients, and stable disease for 52.9% of the sample. The reported median PFS was 13.2 months (95% CI 10.1-NR), with patients who had not previously been exposed to an anti-VEGFR therapy garnering the most benefit.[12]

In the context of mRCC, 5 different VEGFR-TKIs are currently approved as part of guideline-based care: sunitinib, cabozantinib, axitinib, pazopanib, and lenvatinib (in combination with either everolimus or pembrolizumab).[8] Because these trials have included a highly heterogeneous population, we will provide a brief review of the activity of these drugs, as well as the populations that have garnered the greatest benefit.

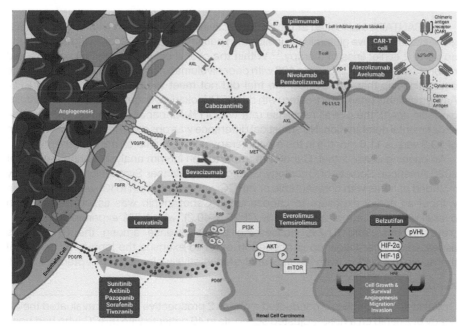

Fig. 1. Sites of action of the different treatment strategies. This figure illustrates the mechanism of action of experimental and Food and Drug Administration-approved drugs. Depicted in this figure illustrates only the major molecules in each pathway. The figure was created by Ameish Govindarajan, MD, Created with Biorender.com. AKT, protein kinase B; APC, antigen-presenting cell; FGF, fibroblast growth factor; FGFR, FGF receptor; HIF, hypoxia-inducible factor; HRE, hypoxia response element; MET, hepatocyte growth factor receptor; mTOR, mechanistic target of rapamycin complex; PD-1, programmed cell death protein; PDGF, platelet derived growth factor; PDGFR, PDGF receptor; PD-L1, PD-1 ligand 1; PD-L2, PD-1 ligand 2; PI3K, phosphoinositide 3-kinase; pVHL, von Hippel–Lindau protein; RTK, receptor tyrosine kinase; VEGF, vascular endothelial growth factor; VEGFR, VEGF receptor.

Fig. 1 displays the primary mechanism of action for therapies with demonstrated clinical activity in this setting.

Cabozantinib

The METEOR trial evaluated the activity of cabozantinib in patients with mRCC who had progressed on an earlier line of treatment, including 32 patients (5%) previously treated with immunotherapy.[13] The overall response rate in the intention-to-treat population was 17% (95% CI 13–22) in the cabozantinib group and 3% (95% CI 2–6) in the everolimus, a mammalian target of rapamycin inhibitor, group. Within the subset of patients with progression on an earlier ICI (N = 18), the median OS was 13.1 months, with a 55% OS rate at 12 months. Similar findings were observed in the BREAKPOINT trial, an open-label, phase 2 single-arm study of cabozantinib in patients with advanced or unresectable mRCC pretreated with an ICI, either as monotherapy (10.0%), in combination with a VEGFR-TKI (26.7%), or as dual ICI therapy (63.3%).[14] Thirty-one patients were included in this trial. The overall response rate was 37.9% (95% CI 20.7–57.7), with an additional 43% presenting with stable disease as their best response. The primary endpoint was met as the median PFS reached 8.3 months (95% CI 3.9–17.4) and a median OS of 13.8 months (95% CI 7.7–29.0).[14]

The CANTATA trial looked at the clinical activity of cabozantinib with or without tela-glenastat (a selective glutaminase inhibitor) in patients with mRCC following progression on up to 2 earlier lines of therapy.[15] Within the overall cohort, 276 (62%) patients had received an earlier ICI, including 128 with prior nivolumab plus ipilimumab and 93 without antiangiogenic therapy. Overall, the trial did not meet the primary endpoint of PFS. Among patients previously treated with dual ICI blockade without exposure to an antian-giogenic agent, the overall response rate was 41% for cabozantinib and 51% for the experimental combination. No statistical difference was observed in PFS, with a median of 10.9 versus 11.6 months in the monotherapy and combination arms, respectively.

An ongoing phase 2 trial, CaboPoint, reported an interim analysis during the recent 2023 American Society of Oncology Genitourinary Cancer Symposium.[16] This study included patients with unresectable or mRCC with progression to ICI-based treatment without an earlier exposure to cabozantinib. Cabozantinib was associated with an overall response rate of 29.5% (95% CI 20.3–40.2), with 1.2% experiencing a complete response and 51.2% possessing stable disease among the 88 patients assessed. Longer follow-up is needed in order to examine the long-term benefit of therapy in this setting, with the final analysis tentatively planned for September 2023.

Axitinib

Ornstein and colleagues[10] conducted a phase 2 prospective trial that evaluated the efficacy of axitinib on a dose-adjusted schedule in 40 patients with mRCC who had been pretreated with ICI therapy. Most patients (48%) had received 2 lines of earlier treatment, whereas 28% had previously received 1 line of treatment, and 26% had previously received 3 to 4 lines of treatment. After a median follow-up of 8.7 months, 45% of patients achieved an objective response, with one patient (3%) achieving a complete response, 17 patients (43%) achieving a partial response, and 18 patients (45%) maintaining stable disease as their best response. The median progression-free survival was 8.8 months (95% CI 5.7–16.6) among the entire cohort. A nonplanned subgroup analysis revealed that patients who discontinued ICI treatment due to progressive disease had a numerically longer PFS of 9.2 months (95% CI 6.2–16.5) in the intention to treat population. However, the trial did not achieve its primary endpoint of a median PFS of 9.5 months or more. Nevertheless, there was suggestion of clinical activity and durability of response (67% of responses sustained for over 12 months) among this cohort.[10]

Tivozanib

Tivozanib is one of the few drugs that have demonstrated activity in a prospective, randomized trial after progression to immunotherapy.[17,18] In the phase 3 TIVO-3 trial, tivozanib was compared with sorafenib among patients with mRCC who had progressed on at least 2 previous lines of systemic treatment, including at least 1 earlier treatment with a VEGFR-TKI.[17,18] Three hundred and fifty patients were randomly assigned to receive either tivozanib or sorafenib. The primary endpoint was met, with PFS favoring the tivozanib group (5.6 months) compared with the sorafenib group (3.9 months; 95% CI 0.56–0.94). In a subgroup analysis of the 91 patients with prior treatment with an ICI (26% of the population), the authors confirmed a greater benefit with tivozanib as compared with sorafenib, with an increase in median PFS of 2.2 months (7.3 vs 5.1 months; 95% CI 0.32–0.94).[18]

Lenvatinib and Everolimus

Based on retrospective evidence, everolimus, in combination with lenvatinib, has demonstrated clinical activity in patients who previously failed immunotherapy.[19] Wiele and colleagues analyzed data from 55 patients who had disease progression after treatment with an ICI, with a median of 4 earlier therapies. The study reported an overall response rate of 21.8% and a disease control rate of 85.4% among the included patients. Among all patients, the median PFS was 6.2 months (95% CI 4.8–9.4), with a median OS of 12.1 months (95% CI 8.8–16.0).[19]

In a further study examining whether VEGFR inhibition may provide benefit after progression on ICI therapy, Pal and colleagues[20] conducted a phase 2 trial in patients with mRCC who had progressed on at least 1 earlier line of VEGFR-TKI therapy. Patients were randomized to receive everolimus in combination with lenvatinib at 2 different starting doses (14 and 18 mg daily), with a primary outcome of overall response rate at week 24. The trial included a total of 343 patients, of whom 26% had received ICIs as an earlier line of therapy. Among patients who had received an earlier ICI therapy, the median PFS was 12.0 months (95% CI 8.9–16.7) in the 14 mg group and 12.9 months (95% CI 8.4-not estimable [NE]) in the 18 mg group.[20] The overall response rate at 24 weeks was 32% (95% CI 25–39) and 35% (95% CI 27–42) for the 14 and 18 mg groups, respectively, with no significant differences noted in the statistical analysis. In the subgroup of patients previously treated with an ICI, the investigator-assessed overall response rate was 30% (95% CI 17–46) and 51% (95% CI 35–68) in the 14 and 18 mg groups, respectively. The median PFS was 12.0 months (95% CI 8.9–16.7) versus 12.9 months (95% CI 8.4-NE) for the 14 versus 18 mg arms, respectively, among those patients in this subgroup. Finally, among ICI pretreated patients, the median OS was 17.1 months (95% CI 10.6–NE) versus 18.0 months (95% CI 13.1–NR) in the 14 and 18 mg arms, respectively.[20]

Sunitinib

Retrospective evidence has shown reasonable clinical activity with sunitinib as a second-line option for patients with prior ICI exposure, with an overall response rate of 22.5% (95% CI 12.6–32.5) and a median overall survival of 15.6 months (95% CI 9.8–21.7).[21] The response rate was most notable among those who had received doublet ICI combination therapy in the first-line setting. Interestingly, 34.5% of patients with prior doublet ICI combination therapy discontinued treatment with sunitinib due to toxicity. In contrast, patients with previous exposure to any VEGFR-TKI treatment appeared to better tolerate this agent, with only 15.0% discontinuing therapy due to toxicity.[21]

IMMUNOTHERAPY

The efficacy associated with rechallenging patients with immunotherapy after disease progression on a first-line ICI-containing regimen is questionable. Ravi and colleagues[22] assessed a cohort of 69 patients with mRCC who had previously received either an ICI monotherapy or the combination of an ICI and a VEGFR-TKI. Of these patients, 31 (45%) experienced any grade of immune-related adverse events after the reintroduction of immunotherapy, and 18 (26%) incurred grade 3 or higher immune-related adverse events. At the time of the immunotherapy rechallenge, the overall response rate was 23%, with a disease control rate of 64%. The median time to progression after immunotherapy rechallenge was 5.7 months (95% CI 3.2–7.6).[22] In this section, we explore retrospective and prospective datasets describing immunotherapy rechallenge in mRCC.

Ipilimumab and Nivolumab

Theoretically, doublet ICI therapy could overcome primary resistance to the anti–programmed death 1 (anti-PD1) pathway targeted therapy by enhancing the stimulation of antitumor immune response through the inhibition of the cytotoxic T-lymphocyte antigen 4 receptor.[23] Gul and colleagues[24] conducted a retrospective cohort study that included 45 patients with mRCC who had progressed on an earlier ICI therapy and had received salvage treatment with nivolumab and ipilimumab. The patients had a median of 3 prior lines of treatment (range, 1–7). The overall response rate to ipilimumab and nivolumab was 20%, with 28 patients (62%) experiencing progressive disease as their best response.[24] Although the study was limited by the small cohort size and retrospective design, these findings suggest a lack of significant clinical efficacy.

The Fast Real-time Assessment of Combination Therapies in Immuno-ONcology Study in Patients With mRCC (FRACTION-RCC) study is another trial assessing the impact of salvage nivolumab/ipilimumab.[25] One arm of this multiarm phase 2 trial was designed to evaluate the clinical activity of nivolumab and ipilimumab in mRCC whose disease had progressed after blockade with a PD-1 or PD-ligand 1 (PD-L1) inhibitor. In total, 46 patients were included. Most had received at least 4 treatment lines (28.3%), all had been previously treated with a PD-(L)1 inhibitor and 89.1% had received prior treatment with a TKI. The overall response rate was 17.4% (95% CI 7.8–31.4), among which no patients achieved a complete response, and 41.3% had stable disease as their best response. Fourteen patients (30.4%) had primary resistance to the treatment combination. Among responders, 75% were previously treated with nivolumab either as monotherapy or in combination, and most (87.5%) preserved and adequate functionality (Karnofsky Performance Score 80–100). The median PFS was 3.7 months (95% CI 2.0–7.3) with a 6-month PFS of 43.2%. In the treatment population with disease control as their best response, the median PFS was 7.2 months (95% CI 3.4–11.0) and the 6-month PFS was 54.5% (27.4 to 75.3).

Furthermore, to address the limited data on salvage immunotherapy in heavily pretreated patients, three phase 2 prospective trials were conducted to evaluate the efficacy of nivolumab and ipilimumab as a salvage regimen for patients with mRCC who had progressed on nivolumab. These trials, particularly the study of Optimized Management of Nivolumab Based on Response in Patients With Advanced Renal Cell Carcinoma (OMNIVORE), cohort A of the the Nivolumab and Salvage Nivolumab/Ipilimumab in Treatment-Naive Patients With Advanced Clear Cell Renal Cell Carcinoma (HCRN GU16–260) awtrial, and the study of Tailored Immunotherapy Approach With Nivolumab in Subjects With Metastatic or Advanced RCC (TITAN-RCC) enrolled a total of 187 patients, with overall response rates of 7.0%, 11.0%, and 13.6%, respectively.[26–28] These studies suggest that patients with symptomatic, progressive disease may not be suitable candidates for dual ICI blockade as salvage therapy and may derive more clinical benefit from therapies that target angiogenesis through VEGFR inhibition.

Lenvatinib and Pembrolizumab

The phase 1b/2 KEYNOTE-146 trial presented an open-label assessment of lenvatinib and pembrolizumab among patients with mRCC who were either treatment-naive or had disease progression after anti-PD-1 therapy.[29] Among the 145 enrolled patients, 104 (72%) were ICI-pretreated, and most had received prior VEGFR-TKI therapy in combination with an ICI. The overall response rate at week 12 was reported to be 51% (95% CI 39.9–61.2), with a median PFS of 11.7 months (95% CI 9.5-NR) and a median duration of response of 9.9 months (95% CI 6.9-NR).[29] The antitumor activity reported with the combination of lenvatinib plus pembrolizumab in ICI-pretreated patients revealed an encouraging disease control rate, with less than 5% of patients experiencing progressive disease as their best response. The authors reported a median PFS of 12.2 months (95% CI 9.5–17.7), whilst the median OS was not yet reached.[29]

Tivozanib and Nivolumab

TiNivo, an open-label phase 1b/2 trial, included 25 patients with mRCC who were both treatment naïve (48%) and previously treated (52%).[30] These patients were treated with tivozanib at 2 different starting doses of 1.0 or 1.5 mg, in combination with nivolumab, every 2 weeks. The combination therapy was well tolerated, with most patients reporting a manageable adverse effect profile. Treatment-related grade 3/4 adverse events were reported in 20 (80%) patients, and 4 (17%) patients experienced adverse events that led to dose reduction. Eight (32%) patients discontinued treatment due to toxicity.[30] The overall response rate for the entire cohort, as assessed by investigators, was 56%, and among the previously treated cohort of 8 patients, the overall response rate was 62%, with a disease control rate of 100%. After a median follow-up of 19.0 months, the PFS for the previously treated cohort had not yet been reached (95% CI 11.0-NR).[30] The TiNivo-2 trial (NCT04987203)[31] is a phase 3, randomized, multicenter, open-label study that seeks to compare the efficacy of tivozanib as monotherapy or in combination with nivolumab among patients with mRCC who have progressed on an earlier ICI. The primary endpoint of this trial is to compare the PFS of patients receiving tivozanib monotherapy to those receiving tivozanib in combination with nivolumab.[32]

Cabozantinib and Atezolizumab

The combination of cabozantinib and atezolizumab was studied in COSMIC 021 in the front line setting with an overall response rate (ORR) approaching 60%.[33] CONTACT-03 (NCT04338269)[34] is a phase 3 trial designed to further evaluate cabozantinib at a daily dose of 60 mg as a monotherapy or in combination with atezolizumab among patients with mRCC who had progressed on either a first-line or second-line treatment.[35] Trial enrollment required an earlier exposure to an ICI regimen that immediately preceded the last line of therapy. With more than 150 global sites and 500 enrolled patients, the primary endpoints were PFS and OS.[35] The study failed to meet its primary endpoint; as we await data from other trials, the result implies that caution should be undertaken in continuing ICI therapy beyond the first-line setting.[36]

NOVEL THERAPIES AND COMBINATIONS
Belzutifan

A hallmark of RCC is dysregulation in the activity of the hypoxia-inducible factor (HIF)-2α. Belzutifan is a small molecule designed to inhibit the heterodimerization of HIF-2α with HIF-1β, thus limiting the transcription of HIF-2α.[37] Currently, belzutifan is being used as monotherapy, or in combination with cabozantinib, among heavily pretreated patients with mRCC or von Hippel-Lindau disease.[37,38]

In the phase 1 LITESPARK-001 trial, the safety of belzutifan was evaluated in a cohort of 55 patients with mRCC who had previously undergone at least 1 line of treatment.[39] Among this cohort, 71% of patients had received a combination of VEGFR-TKI and immunotherapy. The primary endpoint of the study was safety, with the authors reporting a 40% rate of grade 3 treatment-related adverse events. The overall response rate was 25%, with an 80% disease control rate and a confirmed complete response observed in 1 patient (2%). The duration of response was approximately 37.9 months.[39] Based on the International Metastatic RCC Database Consortium risk, favorable-risk patients had the highest overall response rate of 31% and a disease control rate of 92% with belzutifan monotherapy. Among the 39 patients who were previously treated with a combination of VEGFR-TKI and ICI therapy, only 8 patients achieved a partial response, with a subsequent disease control rate of 74%. The median PFS among the entire cohort was 14.5 months (95% CI 7.3–22.1), with further investigation needed to determine the long-term activity of belzutifan in patients with earlier exposure to ICI therapy.[39]

The phase 3 LITESPARK-005 trial (NCT04195750)[40] will address the clinical activity and safety of belzutifan versus everolimus in previously treated patients with mRCC. To be enrolled, patients must have been treated with up to 3 treatment lines, which must include a PD-1/PD-L1 inhibitor (a least 2 doses) and a VEGF-targeted therapy. The dual primary endpoints are PFS and OS. The LITESPARK-005 trial has already completed accrual and results are currently awaited.[40]

Belzutifan and Antiangiogenic Tyrosine Kinase Inhibitors

To investigate the potential synergy between belzutifan and cabozantinib in pretreated patients with mRCC, McDermott and colleagues[38] conducted a phase 1/2 clinical trial. Patients with locally advanced RCC or mRCC, who had previously received immunotherapy and up to 2 lines of treatment, were randomized to receive cabozantinib with or without belzutifan. Most patients (86.5%) experienced a reduction in target lesion size, with a promising median time to response of 2.1 months (95% CI 1.5–13.8) and a median PFS of 16.8 months (95% CI 9.2–22.1).[38] The median duration of response and OS have not been reported as yet.

The LITESPARK-011 trial (NCT04586231)[41] is a phase 3 that is currently enrolling patients with mRCC with disease progression on or after an anti-PD-1/PD-L1 therapy as either first-line or second-line treatment. Patients are randomized to the combination of belzutifan with lenvatinib versus monotherapy with cabozantinib. The dual primary end points are PFS and OS. Investigators are planning to enroll approximately 708 patients.[42]

SUMMARY

Selecting second-line treatment after progression on an ICI-based combination therapy is a challenging task for clinicians treating patients with mRCC. Although VEGFR-TKI or HIF-2α inhibition has demonstrated higher treatment response rates compared with rechallenging with immunotherapy, ongoing research suggests that individualized treatment selection based on clinical and treatment characteristics may be necessary. Novel treatment strategies are currently in development to address these challenging clinical circumstances. For example, clustered regularly interspaced short palindromic repeats chimeric antigen receptor-T (CRISPR CAR-T) cell therapy has shown some clinical activity in heavily pretreated patients with mRCC in a proof of concept phase 1 trial, with 1 of 16 patients achieving a complete response, and the vast majority achieving stable disease.[43] Additionally, monoclonal antibodies designed to induce the activation of lymphocyte activation gene 3, or inhibit the myeloid-specific anti–immunoglobulin-like transcript 4 receptor, are being evaluated in smaller, earlier phase trials, expanding possible targets and treatment options.[44,45] Finally, the assessment of tumor biology at the time of disease progression remains an ongoing area of investigation, with the opportunity to assess serum biomarkers and characterize treatment resistance mechanisms to further tailor treatment selection.[46,47]

FUNDING

None.

DISCLOSURES

S.K. Pal has received travel support from CRISPR Therapeutics and Ipsen.

REFERENCES

1. George S, Faccone J, Huo S, et al. Real-world treatment patterns and sequencing for metastatic renal cell carcinoma (mRCC): Results from the Flatiron database. J Clin Oncol 2021;39(6_suppl):286.
2. Iacovelli R, Ciccarese C, Schutz FA, et al. Complete response to immune checkpoint inhibitors-based therapy in advanced renal cell carcinoma patients. A meta-analysis of randomized clinical trials. Urol Oncol Semin Orig Investig 2020;38(10): 798.e17–24.
3. Motzer RJ, Tannir NM, McDermott DF, et al. Nivolumab plus ipilimumab versus sunitinib in advanced renal-cell carcinoma. N Engl J Med 2018;378(14):1277–90.
4. Rini BI, Plimack ER, Stus V, et al. Pembrolizumab plus axitinib versus sunitinib for advanced renal-cell carcinoma. N Engl J Med 2019;380(12):1116–27.
5. Choueiri TK, Powles T, Burotto M, et al. Nivolumab plus cabozantinib versus sunitinib for advanced renal-cell carcinoma. N Engl J Med 2021;384(9):829–41.
6. Motzer R, Alekseev B, Rha SY, et al. Lenvatinib plus pembrolizumab or everolimus for advanced renal cell carcinoma. N Engl J Med 2021;384(14):1289–300.
7. Giorgione R, Santini D, Stellato M, et al. Active therapy or best supportive care after disease progression to both nivolumab and cabozantinib in metastatic renal cell carcinoma: the BEYOND study (Meet-Uro 19). J Clin Oncol 2021; 39(6_suppl):319.
8. Motzer RJ, Jonasch E, Agarwal N, et al. Kidney cancer, version 3.2022, NCCN clinical practice guidelines in oncology. JNCCN J Natl Compr Cancer Netw 2022;20(1):71–90.
9. Powles T, Albiges L, Bex A, et al. ESMO Clinical Practice Guideline update on the use of immunotherapy in early stage and advanced renal cell carcinoma. Ann Oncol 2021;32(12):1511–9.
10. Ornstein MC, Pal SK, Wood LS, et al. Individualised axitinib regimen for patients with metastatic renal cell carcinoma after treatment with checkpoint inhibitors: a multicentre, single-arm, phase 2 study. Lancet Oncol 2019;20(10):1386–94.
11. Powles T, Plimack ER, Soulières D, et al. Pembrolizumab plus axitinib versus sunitinib monotherapy as first-line treatment of advanced renal cell carcinoma (KEY-NOTE-426): extended follow-up from a randomised, open-label, phase 3 trial. Lancet Oncol 2020;21(12):1563–73.
12. Shah AY, Kotecha RR, Lemke EA, et al. Outcomes of patients with metastatic clear-cell renal cell carcinoma treated with second-line VEGFR-TKI after first-line immune checkpoint inhibitors. Eur J Cancer 2019;114:67–75.
13. Choueiri TK, Escudier B, Powles T, et al. Cabozantinib versus everolimus in advanced renal cell carcinoma (METEOR): final results from a randomised, open-label, phase 3 trial. Lancet Oncol 2016;17(7):917–27.
14. Procopio G, Claps M, Pircher C, et al. A multicenter phase 2 single arm study of cabozantinib in patients with advanced or unresectable renal cell carcinoma pretreated with one immune-checkpoint inhibitor: The BREAKPOINT trial (Meet-Uro trial 03). Tumori J 2022. https://doi.org/10.1177/03008916221138881. 03008916 2211388.
15. Tannir NM, Agarwal N, Porta C, et al. Efficacy and safety of telaglenastat plus cabozantinib vs placebo plus cabozantinib in patients with advanced renal cell carcinoma: the CANTATA randomized clinical Trial. JAMA Oncol 2022;8(10):1411.

16. Albiges L, Powles T, Sharma A, et al. CaboPoint: Interim results from a phase 2 study of cabozantinib after checkpoint inhibitor (CPI) therapy in patients with advanced renal cell carcinoma (RCC). Available at: https://meetings.asco.org/abstracts-presentations/216534. Accessed January 3, 2023.

17. Rini BI, Pal SK, Escudier BJ, et al. Tivozanib versus sorafenib in patients with advanced renal cell carcinoma (TIVO-3): a phase 3, multicentre, randomised, controlled, open-label study. Lancet Oncol 2020;21(1):95–104.

18. Atkins MB, Verzoni E, Escudier B, et al. Long-term PFS from TIVO-3: Tivozanib (TIVO) versus sorafenib (SOR) in relapsed/refractory (R/R) advanced RCC. J Clin Oncol 2022;40(6_suppl):362.

19. Wiele AJ, Bathala TK, Hahn AW, et al. Lenvatinib with or without everolimus in patients with metastatic renal cell carcinoma after immune checkpoint inhibitors and vascular endothelial growth factor receptor-tyrosine kinase inhibitor therapies. Oncol 2021;26(6):476–82.

20. Pal SK, Puente J, Heng DYC, et al. Assessing the safety and efficacy of two starting doses of lenvatinib plus everolimus in patients with renal cell carcinoma: a randomized phase 2 trial. Eur Urol 2022;82(3):283–92.

21. Wells JC, Dudani S, Gan CL, et al. Clinical effectiveness of second-line sunitinib following immuno-oncology therapy in patients with metastatic renal cell carcinoma: a real-world study. Clin Genitourin Cancer 2021;19(4):354–61.

22. Ravi P, Mantia C, Su C, et al. Evaluation of the safety and efficacy of immunotherapy rechallenge in patients with renal cell carcinoma. JAMA Oncol 2020; 6(10):1606.

23. Voron T, Colussi O, Marcheteau E, et al. VEGF-A modulates expression of inhibitory checkpoints on CD8+ T cells in tumors. J Exp Med 2015;212(2):139–48.

24. Gul A, Stewart TF, Mantia CM, et al. Salvage ipilimumab and nivolumab in patients with metastatic renal cell carcinoma after prior immune checkpoint inhibitors. J Clin Oncol 2020;38(27):3088–94.

25. Choueiri TK, Kluger H, George S, et al. FRACTION-RCC: nivolumab plus ipilimumab for advanced renal cell carcinoma after progression on immuno-oncology therapy. J Immunother Cancer 2022;10(11):e005780.

26. McKay RR, McGregor BA, Xie W, et al. Optimized management of nivolumab and ipilimumab in advanced renal cell carcinoma: a response-based phase II study (OMNIVORE). J Clin Oncol 2020;38(36):4240–8.

27. Atkins MB, Jegede OA, Haas NB, et al. Phase II Study of nivolumab and salvage nivolumab/ipilimumab in treatment-naive patients with advanced clear cell renal cell carcinoma (HCRN GU16-260-Cohort A). J Clin Oncol 2022;40(25):2913–23.

28. Grimm MO, Esteban E, Barthélémy P, et al. Efficacy of nivolumab/ipilimumab in patients with initial or late progression with nivolumab: Updated analysis of a tailored approach in advanced renal cell carcinoma (TITAN-RCC). J Clin Oncol 2021;39(15_suppl):4576.

29. Lee CH, Shah AY, Rasco D, et al. Lenvatinib plus pembrolizumab in patients with either treatment-naive or previously treated metastatic renal cell carcinoma (Study 111/KEYNOTE-146): a phase 1b/2 study. Lancet Oncol 2021;22(7):946–58.

30. Albiges L, Barthélémy P, Gross-Goupil M, et al. TiNivo: safety and efficacy of tivozanib-nivolumab combination therapy in patients with metastatic renal cell carcinoma. Ann Oncol 2021;32(1):97–102.

31. U.S National Library of Medicine. Study to Compare Tivozanib in Combination With Nivolumab to Tivozanib Monotherapy in Subjects With Renal Cell Carcinoma.

Available at: https://clinicaltrials.gov/ct2/show/NCT04987203. Accessed April 2, 2023.

32. Choueiri TK, Albiges L, Hammers HJ, et al. TiNivo-2: A phase 3, randomized, controlled, multicenter, open-label study to compare tivozanib in combination with nivolumab to tivozanib monotherapy in subjects with renal cell carcinoma who have progressed following one or two lines of therapy where on. J Clin Oncol 2022;40(6_suppl):TPS405.

33. Pal SK, McGregor B, Suárez C, et al. Cabozantinib in combination with atezolizumab for advanced renal cell carcinoma: results from the COSMIC-021 study. J Clin Oncol 2021;39(33):3725–36.

34. U.S National Library of Medicine. A Study of Atezolizumab in Combination With Cabozantinib Compared to Cabozantinib Alone in Participants With Advanced Renal Cell Carcinoma After Immune Checkpoint Inhibitor Treatment (CONTACT-03). Published April 2, 2023. https://clinicaltrials.gov/ct2/show/NCT04338269. Accessed December 20, 2022.

35. Pal SK, Albiges L, Suarez Rodriguez C, et al. CONTACT-03: Randomized, open-label phase III study of atezolizumab plus cabozantinib versus cabozantinib monotherapy following progression on/after immune checkpoint inhibitor (ICI) treatment in patients with advanced/metastatic renal cell carcinoma. J Clin Oncol 2021;39(6_suppl):TPS370.

36. Exelixis Provides Update on Phase 3 CONTACT-03 Trial Evaluating Cabozantinib in Combination with Atezolizumab in Patients with Previously Treated Advanced Kidney Cancer | Exelixis, Inc. Available at: https://ir.exelixis.com/news-releases/news-release-details/exelixis-provides-update-phase-3-contact-03-trial-evaluating. Accessed March 23, 2023.

37. Jonasch E, Donskov F, Iliopoulos O, et al. Belzutifan for renal cell carcinoma in von hippel–lindau disease. N Engl J Med 2021;385(22):2036–46.

38. McDermott DF, Choueiri TK, Bauer TM, et al. 656MO Phase II study of belzutifan (MK-6482), an oral hypoxia inducible factor 2α (HIF-2α) inhibitor, plus cabozantinib for treatment of advanced clear cell renal cell carcinoma (ccRCC). Ann Oncol 2021;32:S681.

39. Jonasch E, Bauer TM, Papadopoulos KP, et al. Phase 1 LITESPARK-001 (MK-6482-001) study of belzutifan in advanced solid tumors: Update of the clear cell renal cell carcinoma (ccRCC) cohort with more than 3 years of total follow-up. J Clin Oncol 2022;40(16_suppl):4509.

40. U.S National Library of Medicine. A Study of Belzutifan (MK-6482) Versus Everolimus in Participants With Advanced Renal Cell Carcinoma (MK-6482-005). Available at: https://clinicaltrials.gov/ct2/show/NCT04195750. Accessed April 2, 2023.

41. U.S National Library of Medicine. A Study of Belzutifan (MK-6482) in Combination With Lenvatinib Versus Cabozantinib for Treatment of Renal Cell Carcinoma (MK-6482-011). Available at: https://clinicaltrials.gov/ct2/show/NCT04586231. Accessed April 2, 2023.

42. Motzer RJ, Schmidinger M, Eto M, et al. LITESPARK-011: belzutifan plus lenvatinib vs cabozantinib in advanced renal cell carcinoma after anti-PD-1/PD-L1 therapy. Future Oncol 2023. https://doi.org/10.2217/fon-2022-0802. fon-2022-0802.

43. Pal S, Tran B, Haanen J, et al. 558 CTX130 allogeneic CRISPR-Cas9–engineered chimeric antigen receptor (CAR) T cells in patients with advanced clear cell renal cell carcinoma: Results from the phase 1 COBALT-RCC study. J Immunother Cancer 2022;10(Suppl 2):A584.

44. U.S National Library of Medicine. Substudy 03B: A Study of Immune and Targeted Combination Therapies in Participants With Second Line Plus (2L+) Renal

Cell Carcinoma (MK-3475-03B). Available at: https://clinicaltrials.gov/ct2/show/ NCT04626518. Accessed December 2, 2022.

45. Takamatsu K, Tanaka N, Hakozaki K, et al. Profiling the inhibitory receptors LAG-3, TIM-3, and TIGIT in renal cell carcinoma reveals malignancy. Nat Commun 2021;12(1):5547.

46. Heitzer E, van den Broek D, Denis MG, et al. Recommendations for a practical implementation of circulating tumor DNA mutation testing in metastatic non-small-cell lung cancer. ESMO Open 2022;7(2):100399.

47. Geertsen L, Koldby KM, Thomassen M, et al. Circulating tumor DNA in patients with renal cell carcinoma. A systematic review of the literature. Eur Urol Open Sci 2022;37:27–35.

Renal Cell Carcinoma of Variant Histology
Biology and Therapies

Pavlos Msaouel, MD, PhD[a,b,c,]*,
Giannicola Genovese, MD, PhD[a,c,d,e], Nizar M. Tannir, MD[a]

KEYWORDS

- Chromophobe renal cell carcinoma • Collecting duct carcinoma
- Nonclear cell renal cell carcinoma • *MiTF* translocation renal cell carcinoma
- Papillary renal cell carcinoma • Renal medullary carcinoma

KEY POINTS

- Accurate pathologic subclassification is needed to guide management of variant histology renal cell carcinomas.
- Unclassified renal cell carcinoma and collecting duct carcinoma are diagnoses of exclusion.
- Each variant histology renal cell carcinoma (vhRCC) subtype responds differently to cytotoxic chemotherapy, immune checkpoint inhibitors, and targeted therapies.
- Due to its poor response to systemic therapies, local therapies such as metastasectomy may be preferred in certain vhRCC subtypes, in oligometastatic disease.
- Platinum-based cytotoxic chemotherapy is the preferred first-line option for certain rare subtypes such as renal medullary carcinoma and collecting duct cancers.

INTRODUCTION

Renal cell carcinomas (RCCs) are divided into distinct subtypes characterized by specific molecular alterations.[1] Clear cell renal cell carcinoma (ccRCC) constitutes ~75%

[a] Department of Genitourinary Medical Oncology, The University of Texas MD Anderson Cancer Center, Houston, TX 77030, USA; [b] Department of Translational Molecular Pathology, The University of Texas M.D. Anderson Cancer Center, Houston, TX 77030, USA; [c] David H. Koch Center for Applied Research of Genitourinary Cancers, The University of Texas, MD Anderson Cancer Center, Houston, TX 77030, USA; [d] Department of Genomic Medicine, The University of Texas M.D. Anderson Cancer Center, Houston, TX 77030, USA; [e] TRACTION Platform, Division of Therapeutic Discoveries, The University of Texas M.D. Anderson Cancer Center, Houston, TX 77030, USA
* Corresponding author. Department of Genitourinary Medical Oncology, Division of Cancer Medicine, The University of Texas MD Anderson Cancer Center, 1155 Pressler Street, Unit 1374, Houston, TX 77030.
E-mail address: pmsaouel@mdanderson.org

Hematol Oncol Clin N Am 37 (2023) 977–992
https://doi.org/10.1016/j.hoc.2023.04.019
0889-8588/23/© 2023 Elsevier Inc. All rights reserved.
hemonc.theclinics.com

of RCC cases, whereas the remaining 25% are classified under the umbrella term variant histology renal cell carcinomas (vhRCCs).[1] The prognosis and efficacy of therapies can widely vary among vhRCC subtypes, posing a challenge to clinicians managing these tumors. Herein, we provide guidance on how to choose appropriate treatment of vhRCCs based on our evolving clinical and biological evidence. We restrict our focus to RCCs and not non-RCC histologies that can develop from the kidney, and prioritize the more common vhRCC subtypes including papillary RCC (PRCC), chromophobe RCC (CHRCC), microphthalmia transcription factor (MiTF) family RCC (TRCC), renal medullary carcinoma (RMC), fumarate hydratase-deficient RCC (FH-RCC), collecting duct carcinoma (CDC), unclassified RCC (URCC), and vhRCCs with sarcomatoid and rhabdoid dedifferentiation.[1]

SYSTEMIC THERAPIES FOR VARIANT HISTOLOGY RENAL CELL CARCINOMA

There are 3 broad categories of systemic therapies typically used for RCCs: cytotoxic chemotherapies, targeted therapies, and immune checkpoint therapies (ICTs). Each vhRCC histology has a different sensitivity to each of these modalities (Table 1).[1–4] Randomized controlled trials (RCTs) comparing the anti–vascular endothelial growth factor (VEGF) multireceptor tyrosine kinase inhibitor (TKI) sunitinib with mechanistic target of rapamycin (mTOR) inhibitors such as everolimus or temsirolimus in vhRCCs[5–8] were previously reviewed and summarized with the results weakly favoring sunitinib over mTOR inhibition, although the benefit was modest across vhRCC subtypes.[1]

For this article, we have updated the previously reported 2021 meta-analysis[1] of objective response rates (ORR) of ICTs in PRCC and CHRCC, the 2 most common vhRCC subtypes, based on a review of the literature in PubMed, Medline, and abstracts from the Proceedings of the European Society for Medical Oncology and the American Society of Clinical Oncology between September 2012 and January 2023 (Fig. 1).[9–23] The results suggest that although PRCC demonstrates lower response rates (ORR 25.7% with 95% confidence interval [CI] of 17.7%–34.4%) to ICT-based

---

Table 1
Sensitivity of variant histology renal cell carcinoma subtypes to systemic therapy modalities

Histology	Potentially Sensitive to Cytotoxic Chemotherapy	Potentially Sensitive to Targeted Therapies Developed for Clear Cell Renal Cell Carcinomas	Potentially Sensitive to Currently Available Immune Checkpoint Therapies
PRCC	No	Yes	Yes
CHRCC	No	Yes[a]	Yes[a]
FH-RCC	No	Yes	Yes[a]
TRCC	No	Yes[b]	Yes[b]
RMC	Yes	No	No
CDC	Yes	Yes[b]	Yes[b]
URCC	No	Yes[b]	Yes[b]

Abbreviations: ccRCC, clear cell renal cell carcinoma; CDC, collecting duct carcinoma; CHRCC, chromophobe renal cell carcinoma; FH-RCC, fumarate hydratase-deficient renal cell carcinoma; PRCC, papillary renal cell carcinoma; RCC, renal cell carcinoma; RMC, renal medullary carcinoma; vhRCC, variant histology renal cell carcinoma.
[a] Low probability of response based on currently available evidence.
[b] Probability of response may depend on specific biological driver.

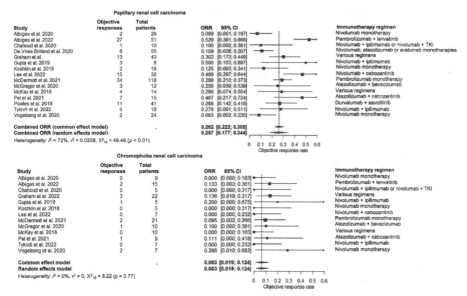

Fig. 1. Forest plots summarizing the reported objective responses to immune checkpoint–based therapies of PRCC and CHRCC.

regimens than what has been observed in ccRCC,[1,24] it is nevertheless far more likely to respond to such therapies than CHRCC (ORR 6.3% with 95% CI of 1.9%–12.4%).

MANAGEMENT OF PAPILLARY RENAL CELL CARCINOMA

PRCC is a heterogeneous malignancy that was previously subclassified into the types 1 and 2 morphologic subtypes. The clinically more indolent type 1 PRCC is associated with activating *MET* mutations and copy number gains of the *MET* gene on chromosome 7, suggesting that c-MET inhibitors such as cabozantinib may be particularly effective for this subtype. The entity formerly defined as type 2 PRCC is clinically more aggressive and more biologically heterogeneous.[1] As mentioned in the article by Matar and colleagues in this issue, there was a major shift following the recent WHO 2022 classification from characterizing PRCC as type 1 or 2, to a therapeutically focused classification based on the potential dependence on the MET pathway.

As reviewed in detail elsewhere,[1] several TKIs targeting c-MET have been investigated in PRCC. The practice-changing randomized, multicenter, 4-arm, phase 2 PAPMET trial was designed to compare cabozantinib versus crizotinib, sunitinib, or the selective c-MET inhibitor savolitinib in patients with PRCC who had received up to one prior systemic therapy excepting VEGF-directed or MET-directed drugs.[25] However, the savolitinib and crizotinib arms were found to underperform during an interim analysis and PAPMET was thus modified into a 2-arm, randomized, phase 2 trial comparing cabozantinib versus sunitinib.[25] Following accrual completion, progression-free survival (PFS) was improved with a covariate-adjusted hazard ratio (HR) of 0.6 and 95% CI 0.37 to 0.97 favoring cabozantinib.[26] The estimates for the secondary endpoint of overall survival were inconclusive, with HR = 0.84, 95% CI 0.47 to 1.51.[25] Cabozantinib is thus a standard for PRCC with responses seen in cases that are resistant to savolitinib.[27]

Although not as effective as in ccRCC, ICT-based combination therapies such as nivolumab + ipilimumab are approved therapies for RCC and can yield responses in patients with PRCC (see **Fig. 1**). ICT + TKI regimens such as nivolumab + cabozantinib that have shown efficacy in PRCC (see **Fig. 1**) should be prioritized in patients with particularly aggressive PRCC that needs to quickly respond to at least one of the drugs in the regimen because it is unlikely that there will be time to administer these therapies sequentially. PAPMET2 (NCT05411081) will help determine whether such a combination would be a robust recommendation for all or most patients with PRCC, whereas SAMETA (NCT05043090) is exploring savolitinib with durvalumab. Emerging data also suggest that lenvatinib + pembrolizumab can yield high response rates in PRCC (see **Fig. 1**).[23]

The combination of lenvatinib + everolimus yielded ORR of 15% (3/20) of patients with treatment-naïve PRCC.[28] This combination has shown efficacy in ccRCC refractory to earlier anti-VEGF TKIs, including cabozantinib.[29] Combining bevacizumab with the antiepidermal growth factor receptor (anti-EGFR) TKI erlotinib produced objective responses in 35% of patients with PRCC (95% CI 22.1%–50.6%).[30] Molecular testing may also help further subclassify PRCC tumors and guide tailored management. For example, heavily pretreated patients with PRCC harboring anaplastic lymphoma kinase (ALK)- echinoderm microtubule-associated protein-like 4 (EML4) fusions have shown responses to the ALK inhibitor alectinib.[31]

MANAGEMENT OF CHROMOPHOBE RENAL CELL CARCINOMA

Although typically indolent, between 5% and 10% of patients with CHRCC will develop metastatic disease.[1,32–34] The presence of sarcomatoid dedifferentiation, noted in ~20% of patients with metastatic CHRCC,[34] is associated with a particularly aggressive and treatment-refractory clinical course[1,35] (see **Fig. 1**).[32,35]

TKIs such as sunitinib and cabozantinib are generally less effective against CHRCC but occasionally produce responses.[4,27,36] The mutation landscape of metastatic CHRCC includes a large proportion of *TP53* mutations (58% of cases), *PTEN* mutations (24%), and imbalanced chromosome duplications.[33] Other mTOR pathway mutations can be found less commonly in CHRCC,[33] providing a mechanistic rationale for using mTOR inhibitors such as everolimus.[5,8] To that end, lenvatinib + everolimus has provided a signal of increased efficacy against CHRCC, with 4 of 9 patients responding to therapy.[28] Notably, in a retrospective report of 5 patients with sarcomatoid CHRCC lenvatinib + everolimus did not produce responses.[32] Furthermore, emerging data suggest that the combination of lenvatinib + pembrolizumab yields far fewer responses in CHRCC with ORR of only 13% (see **Fig. 1**).[23] Novel pathways of interest include the targeting of ferroptosis as a metabolic vulnerability of CHRCC.[37]

MANAGEMENT OF MICROPHTHALMIA TRANSCRIPTION FACTOR RENAL CELL CARCINOMAS

The MiTF family of transcription factors comprises transcription factor E3 (TFE3), transcription factor EB (TFEB), transcription factor EC (TFEC), and MiTF.[38] Aberrant activation of these proteins can happen either via translocations producing oncogenic fusions or copy number amplifications.[39] TRCCs occur most commonly due to *TFE3* translocations, *TFEB* amplifications (second most common), and *TFEB* translocations (third most common).[40] The list of fusion partner genes for *TFE3/TFEB* continues to be expanded, and each fusion partner confers distinct histomorphological and biological features.[39] TRCCs can be challenging to diagnose because they can mimic ccRCC and PRCC on histologic examination.[39] TRCC should be suspected in children and young adults, particularly women, and in tumors that contain mixed morphologies—especially if they have a history of chemotherapy during childhood, as 20% of TFE3 TRCC cases are associated with childhood malignancies.

Responses to dual ICT therapies are typically low with one retrospective study reporting ORR to dual ICT in 1 out of 18 patients with TRCC (5.5%), whereas ICT + TKI yielded responses in 4 out of 11 patients (36%).[41] Conversely, another retrospective study of 23 patients with TRCC who received either ICT monotherapy or dual ICTs as salvage therapy noted PR in 3 patients (13%) and stable disease (SD) in 3 patients (13%) for a disease control rate of 26%.[42]

Oncogenic *TFE3* fusions can upregulate the MET pathway. One recent multicenter retrospective study of 52 patients with TRCC reported ORR 17.3% with cabozantinib, including 2 CRs.[43] A retrospective study of salvage therapy with mTOR inhibitor monotherapy showed a durable response in one heavily pretreated patient with TRCC and SD in the remaining 6 patients, with a median PFS of 3 months.[44] Therefore, mTOR inhibition may have a role in TRCC therapy.

MANAGEMENT OF FUMARATE HYDRATASE-DEFICIENT RENAL CELL CARCINOMA

FH-RCC is an aggressive RCC that most commonly develops in individuals with germline inactivating mutations in the fumarate hydratase (*FH*) gene.[45,46] Up to 35% of individuals with a pathogenic germline *FH* mutation will develop FH-RCC.[47] Less than 20% of FH-RCC cases occur due to sporadic *FH* mutations.[45,48] Because FH inactivation results in aberrant succination of cellular proteins due the high fumarate levels, FH-RCC can be detected by immunohistochemistry (IHC) staining for S-(2-succino)-cysteine (2SC).[47] All cases will show strong cytoplasmic and nuclear 2SC expression, with negative IHC staining in the background nontumor cells making this another highly sensitive assay for FH-RCC.[47,49]

The combination of bevacizumab with erlotinib showed an ORR of 72.1% (95% CI 57.2%–83.4%) and a median PFS of 21.1 months (95% CI 15.6–26.6) in patients with FH-RCC.[30] FH-RCC also often harbors copy number gains of chromosome 7q where *MET* is located,[50,51] and retrospective data suggest that cabozantinib can provide higher efficacy than ICTs or mTOR inhibitors in FH-RCC.[52] Furthermore, cabozantinib in combination with nivolumab yielded responses in 5 out of 5 patients with FH-RCC treated in a single-center phase 2 study.[20] Emerging retrospective data also suggest that lenvatinib in combination with either everolimus or pembrolizumab can yield responses in patients with FH-RCC.[48] Given that bevacizumab + erlotinib has shown excellent efficacy in anti-VEGF TKI-refractory FH-RCC,[30] it may be reasonable to start with first-line ICT combinations and use bevacizumab + erlotinib as a salvage regimen.

MANAGEMENT OF RENAL MEDULLARY CARCINOMA

RMC is a highly aggressive malignancy that mainly occurs in young individuals with sickle hemoglobinopathies such as sickle cell trait, Sβ, SC, or sickle cell disease.[2,53] RMC is more common in men than women (~2:1 ratio) and originates from the right kidney in ~75% of cases due to the increased risk of renal medullary infarcts in the right kidney in the setting of sickle hemoglobinopathies.[53,54] High-intensity exercise may increase RMC risk by aggravating renal medullary hypoxia induced by red blood cell sickling.[54] Less than 10% of RMC cases occur in patients without sickle hemoglobinopathies, which are designated as RCC unclassified with medullary phenotype to distinguish from typical RMC associated with sickle hemoglobinopathies.[2] All RMC tumors demonstrate loss of INI1 (encoded by the *SMARCB1* gene) by IHC.[2,55]

Platinum-based cytotoxic chemotherapy such as carboplatin + paclitaxel is the preferred first-line therapy for RMC because it has occasionally led to CRs in patients with metastatic RMC.[2] Due to the high propensity of RMC to metastasize even when the primary tumor is small, upfront cytotoxic chemotherapy is strongly recommended even in localized RMC. The only exception may be in rare cases where the primary tumor is 4 cm or lesser in greatest dimension and the disease is clearly confined to the kidney.[2]

Responses to platinum-based cytotoxic chemotherapy in RMC are approximately 29% and often brief.[56] Retrospective data reported that gemcitabine in combination with doxorubicin yielded PRs in 3 out of 16 (19%) patients with platinum-refractory RMC making this a viable second-line option.[3] A recently completed clinical trial (NCT03587662) will report on the efficacy of adding the proteasome inhibitor ixazomib to gemcitabine + doxorubicin. The EGFR pathway is significantly upregulated in RMC,[55] and retrospective experience shows that erlotinib + bevacizumab can produce responses in heavily pretreated patients with RMC who progressed on earlier platinum-based chemotherapy followed by gemcitabine + doxorubicin.[57] This approach is therefore a reasonable third-line option for patients with RMC. Regarding ICT, the efficacy of nivolumab + ipilimumab in RMC was prospectively investigated in a clinical trial that stopped early for futility (NCT03274258). Due to the notably high upregulation of LAG3 in RMC, an ongoing phase 2 clinical trial is testing high doses of the anti-LAG3 ICT relatlimab in combination with nivolumab in patients with RMC (NCT05347212).

MANAGEMENT OF COLLECTING DUCT CARCINOMA

Other malignancies should be excluded before making a diagnosis of CDC.[45] Platinum-based cytotoxic chemotherapy such as gemcitabine plus cisplatin or carboplatin plus paclitaxel can be effective in CDC.[1,58] CDCs can be sensitive to VEGF inhibition with cabozantinib demonstrating ORR of 35% (including one CR) in a phase 2 single-center trial of 23 patients with CDC (BONSAI).[59] The addition of bevacizumab to platinum-based chemotherapy may also improve outcomes but increase toxicity.[60] ICTs have anecdotally produced responses in patients with CDC.[12,14] HER2 amplification has been noted in up to 45% of CDC tumors and the combination of capecitabine + lapatinib + trastuzumab produced a PR in a case report of a patient with CDC.[61,62] Loss of chromosome 9p, where CDKN2A/B are located, confers poor prognosis in CDC.[63] A PR lasting more than 6 months with the CDK4/6 inhibitor palbociclib was reported in a patient with metastatic CDC harboring homozygous CDKN2A/B deletion.[64]

MANAGEMENT OF UNCLASSIFIED RENAL CELL CARCINOMA

Aggressive URCC variants frequently harbor mutations in NF2 (18%), SETD2 (18%), BAP1 (13%), KMT2C (10%), and mTOR (8%).[65] URCCs with NF2 mutations are nowadays considered a distinct subtype of NF2-mutated RCCs that can occasionally show dramatic response to ICT[66] and may be susceptible to therapeutic targeting of the Hippo pathway. NF2-mutated RCCs may also respond to mTOR[67–69] and EGFR[70] pathway inhibitors. Before making a diagnosis of URCC, clinicians should look for clues in the patient's clinical and family history that can point to a specific vhRCC subtype.

SARCOMATOID OR/AND RHABDOID DEDIFFERENTIATION

Sarcomatoid or rhabdoid dedifferentiation is associated with worse prognosis than RCCs without such morphologic features and occurs across vhRCC subtypes.[35,71]

Table 2
Specific considerations for each variant histology renal cell carcinoma subtype

Histologic Subtype	Incidence Among all RCCs	Median Age	Common Molecular Alterations	Clinical Considerations	Systemic Therapy Options
PRCC	10%–20%	62	c-MET pathway: • MET amplifications • Chromosome 7 gain • HGF amplifications • MET kinase domain mutations 9p loss NF2 loss (may be included in NF2-RCC subtype) ALK translocations (ALK translocation RCC subtype)	• Clinically and molecular heterogeneous • "PRCC of classic pattern" (formerly type 1 PRCC) is more frequently associated with c-MET pathway alterations	• Cabozantinib ± ICT • ICT alone • Lenvatinib + everolimus after cabozantinib • Bevacizumab + erlotinib (less response than FH-RCC)
CHRCC	5%	58	PTEN and TP53 mutations Imbalanced chromosome duplications mTOR pathway alterations Low TMB	• 5%–10% of patients with CHRCC will develop metastatic disease • Metastatic CHRCC with sarcomatoid features is highly aggressive	• Sunitinib or cabozantinib have limited efficacy • Lenvatinib + everolimus yields high ORR though efficacy in presence of sarcomatoid features unknown • Currently available ICTs are not effective • Local definitive therapies such as surgical metastasectomy are preferred whenever feasible in oligometastatic CHRCC

(continued on next page)

Table 2
(continued)

Histologic Subtype	Incidence Among all RCCs	Median Age	Common Molecular Alterations	Clinical Considerations	Systemic Therapy Options
TRCC	Up to 1%	31–49	Defined by MiTF alterations. Most commonly in *TFE3* and less commonly in *TFEB* • 9p21.3 homozygous deletions found in ~20% of cases • *TFEB* translocation confers a better prognosis compared with *TFE3* translocation • *TFEB* amplification is common and more aggressive • *TFE3* fusions upregulate the MET pathway • *TFE3* fusions may upregulate the PI3K/AKT/mTOR pathway • Typically low TMB	• Most common RCC in children and young adults. Adults may have worse prognosis • More common in women • Prior chemotherapy during childhood is a risk factor • Should always be considered in RCC cases with histomorphological features of both clear cell and papillary histologies • The FISH assay used to detect *TFE3* alterations is different from the one used to detect *TFEB* alterations. These assays cannot provide information on the specific fusion partners in *TFE3* or *TFEB* translocation cases	• TKIs such as cabozantinib • mTOR inhibitors alone or in combination with lenvatinib • ICTs have shown heterogeneous albeit generally modest efficacy
FH-RCC	< 1%	39–45	FH inactivation in all cases 7q gain 9p loss NF2 loss Low TMB	• Between 20% and 35% of patients with germline *FH* mutations (HLRCC syndrome) will develop FH-RCC. Between 11% and 16% of FH-RCC cases will occur due to sporadic FH mutations • Loss of FH by IHC is highly specific but not as sensitive as positive 2SC staining by IHC in diagnosing FH-RCC	• Cabozantinib alone or in combination with ICT appears • Lenvatinib in combination either ICT or everolimus • Bevacizumab + erlotinib can be used either in first-line or in the salvage setting

	%	Median age	Molecular features	Diagnosis/clinical features	Treatment
RMC	<1%	27	All RMC cases are characterized by loss of INI1 encoded by the SMARCB1 gene 8q gain Low TMB but high focal copy number alterations	• Highly aggressive • Right kidney is more commonly involved • More often in men than women • Mainly afflicts young individuals with sickle cell trait or other sickle hemoglobinopathies • Often associated with history of high-intensity exercise	• Refractory to anti-VEGF TKIs • Refractory to standard ICT Regimens • Carboplatin + paclitaxel is the preferred first-line therapy • Gemcitabine + doxorubicin effective second line • EGFR pathway targeting with erlotinib can yield responses in heavily pretreated patients
CDC	Very rare	65	HER2 amplification can be found in up to 45% of cases Loss of CDKN2A gene located in chromosome 9p is found in up to 62% of cases	• Diagnosis of exclusion. Necessary to rule out specific subtypes such as RMC and FH-RCC • Occurs in older individuals than RMC • Expresses INI1 and FH by IHC and is not associated with sickle hemoglobinopathies	• Platinum-based cytotoxic chemotherapy or anti-VEGF TKIs such as cabozantinib are reasonable options • Addition of bevacizumab to cytotoxic chemotherapy may improve responses but increase toxicity • ICTs can anecdotally produce responses in some CDC cases • Capecitabine + lapatinib + trastuzumab can be considered in CDCs with HER2 overexpression • CDK4/6 inhibitors such as palbociclib can be considered in CDCs with 9p loss
URCC	< 5%	50–55	Molecularly heterogeneous NF2, SETD2, BAP1, KMT2C, and/or mTOR mutations are found in aggressive URCC variants	• Diagnosis of exclusion. Necessary to rule out specific vhRCC subtypes such as TRCC • IHC for ALK may establish the diagnosis of ALK-translocation RCC	• ICTs and targeted therapies are the therapeutic mainstays • NF2-mutated RCCs are emerging as a distinct subtype that may respond to ICTs and targeting of the mTOR and EGFR pathways • ALK-translocation RCC may respond to ALK inhibitors

Abbreviations: 2SC, S-(2-succino)-cysteine; ALK, anaplastic lymphoma kinase; ccRCC, clear cell renal cell carcinoma; CDC, collecting duct carcinoma; CHRCC, chromophobe renal cell carcinoma; EGFR, epithelial growth factor receptor; FH, fumarate hydratase; FH-RCC, fumarate hydratase-deficient RCC; FISH, fluorescence *in situ* hybridization; HLRCC, hereditary leiomyomatosis and renal cell carcinoma; ICT, immune checkpoint therapy; IHC, immunohistochemistry; MiTF, microphthalmia transcription factor family; PD-L1, programmed death-ligand 1; PRCC, papillary renal cell carcinoma; Pt, patient; RCC, renal cell carcinoma; RMC, renal medullary carcinoma; TKIs, tyrosine kinase inhibitors; TMB, Tumor mutation burden; TRCC, MiTF family renal cell carcinoma; URCC, unclassified renal cell carcinoma; VEGF, vascular endothelial growth factor; vhRCC, variant histology rena cell carcinoma.

The presence of sarcomatoid dedifferentiation attenuates responses to mTOR inhibitors and TKIs.[71,72] The addition of cytotoxic chemotherapy agents such as gemcitabine to TKIs such as sunitinib or axitinib increases toxicity and is typically not favored.[73] These tumors often harbor higher PD-L1 expression and increased density of tumor-infiltrating lymphocytes.[74,75] Accordingly, ICT combinations such as nivolumab + ipilimumab can produce durable CRs in up to 18% of patients with sarcomatoid ccRCC,[76] making such regimens the contemporary therapeutic mainstay for this histology. However, the role of ICT is less well defined in vhRCCs with sarcomatoid or rhabdoid dedifferentiation. There is anecdotal evidence of deep, durable responses to ICT in PRCCs with sarcomatoid and rhabdoid dedifferentiation.[77] Conversely, sarcomatoid CHRCC typically responds poorly to currently available ICT regimens, consistent with the overall experience in this subtype (see **Fig. 1**).[32]

ADJUVANT THERAPY CONSIDERATIONS

Data are urgently needed on the efficacy of adjuvant immunotherapy in vhRCC histologies. In the absence of such data, clinicians can use structured frameworks reviewed extensively elsewhere and may occasionally extrapolate from Keynote-427, a first-line study of single agent pembrolizumab in vhRCC to inform patient-centered decisions.[13,78]

SUMMARY

Each vhRCC subtype has distinct clinical and biological characteristics that influence management as summarized in **Table 2**. Accurate diagnosis is therefore critical because certain histologies are refractory to established therapies for ccRCC and are instead sensitive to cytotoxic chemotherapy. Trials dedicated to each vhRCC subtype should emphasize RCTs for the more heterogeneous and common entities such as PRCC requiring robust inferences, and biology-driven interventional studies, including umbrella and basket trials,[79] for the more rare and homogeneous vhRCCs with well-defined biological drivers.

CLINICS CARE POINTS

- Identifying the specific vhRCC subtype for each patient is critical for proper management.
- Although most vhRCC histologies are refractory to cytotoxic chemotherapy, it is the preferred treatment strategy for certain rare subtypes such as RMC.
- Certain vhRCC subtypes such as RMC are refractory to the targeted therapies and ICT strategies developed for ccRCC.

DISCLOSURES

P. Msaouel reports honoraria for scientific advisory boards membership for Mirati Therapeutics, United States, Bristol Myers Squibb, United States, and Exelixis, United States; consulting fees from Axiom Healthcare; nonbranded educational programs supported by Exelixis and Pfizer; leadership or fiduciary roles as a Medical Steering Committee member for the Kidney Cancer Association, United States and a Kidney Cancer Scientific Advisory Board member for KCCure; and research funding from Takeda, United States, Bristol Myers Squibb, Mirati Therapeutics, and Gateway for Cancer Research, United States. G. Genovese has no disclosures. N.M. Tannir has received honoraria for service on Scientific Advisory Boards for Eisai Medical

Research; Bristol-Myers-Squibb; Intellisphere; Oncorena; Merck Sharp & Dohme; Neoleukin; Exelixis; and AstraZeneca; for strategic council meetings with Eisai Inc.; steering committee meetings with Pfizer, Inc.; as well as research funding for clinical trials from Bristol-Myers Squibb; Nektar Therapeutics; Arrowhead Pharmaceuticals, United States; Novartis, Switzerland, Calithera Biosciences, United States, and Exelixis, United States.

ACKNOWLEDGMENTS

The authors would like to thank Dr Jeffrey Graham for providing the exact numbers of PRCC and CHRCC responders in the Graham and colleagues study used in our meta-analysis.[21] P. Msaouel is supported by the MD Anderson Khalifa Scholar Award, the Andrew Sabin Family Foundation Fellowship, a Translational Research Partnership Award (KC200096P1) by the United States Department of Defense, an Advanced Discovery Award by the Kidney Cancer Association, a Translational Research Award by the V Foundation, the MD Anderson Physician-Scientist Award, donations from the Renal Medullary Carcinoma Research Foundation in honor of Ryse Williams, as well as philanthropic donations by the Chris "CJ" Johnson Foundation, and by the family of Mike and Mary Allen. G. Genovese is supported by the NIH, United States R01CA258226, the NIH R21 CA259799-01A1 and Translational Research Partnership Award (KC200096P1) by the United States Department of Defense.

REFERENCES

1. Zoumpourlis P, Genovese G, Tannir NM, et al. Systemic Therapies for the Management of Non-Clear Cell Renal Cell Carcinoma: What Works, What Doesn't, and What the Future Holds. Clin Genitourin Cancer 2021;19(2):103–16.
2. Msaouel P, Hong AL, Mullen EA, et al. Updated Recommendations on the Diagnosis, Management, and Clinical Trial Eligibility Criteria for Patients With Renal Medullary Carcinoma. Clin Genitourin Cancer 2019;17(1):1–6.
3. Wilson NR, Wiele AJ, Surasi DS, et al. Efficacy and safety of gemcitabine plus doxorubicin in patients with renal medullary carcinoma. Clin Genitourin Cancer 2021;19(6):e401–8.
4. Tannir NM, Plimack E, Ng C, et al. A phase 2 trial of sunitinib in patients with advanced non-clear cell renal cell carcinoma. Eur Urol 2012;62(6):1013–9.
5. Armstrong AJ, Halabi S, Eisen T, et al. Everolimus versus sunitinib for patients with metastatic non-clear cell renal cell carcinoma (ASPEN): a multicentre, open-label, randomised phase 2 trial. Lancet Oncol 2016;17(3):378–88.
6. Bergmann L, Grunwald V, Maute L, et al. A Randomized Phase IIa Trial with Temsirolimus versus Sunitinib in Advanced Non-Clear Cell Renal Cell Carcinoma: An Intergroup Study of the CESAR Central European Society for Anticancer Drug Research-EWIV and the Interdisciplinary Working Group on Renal Cell Cancer (IAGN) of the German Cancer Society. Oncol Res Treat 2020;43(7–8):333–9.
7. Motzer RJ, Barrios CH, Kim TM, et al. Phase II randomized trial comparing sequential first-line everolimus and second-line sunitinib versus first-line sunitinib and second-line everolimus in patients with metastatic renal cell carcinoma. J Clin Oncol 2014;32(25):2765–72.
8. Tannir NM, Jonasch E, Albiges L, et al. Everolimus Versus Sunitinib Prospective Evaluation in Metastatic Non-Clear Cell Renal Cell Carcinoma (ESPN): A Randomized Multicenter Phase 2 Trial. Eur Urol 2016;69(5):866–74.
9. Chahoud J, Msaouel P, Campbell MT, et al. Nivolumab for the Treatment of Patients with Metastatic Non-Clear Cell Renal Cell Carcinoma (nccRCC): A

Single-Institutional Experience and Literature Meta-Analysis. Oncol 2020;25(3): 252–8.

10. de Vries-Brilland M, Gross-Goupil M, Seegers V, et al. Are immune checkpoint inhibitors a valid option for papillary renal cell carcinoma? A multicentre retrospective study. Eur J Cancer 2020;136:76–83.

11. Gupta R, Ornstein MC, Li H, et al. Clinical Activity of Ipilimumab Plus Nivolumab in Patients With Metastatic Non-Clear Cell Renal Cell Carcinoma. Clin Genitourin Cancer 2019. https://doi.org/10.1016/j.clgc.2019.11.012.

12. Koshkin VS, Barata PC, Zhang T, et al. Clinical activity of nivolumab in patients with non-clear cell renal cell carcinoma. J Immunother Cancer 2018;6(1):9.

13. McDermott DF, Lee JL, Ziobro M, et al. Open-Label, Single-Arm, Phase II Study of Pembrolizumab Monotherapy as First-Line Therapy in Patients With Advanced Non-Clear Cell Renal Cell Carcinoma. J Clin Oncol 2021;39(9):1029–39.

14. McGregor BA, McKay RR, Braun DA, et al. Results of a Multicenter Phase II Study of Atezolizumab and Bevacizumab for Patients With Metastatic Renal Cell Carcinoma With Variant Histology and/or Sarcomatoid Features. J Clin Oncol 2020; 38(1):63–70.

15. McKay RR, Bosse D, Xie W, et al. The Clinical Activity of PD-1/PD-L1 Inhibitors in Metastatic Non-Clear Cell Renal Cell Carcinoma. Cancer Immunol Res 2018;6(7): 758–65.

16. Powles T, Larkin JMG, Patel P, et al. A phase II study investigating the safety and efficacy of savolitinib and durvalumab in metastatic papillary renal cancer (CALYPSO). J Clin Oncol 2019;37(7_suppl):545.

17. Vogelzang NJ, Olsen MR, McFarlane JJ, et al. Safety and Efficacy of Nivolumab in Patients With Advanced Non-Clear Cell Renal Cell Carcinoma: Results From the Phase IIIb/IV CheckMate 374 Study. Clin Genitourin Cancer 2020. https://doi.org/10.1016/j.clgc.2020.05.006.

18. Tykodi SS, Gordan LN, Alter RS, et al. Safety and efficacy of nivolumab plus ipilimumab in patients with advanced non-clear cell renal cell carcinoma: results from the phase 3b/4 CheckMate 920 trial. J Immunother Cancer 2022;10(2). https://doi.org/10.1136/jitc-2021-003844.

19. Pal SK, McGregor B, Suarez C, et al. Cabozantinib in Combination With Atezolizumab for Advanced Renal Cell Carcinoma: Results From the COSMIC-021 Study. J Clin Oncol 2021;39(33):3725–36.

20. Lee CH, Voss MH, Carlo MI, et al. Phase II Trial of Cabozantinib Plus Nivolumab in Patients With Non-Clear-Cell Renal Cell Carcinoma and Genomic Correlates. J Clin Oncol 2022;40(21):2333–41.

21. Graham J, Wells JC, Dudani S, et al. Outcomes of patients with advanced non-clear cell renal cell carcinoma treated with first-line immune checkpoint inhibitor therapy. Eur J Cancer 2022;171:124–32.

22. Albiges L, Pouessel D, Beylot-Barry M, et al. Nivolumab in metastatic nonclear cell renal cell carcinoma: First results of the AcSe prospective study. J Clin Oncol 2020;38(6_suppl):699.

23. Albiges L, Gurney HP, Atduev C, et al. Phase II KEYNOTE-B61 study of pembrolizumab (Pembro) + lenvatinib (Lenva) as first-line treatment for non-clear cell renal cell carcinoma (nccRCC). Ann Oncol 2022;33(suppl_7):S660–80.

24. Adashek JJ, Genovese G, Tannir NM, et al. Recent advancements in the treatment of metastatic clear cell renal cell carcinoma: A review of the evidence using second-generation p-values. Cancer Treat Res Commun 2020;23:100166.

25. Pal SK, Tangen C, Thompson IM Jr, et al. A comparison of sunitinib with cabozantinib, crizotinib, and savolitinib for treatment of advanced papillary renal cell

carcinoma: a randomised, open-label, phase 2 trial. Lancet (London, England) 2021;397(10275):695–703.

26. Rafi Z, Greenland S. Semantic and cognitive tools to aid statistical science: replace confidence and significance by compatibility and surprise. BMC Med Res Methodol 2020;20(1):244.

27. Campbell MT, Bilen MA, Shah AY, et al. Cabozantinib for the treatment of patients with metastatic non-clear cell renal cell carcinoma: A retrospective analysis. Eur J Cancer 2018;104:188–94.

28. Hutson TE, Michaelson MD, Kuzel TM, et al. A Single-arm, Multicenter, Phase 2 Study of Lenvatinib Plus Everolimus in Patients with Advanced Non-Clear Cell Renal Cell Carcinoma. Eur Urol 2021;80(2):162–70.

29. Wiele AJ, Bathala TK, Hahn AW, et al. Lenvatinib with or Without Everolimus in Patients with Metastatic Renal Cell Carcinoma After Immune Checkpoint Inhibitors and Vascular Endothelial Growth Factor Receptor-Tyrosine Kinase Inhibitor Therapies. Oncol 2021;26(6):476–82.

30. Srinivasan R, Gurram S, Harthy MA, et al. Results from a phase II study of bevacizumab and erlotinib in subjects with advanced hereditary leiomyomatosis and renal cell cancer (HLRCC) or sporadic papillary renal cell cancer. J Clin Oncol 2020;38(15_suppl):5004.

31. Pal SK, Bergerot P, Dizman N, et al. Responses to Alectinib in ALK-rearranged Papillary Renal Cell Carcinoma. Eur Urol 2018;74(1):124–8.

32. Ged Y, Chen YB, Knezevic A, et al. Metastatic Chromophobe Renal Cell Carcinoma: Presence or Absence of Sarcomatoid Differentiation Determines Clinical Course and Treatment Outcomes. Clin Genitourin Cancer 2019;17(3):e678–88.

33. Casuscelli J, Becerra MF, Seier K, et al. Chromophobe Renal Cell Carcinoma: Results From a Large Single-Institution Series. Clin Genitourin Cancer 2019;17(5): 373–379 e4.

34. Casuscelli J, Weinhold N, Gundem G, et al. Genomic landscape and evolution of metastatic chromophobe renal cell carcinoma. JCI Insight 2017;(12):2. https://doi.org/10.1172/jci.insight.92688.

35. Hahn AW, Lebenthal J, Genovese G, et al. The significance of sarcomatoid and rhabdoid dedifferentiation in renal cell carcinoma. Cancer Treat Res Commun 2022;33:100640. https://doi.org/10.1016/j.ctarc.2022.100640.

36. Martinez Chanza N, Xie W, Asim Bilen M, et al. Cabozantinib in advanced non-clear-cell renal cell carcinoma: a multicentre, retrospective, cohort study. Lancet Oncol 2019;20(4):581–90.

37. Zhang L, Hobeika CS, Khabibullin D, et al. Hypersensitivity to ferroptosis in chromophobe RCC is mediated by a glutathione metabolic dependency and cystine import via solute carrier family 7 member 11. Proc Natl Acad Sci U S A 2022; 119(28). e2122840119.

38. Srigley JR, Delahunt B, Eble JN, et al. The International Society of Urological Pathology (ISUP) Vancouver Classification of Renal Neoplasia. Am J Surg Pathol 2013;37(10):1469–89.

39. Tretiakova MS. Chameleon TFE3-translocation RCC and How Gene Partners Can Change Morphology: Accurate Diagnosis Using Contemporary Modalities. Adv Anat Pathol 2022;29(3):131–40.

40. Skala SL, Xiao H, Udager AM, et al. Detection of 6 TFEB-amplified renal cell carcinomas and 25 renal cell carcinomas with MITF translocations: systematic morphologic analysis of 85 cases evaluated by clinical TFE3 and TFEB FISH assays. Mod Pathol 2018;31(1):179–97.

41. Alhalabi O, Thouvenin J, Negrier S, et al. Immune Checkpoint Therapy Combinations in Adult Advanced MiT Family Translocation Renal Cell Carcinomas. Oncol 2023. https://doi.org/10.1093/oncolo/oyac262.

42. Boileve A, Carlo MI, Barthelemy P, et al. Immune checkpoint inhibitors in MITF family translocation renal cell carcinomas and genetic correlates of exceptional responders. J Immunother Cancer 2018;6(1):159.

43. Thouvenin J, Alhalabi O, Carlo M, et al. Efficacy of Cabozantinib in Metastatic MiT Family Translocation Renal Cell Carcinomas. Oncol 2022;27(12):1041–7.

44. Malouf GG, Camparo P, Oudard S, et al. Targeted agents in metastatic Xp11 translocation/TFE3 gene fusion renal cell carcinoma (RCC): a report from the Juvenile RCC Network. Ann Oncol 2010;21(9):1834–8.

45. Baniak N, Tsai H, Hirsch MS. The Differential Diagnosis of Medullary-Based Renal Masses. Arch Pathol Lab Med 2021;145(9):1148–70.

46. Linehan WM, Ricketts CJ. The Cancer Genome Atlas of renal cell carcinoma: findings and clinical implications. Nat Rev Urol 2019;16(9):539–52.

47. Skala SL, Dhanasekaran SM, Mehra R. Hereditary Leiomyomatosis and Renal Cell Carcinoma Syndrome (HLRCC): A Contemporary Review and Practical Discussion of the Differential Diagnosis for HLRCC-Associated Renal Cell Carcinoma. Arch Pathol Lab Med 2018;142(10):1202–15.

48. Gleeson JP, Nikolovski I, Dinatale R, et al. Comprehensive Molecular Characterization and Response to Therapy in Fumarate Hydratase-Deficient Renal Cell Carcinoma. Clin Cancer Res 2021;27(10):2910–9.

49. Mannan R, Wang X, Bawa PS, et al. Characterization of Protein (2SC) Succination as a Biomarker for Fumarate Hydratase-deficient Renal Cell Carcinoma. Hum Pathol 2022. https://doi.org/10.1016/j.humpath.2022.12.013.

50. Sun G, Zhang X, Liang J, et al. Integrated Molecular Characterization of Fumarate Hydratase-deficient Renal Cell Carcinoma. Clin Cancer Res 2021;27(6):1734–43.

51. Xu Y, Kong W, Cao M, et al. Genomic Profiling and Response to Immune Checkpoint Inhibition plus Tyrosine Kinase Inhibition in FH-Deficient Renal Cell Carcinoma. Eur Urol 2022. https://doi.org/10.1016/j.eururo.2022.05.029.

52. Carril-Ajuria L, Colomba E, Cerbone L, et al. Response to systemic therapy in fumarate hydratase-deficient renal cell carcinoma. Eur J Cancer 2021;151:106–14.

53. Msaouel P, Tannir NM, Walker CL. A Model Linking Sickle Cell Hemoglobinopathies and SMARCB1 Loss in Renal Medullary Carcinoma. Clin Cancer Res 2018;24(9):2044–9.

54. Shapiro DD, Soeung M, Perelli L, et al. Association of High-Intensity Exercise with Renal Medullary Carcinoma in Individuals with Sickle Cell Trait: Clinical Observations and Experimental Animal Studies. Cancers 2021;(23):13. https://doi.org/10.3390/cancers13236022.

55. Msaouel P, Malouf GG, Su X, et al. Comprehensive Molecular Characterization Identifies Distinct Genomic and Immune Hallmarks of Renal Medullary Carcinoma. Cancer Cell 2020;37(5):720–734 e13.

56. Shah AY, Karam JA, Malouf GG, et al. Management and outcomes of patients with renal medullary carcinoma: a multicentre collaborative study. BJU Int 2017;120(6):782–92.

57. Wiele AJ, Surasi DS, Rao P, et al. Efficacy and Safety of Bevacizumab Plus Erlotinib in Patients with Renal Medullary Carcinoma. Cancers 2021;13(9). https://doi.org/10.3390/cancers13092170.

58. Oudard S, Banu E, Vieillefond A, et al. Prospective multicenter phase II study of gemcitabine plus platinum salt for metastatic collecting duct carcinoma: results

of a GETUG (Groupe d'Etudes des Tumeurs Uro-Genitales) study. J Urol 2007; 177(5):1698–702.

59. Procopio G, Sepe P, Claps M, et al. Cabozantinib as First-line Treatment in Patients With Metastatic Collecting Duct Renal Cell Carcinoma: Results of the BONSAI Trial for the Italian Network for Research in Urologic-Oncology (Meet-URO 2 Study). JAMA Oncol 2022;8(6):910–3.

60. Pecuchet N, Bigot F, Gachet J, et al. Triple combination of bevacizumab, gemcitabine and platinum salt in metastatic collecting duct carcinoma. Ann Oncol 2013;24(12):2963–7.

61. Bronchud MH, Castillo S, Escriva de Romani S, et al. HER2 blockade in metastatic collecting duct carcinoma (CDC) of the kidney: a case report. Onkologie 2012; 35(12):776–9.

62. Selli C, Amorosi A, Vona G, et al. Retrospective evaluation of c-erbB-2 oncogene amplification using competitive PCR in collecting duct carcinoma of the kidney. J Urol 1997;158(1):245–7.

63. Wang J, Papanicolau-Sengos A, Chintala S, et al. Collecting duct carcinoma of the kidney is associated with CDKN2A deletion and SLC family gene up-regulation. Oncotarget 2016;7(21):29901–15.

64. Pal SK, Ali SM, Ross J, et al. Exceptional Response to Palbociclib in Metastatic Collecting Duct Carcinoma Bearing a CDKN2A Homozygous Deletion. JCO Precision Oncology 2017;1:1–5.

65. Chen YB, Xu J, Skanderup AJ, et al. Molecular analysis of aggressive renal cell carcinoma with unclassified histology reveals distinct subsets. Nat Commun 2016;7:13131.

66. Paintal A, Tjota MY, Wang P, et al. NF2-mutated Renal Carcinomas Have Common Morphologic Features Which Overlap With Biphasic Hyalinizing Psammomatous Renal Cell Carcinoma: A Comprehensive Study of 14 Cases. Am J Surg Pathol 2022;46(5):617–27.

67. Ali SM, Miller VA, Ross JS, et al. Exceptional Response on Addition of Everolimus to Taxane in Urothelial Carcinoma Bearing an NF2 Mutation. Eur Urol 2015;67(6): 1195–6.

68. Lopez-Lago MA, Okada T, Murillo MM, et al. Loss of the tumor suppressor gene NF2, encoding merlin, constitutively activates integrin-dependent mTORC1 signaling. Mol Cell Biol 2009;29(15):4235–49.

69. Pal SK, Choueiri TK, Wang K, et al. Characterization of Clinical Cases of Collecting Duct Carcinoma of the Kidney Assessed by Comprehensive Genomic Profiling. Eur Urol 2016;70(3):516–21.

70. Morris ZS, McClatchey AI. Aberrant epithelial morphology and persistent epidermal growth factor receptor signaling in a mouse model of renal carcinoma. Proc Natl Acad Sci U S A 2009;106(24):9767–72.

71. Blum KA, Gupta S, Tickoo SK, et al. Sarcomatoid renal cell carcinoma: biology, natural history and management. Nat Rev Urol 2020;17(12):659–78.

72. Keskin SK, Msaouel P, Hess KR, et al. Outcomes of Patients with Renal Cell Carcinoma and Sarcomatoid Dedifferentiation Treated with Nephrectomy and Systemic Therapies: Comparison between the Cytokine and Targeted Therapy Eras. J Urol 2017;198(3):530–7.

73. Michaelson MD, McKay RR, Werner L, et al. Phase 2 trial of sunitinib and gemcitabine in patients with sarcomatoid and/or poor-risk metastatic renal cell carcinoma. Cancer 2015;121(19):3435–43.

74. Kawakami F, Sircar K, Rodriguez-Canales J, et al. Programmed cell death ligand 1 and tumor-infiltrating lymphocyte status in patients with renal cell carcinoma and sarcomatoid dedifferentiation. Cancer 2017;123(24):4823–31.

75. Kiyozawa D, Takamatsu D, Kohashi K, et al. Programmed death ligand 1/indoleamine 2,3-dioxygenase 1 expression and tumor-infiltrating lymphocyte status in renal cell carcinoma with sarcomatoid changes and rhabdoid features. Hum Pathol 2020;101:31–9.

76. Tannir NM, Signoretti S, Choueiri TK, et al. Efficacy and Safety of Nivolumab Plus Ipilimumab versus Sunitinib in First-line Treatment of Patients with Advanced Sarcomatoid Renal Cell Carcinoma. Clin Cancer Res 2021;27(1):78–86.

77. Schvartsman G, Carneiro A, Filippi RZ, et al. Rapid Deep Responses With Nivolumab Plus Ipilimumab in Papillary Renal Cell Carcinoma With Sarcomatoid Dedifferentiation. Clin Genitourin Cancer 2019;17(4):315–8.

78. Msaouel P, Lee J, Karam JA, et al. A Causal Framework for Making Individualized Treatment Decisions in Oncology. Cancers 2022;(16):14. https://doi.org/10.3390/cancers14163923.

79. Subbiah V. The next generation of evidence-based medicine. Nat Med 2023; 29(1):49–58.

Toxicity Management of Systemic Kidney Cancer Therapies

Qian Qin, MD[a,b], Ellen Nein, MD[a], Andrea Flaten[a,b], Tian Zhang, MD, MHS[a,b],*

KEYWORDS

- Renal cell carcinoma • Adverse events • Toxicity management
- Immune-related adverse events

KEY POINTS

- As a class vascular endothelial growth factor receptor-tyrosine kinase inhibitors commonly cause adverse events (AEs) include fatigue, hypertension, delayed wound healing, hand-foot syndrome, mucositis, nausea, diarrhea, and elevation in liver function enzymes, thyroid dysfunction, and cytopenias. Most of these AEs can be managed with treatment interruption and dose reduction.
- Immune checkpoint inhibitors have improved outcomes for metastatic renal cell carcinoma; common adverse reactions include rashes, diarrhea/colitis, endocrinopathies, and rarer ones such as pneumonitis, myocarditis, myasthenia gravis—which can be severe and life-threatening if not recognized early and treated.
- Hypoxia inducible factor-2a inhibitors are also now approved for von Hippel–Lindau syndrome patients with clear cell renal cell carcinoma and other tumor types; on-target toxicities include hypoxia and anemia and can also be managed.
- Treatment toxicities must be managed early and well to result in the most efficacy for that particular treatment.

BACKGROUND ON METASTATIC RENAL CELL CARCINOMA AND RELEVANCE OF TOPIC

Multiple systemic therapies are available for the treatment of metastatic renal cell carcinoma (mRCC), including mammalian target of rapamycin (mTOR), vascular endothelial growth factor receptor-tyrosine kinase inhibitors (VEGFR-TKIs), immune checkpoint inhibitors (ICIs), and combination regimens incorporating ICI/ICI or ICI/VEGFR-TKI.

[a] Division of Hematology and Oncology, Department of Internal Medicine, UT Southwestern Medical Center, 5323 Harry Hines Boulevard, Dallas, TX 75390-8852, USA; [b] Harold C. Simmons Comprehensive Cancer Center
* Corresponding author. University of Texas Southwestern Medical Center, 5323 Harry Hines Boulevard, Dallas, TX 75390-8852.
E-mail address: tian.zhang@utsouthwestern.edu

Hematol Oncol Clin N Am 37 (2023) 993–1003
https://doi.org/10.1016/j.hoc.2023.05.006
0889-8588/23/© 2023 Elsevier Inc. All rights reserved.

Most recently, the hypoxia inducible factor 2α (HIF2 α) inhibitor, belzutifan, showed excellent clinical activity in patients with von Hippel–Lindau hereditary syndrome with tumor types including clear cell renal cell carcinoma (ccRCC) and is in active investigation for patients with sporadic ccRCC.[1–8] Each therapy and combination has associated short-term and/or long-term toxicities that can impact patients' quality of life, and some have overlapping toxicities that pose management challenges. The authors provide an overview of potential toxicities and management strategies for ccRCC therapy-associated toxicities.

SMALL MOLECULE INHIBITORS OF VASCULAR ENDOTHELIAL GROWTH FACTOR RECEPTORS AND MAMMALIAN TARGET OF RAPAMYCIN

VEGFR-TKIs and mTOR inhibitors have improved clinical outcomes for mRCC. Common adverse events (AEs) of VEGFR-TKI and mTOR inhibitors are often class effects (**Table 1**), severity is generally graded per Common Terminology Criteria for Adverse Events (CTCAE), and management depends on type, severity, and recovery from the AE.[9–11]

One of the most common class effect of VEGFR-TKIs is hypertension, with systematic reviews and meta-analyses indicating incidence of all-grade hypertension in the 20% to 40% range; a minority of patients present with severe hypertension (approximately 5%–10%).[12–18] Treatment of hypertension should follow the Cardiovascular Toxicities Panel recommendations for risk assessment, monitoring, and management of blood pressure with an ideal goal of keeping blood pressure less than 130/80 mm Hg.[19] Specifically, oral antihypertensives should be started in patients who develop stage 1 hypertension (140/90) or those who have an increase in diastolic blood pressure by more than 20 mm Hg from baseline. Preferred agents are dependent on organ function and comorbidities. For persistent uncontrolled hypertension (defined as > 140/90 despite optimal medical management or hypertensive urgency or emergency), VEGFR-TKIs should be held. On the resolution of symptoms with controlled blood pressures, dose reduction of the VEGFR-TKI should be pursued with discontinuation considered based on the severity of the event. Other less common, but potentially more life-threatening, cardiovascular complications of VEGFR-TKIs include arterial/venous thromboembolism, heart failure, aortic dissection/aneurysms, delayed wound healing/fistula formation, and bleeding.[20,21] Threshold to reintroduce the VEGFR-TKI should be considered cautiously in selected cases if the patient is deriving significant benefit from the drug.

Another common side effect of VEGFR-TKIs is proteinuria (20%–60% depending on trial), although nephrotic range (>3.5 g/24 hours) or nephrotic syndrome is uncommon (<10%).[22] Baseline and periodic urinalysis for urine protein creatinine ratio (UPCR) should be performed. Evidence-based guideline for the management of asymptomatic proteinuria is lacking, though in general, the VEGFR-TKI can be continued for UPCR less than 1 mg/mg. For UPCR greater than 1 and less than 3.5 mg/mg, confirmatory 24-hour protein assessment should be considered. VEGFR-TKI can be continued for UCPR less than 2 mg/mg and/or 24-hour urine less than 2 g/24 hour, whereas dose interruption and subsequent dose reduction at reinitiation should be considered for UCPR greater than 2 mg/mg and/or 24-hour urine greater than 2 g/24 hour. For UPCR greater than 3.5 mg/mg, the VEGFR-TKI should be held until UPCR decreases to less than 2 mg/mg and restarted at a reduced dose with close monitoring. For any patient who develops nephrotic syndrome (proteinuria > 3.5 grams per day in combination with hypoalbuminemia, peripheral edema, with or without hyperlipidemia), consider discontinuation of the VEGFR-TKI.[23,24]

Table 1
Common and uncommon but significant toxicities associated with vascular endothelial growth factor receptor-tyrosine kinase inhibitors, mammalian target of rapamycin inhibitors, and ICI therapies

Organ/System Affected by AEs	VEGFR-TKI	ICI Therapies	mTOR Inhibitor
Nervous system or systemic	Fatigue, headache, weight loss, reversible posterior leukoencephalopathy syndrome	Fatigue, infusion reaction, peripheral neuropathy, aseptic meningitis/encephalitis, transverse myelitis, myasthenia gravis, reversible posterior leukoencephalopathy syndrome, Guillain–Barre syndrome	Fatigue
Cardiovascular	HTN (including hypertensive crisis), heart failure, peripheral edema, thromboembolism	Myocarditis, pericarditis, vasculitis, arrythmias, heart failure	HTN, peripheral edema
Dermatologic	HFS, xeroderma	Severity varies from inflammatory skin reactions (pruritis, vitiligo, skin rash) to immunobullous disease (bullous pemphigoid) and cutaneous drug reaction (such as Steven–Johnson syndrome, toxic epidermal necrolysis)	Pruritis, skin rash, xeroderma, acne vulgaris, nail changes, HFS
Endocrine/metabolic	Thyroid dysfunction, electrolyte changes, hypoglycemia	Hypo/hyperthyroidism, Hypophysitis, adrenocortical insufficiency (primary and secondary, including adrenal crisis), type 1 diabetes mellitus (including diabetic ketoacidosis), electrolyte changes	Diabetes mellitus, electrolyte changes, hyperlipidemia
Gastrointestinal/mucosal	Anorexia, nausea/vomiting, abdominal pain, diarrhea, stomatitis/mucositis, elevation in amylase/lipase (including overt pancreatitis)	Colitis, stomatitis	Nausea/vomiting, abdominal pain, diarrhea/constipation, stomatitis/mucositis, gastroenteritis
Hematologic	Myelosuppression/cytopenias, bleeding	Severity varies from mild, asymptomatic cytopenias to immune-mediated toxicities such as ITP, AIHA, acquired hemophilia, DIC	cytopenias

(continued on next page)

Table 1
(continued)

Organ/ System Affected by AEs	VEGFR-TKI	ICI Therapies	mTOR Inhibitor
Hepatic	Liver enzyme elevation, liver dysfunction	Hepatitis	Liver enzyme elevation, liver dysfunction
Musculoskeletal	Arthralgia, myalgia, muscle spasm, asthenia, osteonecrosis of the jaw	Arthralgia, myalgia, asthenia, immune-mediated rheumatologic manifestations (such as myositis, inflammatory arthritis)	Arthralgia, myalgia, muscle spasm, asthenia
Pulmonary	Cough, dyspnea	pneumonitis	Cough, dyspnea, pneumonitis/ pulmonary disease, nasopharyngitis, epistaxis
Renal	Elevation in serum creatinine, proteinuria (including nephrotic syndrome)	Elevation in serum creatinine, nephritis	Elevation in serum creatinine, proteinuria
Others	Delayed wound healing, intestinal perforation/fistula formation	Ophthalmic toxicity (such as uveitis, dry eye syndrome, ocular myasthenia, optic neuritis)	Delayed wound healing, ocular (conjunctivitis, eyelid edema), reproductive endocrine dysfunction (such as gonadal dysfunction in men and menstrual disturbances in women)

Abbreviations: AIHA, autoimmune hemolytic anemia; AE, adverse event; DIC, disseminated intravascular coagulation; HFS, hand-foot syndrome; HTN, hypertension; ICI, immune checkpoint inhibitor; irAEs, immune-related adverse events; ITP, immune thrombocytopenia; mTOR, mammalian target of rapamycin; VEGFR-TKI, vascular endothelial growth factor receptor-tyrosine kinase inhibitors.

HFS caused by VEGFR-TKIs differs from HFS caused by cytotoxic chemotherapy with focal hyperkeratotic, callous such as lesions on hands and feet rather than diffuse erythema. Treatment includes topical urea, topical steroids, topical analgesics, and oral analgesics.[25,26] Grade 3 HFS interfering with daily activity require VEGFR-TKI therapy interruption and reintroduction at lower dose once symptoms improve.

mTOR is a regulator of signaling pathways in the increased metabolic (lipid and glucose metabolism) and angiogenic needs of RCC. mTOR inhibition through everolimus is often combined with a VEGFR-TKI (lenvatinib) in contemporary treatment of mRCC with both distinct and overlapping toxicities (see **Table 1**).[27,28] Particularly, stomatitis/mucositis are common, overlapping AEs. For mild stomatitis/mucositis (grade 1), dose reduction or cessation is not recommended. Treatment interruption should be considered for grade 2 or higher stomatitis/mucositis. Avoiding spicy foods and using mouthwashes that contain topical corticosteroids, nonsteroidal anti-inflammatory drugs, and/or anesthetics may help alleviate symptoms. Other overlapping toxicities of VEGFR-TKI and mTOR inhibitor, such as hypertension and proteinuria, should be managed in a similar fashion as detailed above.

Pneumonitis is a potential complication of mTOR inhibitors not usually seen with VEGFR-TKIs. Presentation can range from asymptomatic with ground-glass opacities/focal consolidation on imaging to pulmonary symptoms including cough, exertional dyspnea, respiratory distress, and hypoxia.[28] For grade 1 toxicity, continuing treatment with monitoring is appropriate. For grade greater than 2 toxicity, corticosteroid could be considered. For grade 2 to 3 toxicity, consider drug interruption until symptom improvement to grade less than 1 and reinitiate at a reduced dose; for grade 4 toxicity, consider permanent discontinuation of therapy.[29]

IMMUNE CHECKPOINT INHIBITORS

Although significant clinical benefits have been observed, ICIs also carry unique spectrum of side effects known as immune-related adverse events (irAEs).[30] Class effect is observed across ICIs, with manifestations likely a result of general immunologic enhancement across organ systems (see **Table 1**).[30] Data suggest anti-cytotoxic T-lymphocyte antigen 4 therapy may result in higher incidence or severity of irAEs when compared with anti-programmed cell death 1 /PD-L1 therapies.[30,31] Although most irAEs are reversible and resolve with time and supportive treatment, some can be fatal. Endocrinopathies usually require lifelong treatment with hormone replacement or suppressive therapy.[30-32]

Recommendations for the management of irAEs are detailed by the American Society of Clinical Oncology and the Society of Immunotherapy of Cancer guidelines.[33-35] In general, with grade 1 toxicity, ICI therapy should be continued, and treatment is supportive. In cases of grade 2 toxicity, ICI therapy should be held until symptoms or toxicity is grade 1 or less. In cases of grade 3 or 4 toxicity, permanent discontinuation of ICI should be considered. Systemic steroids should be prescribed for patients with grade 2 (prednisone 0.5 mg/kg/day or equivalent) or grade 3 or 4 (prednisone 1–2 mg/kg/day or equivalent) toxicities. For refractory cases, additional immunosuppressive agents, such as infliximab, vedolizumab, and mycophenolate mofetil should be administered. Consultation with specialists should also be considered for grade 2 or higher and/or persistent/worsening toxicities.

ICIs can cause life-altering endocrinopathy AEs, involving the pituitary, thyroid, pancreas, and/or adrenal glands.[36] Patients often present with nonspecific symptoms, and high levels of clinical suspicion are required. Manifestations include thyroiditis/hyperthyroidism followed by hypothyroidism, hypophysitis, adrenal insufficiency, and/or type I diabetes mellitus. Endocrine replacement therapy is the mainstay treatment approach (levothyroxine, hydrocortisone, and/or insulin). Except for adrenal crisis or pituitary compressive symptoms, glucocorticoids (and other immunosuppressive agents) are usually not indicated.

Less common but potentially severe or fatal complications of ICI therapy include cardiovascular (such as myocarditis, pericarditis, heart failure, arrythmias, vasculitis), neurologic (such as Guillain–Barre syndrome and myasthenia gravis) and hematologic (such as immune thrombocytopenic purpura and autoimmune hemolytic anemia) toxicities. Early detection and management, often in the hospital setting in consultation with specialists, are warranted to optimize immunosuppression/supportive measures and aid recovery.[33–35] Often these toxicities require permanent discontinuation of the ICI.

IMMUNE CHECKPOINT INHIBITOR/VASCULAR ENDOTHELIAL GROWTH FACTOR RECEPTOR-TYROSINE KINASE INHIBITOR COMBINATION THERAPIES

Toxicities of ICI/VEGFR-TKI are usually reflective of the AEs of individual drugs with grade $\geq$ 3 AEs occurring in 50% to 70% of patients treated with combination regimens.[37–50] Although no overt, synergistic toxicities, overlapping toxicities can make management a challenge. These include AEs such as dermatologic reactions, diarrhea, fatigue, thyroid disorder, and hepatic toxicities (**Fig. 1**; see **Table 1**).[23]

Onset and specific symptoms may cue to the culprit drug. For example, the dermatologic AE associated with VEGFR-TKI is most often HFS, where supportive management with or without drug interruption/dose reduction is usually sufficient.[25,26] Conversely, dermatologic AEs associated with ICI are immune-mediated with a spectrum of manifestation and severity (from pruritis to life-threatening AEs such as Stevens–Johnson syndrome and toxic epidermal necrolysis).[31] For renal toxicities, VEGFR-TKIs cause proteinuria, whereas ICIs cause nephritis with differing clinical symptoms and laboratory abnormalities.

In other cases, such as fatigue, diarrhea, and liver enzyme elevation, differentiation is a challenge and holding of one or both agents with or without the addition of immunosuppressive therapy may be indicated.[23] Focusing on diarrhea, diarrhea associated

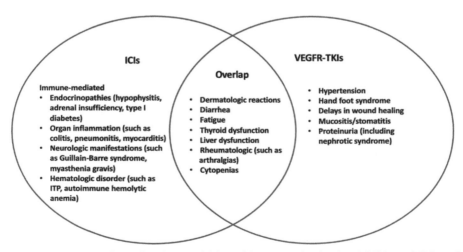

Fig. 1. Common and overlapping toxicities of immune checkpoint inhibitors (ICIs) and vascular endothelial growth factor receptor-tyrosine kinase inhibitors (VEGFR-TKIs).

with VEGFR-TKIs tend to occur early (within weeks), have a gradual onset, and associated with small frequent stools, whereas colitis associated with ICIs tends to occur later with more sudden onset and large-volume watery stools.[51] If the causative agent cannot be determined and patient experiences grade greater than 2 toxicities, consider holding both agents; rapid resolution of symptoms (within 1–2 weeks, without corticosteroid) suggests VEGFR-TKI as the offending agent, whereas persistent diarrhea suggests that colitis and initiation of corticosteroid should be considered. For non-several diarrhea, consider corticosteroids that are locally absorbed, such as budesonide. Rule out infectious causes and consulting gastroenterology for endoscopic workup are also important in the management paradigm. Similarly, for grade greater than 2 liver enzyme elevation, consider holding both agents until improvement to grade less than 1. If liver enzyme elevation persists beyond 2 weeks, consider ICI as the likely cause and initiate appropriate immunosuppressive therapy. Fatigue is a common AE both VEGFR-TKIs and ICIs, but often mild with no intervention needed. However, endocrinopathies should be ruled out.

In general, when managing toxicities in this setting, both agents can likely be continued for grade 1 toxicity. If tolerable grade 2 toxicities occur, most consensus statements support holding VEGFR-TKI therapy initially. If symptoms do not improve or stabilize off the TKI, this is concerning for an irAE and appropriate immunosuppressive therapy (such as corticosteroid) should be initiated while holding the ICI. If intolerable grade 2, grade 3 or 4 toxicity develops, consider holding both VEGFR-TKI and ICI treatments and initiating appropriate immunosuppressive therapy. Reintroduction of one or both should occur in a stepwise approach.

HYPOXIA-INDUCIBLE FACTOR-2ALPHA INHIBITORS

From a toxicity perspective, belzutifan, the first approved HIF2α, in RCC, exhibits a favorable safety profile, with anemia, fatigue, and headache, dizziness, and nausea being the most common AEs; the majority were grades 1 and 2.[7] An intriguing AE is hypoxia, which usually resolves with dose interruption. Mechanisms of hypoxia remain obscure with one study suggesting impaired ventilatory responses to hypoxia and potential involvement of the carotid physiology.[52] Similar to the management of other drug-induced toxicities, AEs should be graded per CTCAE and managed per type, severity, and respective guidelines. Of note, anemia can be significant (due to on-target inhibition of erythropoietin [EPO] gene), managed with belzutifan dose interruption/reduction, addition of erythropoietin mimetics, and/or blood transfusion.

CONCLUDING REMARKS

Optimal approaches on toxicity management should consider the type of drug, severity of AE, available supportive and therapeutic options, and consultation with organ-specific experts for rare and/or severe AEs. Ultimately, the goal is managing toxicities to minimize disruption on patients' quality of life while maximizing drug exposure and optimizing therapeutic efficacy.

CLINICS CARE POINTS

- As treatments for metastatic renal cell carcinoma expand with both antiangiogenic and immune checkpoint inhibitor therapies, prompt and appropriate management of toxicities is particularly important.

- Common toxicities of anti-VEGF targeting therapies include hypertension, palmar-plantar erythrodysesthesia, diarrhea, and stomatitis. Common immune-mediated toxicities include rashes, diarrhea, hepatitis, pneumonitis, and endocrinopathies. Overlapping toxicities of rashes, diarrhea, and elevation of liver enzymes/hepatitis should be managed by early hold of anti-VEGF therapies and adding steroids early for the right patient population.

- Of note for severe immune-mediated toxicities, steroid doses of prednisone equivalent 1 to 2 mg/kg daily are generally recommended, and disease-modifying agents are subsequently given if high-dose steroids are not effective in controlling adverse events.

DISCLOSURE

Q Qin reports consulting for Exelixis and MJH Associates. T Zhang reports the following: Research funding: Novartis, Switzerland, Merck, United States, Regeneron, United States, Mirati Therapeutics, United States, Janssen, United States, AstraZeneca, Pfizer, United States, Astellas, Eli Lilly & Co, United States, and Tempus; Advisory/Consulting fees: Merck, Exelixis, Sanofi-Aventis, BMS, Janssen, Astra Zeneca, United States, Pfizer, Amgen, Pharmacyclics, SeaGen, QED Therapeutics, Eisai, Aveo, Eli Lilly, Bayer, Aravive, Caris, MJH Associates, Vaniam, Aptitude Health, and Peerview. E. Nein and A. Flaten have no disclosures.

REFERENCES

1. Rogers JL, Bayeh L, Scheuermann TH, et al. Development of inhibitors of the PAS-B domain of the HIF-2alpha transcription factor. J Med Chem 2013;56(4):1739–47.
2. Scheuermann TH, Li Q, Ma HW, et al. Allosteric inhibition of hypoxia inducible factor-2 with small molecules. Nat Chem Biol 2013;9(4):271–6.
3. Wallace EM, Rizzi JP, Han G, et al. A small-molecule antagonist of HIF2alpha is efficacious in preclinical models of renal cell carcinoma. Cancer Res 2016;76(18):5491–500.
4. Courtney KD, Infante JR, Lam ET, et al. Phase I dose-escalation trial of PT2385, a first-in-class hypoxia-inducible factor-2alpha antagonist in patients with previously treated advanced clear cell renal cell carcinoma. J Clin Oncol 2018;36(9):867–74.
5. Xu R, Wang K, Rizzi JP, et al. 3-[(1S,2S,3R)-2,3-Difluoro-1-hydroxy-7-methylsulfonylindan-4-yl]oxy-5-fluorobenzo nitrile (PT2977), a hypoxia-inducible factor 2alpha (HIF-2alpha) inhibitor for the treatment of clear cell renal cell carcinoma. J Med Chem 2019;62(15):6876–93.
6. Choueiri TK, Bauer TM, Papadopoulos KP, et al. Inhibition of hypoxia-inducible factor-2alpha in renal cell carcinoma with belzutifan: a phase 1 trial and biomarker analysis. Nat Med 2021;27(5):802–5.
7. Jonasch E, Donskov F, Iliopoulos O, et al. Belzutifan for renal cell carcinoma in von Hippel-Lindau disease. N Engl J Med 2021;385(22):2036–46.
8. Iacovelli R, Arduini D, Ciccarese C, et al. Targeting hypoxia-inducible factor pathways in sporadic and Von Hippel-Lindau syndrome-related kidney cancers. Crit Rev Oncol Hematol 2022;176:103750.
9. Eskens FA, Verweij J. The clinical toxicity profile of vascular endothelial growth factor (VEGF) and vascular endothelial growth factor receptor (VEGFR) targeting angiogenesis inhibitors; a review. Eur J Cancer 2006;42(18):3127–39.
10. Master SR, Findakly D. Toxicities of anti-VEGF therapies used in metastatic renal cell carcinoma: a real-world experience. J Clin Oncol 2022;40(16_suppl):e16533.

11. Hayman SR, Leung N, Grande JP, et al. VEGF inhibition, hypertension, and renal toxicity. Curr Oncol Rep 2012;14(4):285–94.
12. Sica DA. Angiogenesis inhibitors and hypertension: an emerging. J Clin Oncol 2006;24(9):1329–31.
13. Izzedine H, Ederhy S, Goldwasser F, et al. Management of hypertension in angiogenesis inhibitor-treated patients. Ann Oncol 2009;20(5):807–15.
14. Liu B, Ding F, Liu Y, et al. Incidence and risk of hypertension associated with vascular endothelial growth factor receptor tyrosine kinase inhibitors in cancer patients: a comprehensive network meta-analysis of 72 randomized controlled trials involving 30013 patients. Oncotarget 2016;7(41):67661–73.
15. Zhu X, Stergiopoulos K, Wu S. Risk of hypertension and renal dysfunction with an angiogenesis inhibitor sunitinib: systematic review and meta-analysis. Acta Oncol 2009;48(1):9–17.
16. Wu S, Chen JJ, Kudelka A, et al. Incidence and risk of hypertension with sorafenib in patients with cancer: a systematic review and meta-analysis. Lancet Oncol 2008;9(2):117–23.
17. Qi WX, Lin F, Sun YJ, et al. Incidence and risk of hypertension with pazopanib in patients with cancer: a meta-analysis. Cancer Chemother Pharmacol 2013;71(2):431–9.
18. Rini BI, Escudier B, Tomczak P, et al. Comparative effectiveness of axitinib versus sorafenib in advanced renal cell carcinoma (AXIS): a randomised phase 3 trial. Lancet 2011;378(9807):1931–9.
19. Maitland ML, Bakris GL, Black HR, et al. Initial assessment, surveillance, and management of blood pressure in patients receiving vascular endothelial growth factor signaling pathway inhibitors. J Natl Cancer Inst 2010;102(9):596–604.
20. Abdel-Qadir H, Ethier JL, Lee DS, et al. Cardiovascular toxicity of angiogenesis inhibitors in treatment of malignancy: a systematic review and meta-analysis. Cancer Treat Rev 2017;53:120–7.
21. Totzeck M, Mincu RI, Mrotzek S, et al. Cardiovascular diseases in patients receiving small molecules with anti-vascular endothelial growth factor activity: A meta-analysis of approximately 29,000 cancer patients. Eur J Prev Cardiol 2018;25(5):482–94.
22. Izzedine H, Massard C, Spano JP, et al. VEGF signalling inhibition-induced proteinuria: Mechanisms, significance and management. Eur J Cancer 2010;46(2):439–48.
23. McGregor B, Mortazavi A, Cordes L, et al. Management of adverse events associated with cabozantinib plus nivolumab in renal cell carcinoma: a review. Cancer Treat Rev 2022;103:102333.
24. Exelixis, Inc. Cabometyx (cabozantinib) package insert. U.S. Food and Drug Administration. Available at: https://www.accessdata.fda.gov/drugsatfda_docs/label/2021/208692s010lbl.pdf. Revised Janurary 2021. Accessed April 30, 2023.
25. McLellan B, Ciardiello F, Lacouture ME, et al. Regorafenib-associated hand-foot skin reaction: practical advice on diagnosis, prevention, and management. Ann Oncol 2015;26(10):2017–26.
26. Lacouture ME, Wu S, Robert C, et al. Evolving strategies for the management of hand-foot skin reaction associated with the multitargeted kinase inhibitors sorafenib and sunitinib. Oncol 2008;13(9):1001–11.
27. Motzer RJ, Hutson TE, Glen H, et al. Lenvatinib, everolimus, and the combination in patients with metastatic renal cell carcinoma: a randomised, phase 2, open-label, multicentre trial. Lancet Oncol 2015;16(15):1473–82.

28. Kaplan B, Qazi Y, Wellen JR. Strategies for the management of adverse events associated with mTOR inhibitors. Transplant Rev 2014;28(3):126–33.

29. White DA, Camus P, Endo M, et al. Noninfectious pneumonitis after everolimus therapy for advanced renal cell carcinoma. Am J Respir Crit Care Med 2010; 182(3):396–403.

30. Naidoo J, Page DB, Li BT, et al. Toxicities of the anti-PD-1 and anti-PD-L1 immune checkpoint antibodies. Ann Oncol 2016;27(7):1362.

31. Geisler AN, Phillips GS, Barrios DM, et al. Immune checkpoint inhibitor-related dermatologic adverse events. J Am Acad Dermatol 2020;83(5):1255–68.

32. Wang DY, Salem JE, Cohen JV, et al. Fatal toxic effects associated with immune checkpoint inhibitors: a systematic review and meta-analysis. JAMA Oncol 2018; 4(12):1721–8.

33. Schneider BJ, Naidoo J, Santomasso BD, et al. Management of immune-related adverse events in patients treated with immune checkpoint inhibitor therapy: ASCO guideline update. J Clin Oncol 2021;39(36):4073–126.

34. Schneider BJ, Lacchetti C, Bollin K. Management of the Top 10 most common immune-related adverse events in patients treated with immune checkpoint inhibitor therapy. JCO Oncol Pract 2022;18(6):431–44.

35. Available at: https://www.sitcancer.org/research/cancer-immunotherapy-guide lines. Society for Immunotherapy of Cancer (SITC) Cancer Immunotherapy Guide lines.(Accessed on January 10, 2022).

36. Barroso-Sousa R, Barry WT, Garrido-Castro AC, et al. incidence of endocrine dysfunction following the use of different immune checkpoint inhibitor regimens: a systematic review and meta-analysis. JAMA Oncol 2018;4(2):173–82.

37. Motzer RJ, Tannir NM, McDermott DF, et al. Nivolumab plus ipilimumab versus sunitinib in advanced renal-cell carcinoma. N Engl J Med 2018;378(14):1277–90.

38. Motzer RJ, Rini BI, McDermott DF, et al. Nivolumab plus ipilimumab versus suni-tinib in first-line treatment for advanced renal cell carcinoma: extended follow-up of efficacy and safety results from a randomised, controlled, phase 3 trial. Lancet Oncol 2019;20(10):1370–85.

39. Albiges L, Tannir NM, Burotto M, et al. Nivolumab plus ipilimumab versus sunitinib for first-line treatment of advanced renal cell carcinoma: extended 4-year follow-up of the phase III CheckMate 214 trial. ESMO Open 2020;5(6):e001079.

40. Rini BI, Plimack ER, Stus V, et al. Pembrolizumab plus axitinib versus sunitinib for advanced renal-cell carcinoma. N Engl J Med 2019;380(12):1116–27.

41. Motzer RJ, Penkov K, Haanen J, et al. Avelumab plus axitinib versus sunitinib for advanced renal-cell carcinoma. N Engl J Med 2019;380(12):1103–15.

42. Powles T, Plimack ER, Soulieres D, et al. Pembrolizumab plus axitinib versus su-nitinib monotherapy as first-line treatment of advanced renal cell carcinoma (KEY-NOTE-426): extended follow-up from a randomised, open-label, phase 3 trial. Lancet Oncol 2020;21(12):1563–73.

43. Motzer R, Alekseev B, Rha SY, et al. Lenvatinib plus Pembrolizumab or Everoli-mus for Advanced Renal Cell Carcinoma. N Engl J Med 2021;384(14):1289–300.

44. Motzer RJ, Robbins PB, Powles T, et al. Avelumab plus axitinib versus sunitinib in advanced renal cell carcinoma: biomarker analysis of the phase 3 JAVELIN Renal 101 trial. Nat Med 2020;26(11):1733–41.

45. Choueiri TK, Motzer RJ, Rini BI, et al. Updated efficacy results from the JAVELIN Renal 101 trial: first-line avelumab plus axitinib versus sunitinib in patients with advanced renal cell carcinoma. Ann Oncol 2020;31(8):1030–9.

46. Choueiri TK, Powles T, Burotto M, et al. Nivolumab plus cabozantinib versus su-nitinib for advanced renal-cell carcinoma. N Engl J Med 2021;384(9):829–41.

47. Rini BI, Plimack ER, Stus V, et al. Pembrolizumab (pembro) plus axitinib (axi) versus sunitinib as first-line therapy for advanced clear cell renal cell carcinoma (ccRCC): Results from 42-month follow-up of KEYNOTE-426. J Clin Oncol 2021; 39(15_suppl):4500.
48. Motzer RJ, Choueiri TK, Powles T, et al. Nivolumab + cabozantinib (NIVO+CABO) versus sunitinib (SUN) for advanced renal cell carcinoma (aRCC): Outcomes by sarcomatoid histology and updated trial results with extended follow-up of Check-Mate 9ER. J Clin Oncol 2021;39(6_suppl):308.
49. Apolo AB, Powles T, Burotto M, et al. Nivolumab plus cabozantinib (N+C) versus sunitinib (S) for advanced renal cell carcinoma (aRCC): Outcomes by baseline disease characteristics in the phase 3 CheckMate 9ER trial. J Clin Oncol 2021; 39(15_suppl):4553.
50. Choueiri TK, Eto M, Kopyltsov E, et al. Phase III CLEAR trial in advanced renal cell carcinoma (aRCC): Outcomes in subgroups and toxicity update. Ann Oncol 2021;32(suppl_5):S678–724.
51. Apolo AB, Nadal R, Girardi DM, et al. Phase I study of cabozantinib and nivolumab alone or with ipilimumab for advanced or metastatic urothelial carcinoma and other genitourinary tumors. J Clin Oncol 2020;38(31):3672–84.
52. Cheng X, Prange-Barczynska M, Fielding JW, et al. Marked and rapid effects of pharmacological HIF-2alpha antagonism on hypoxic ventilatory control. J Clin Invest 2020;130(5):2237–51.

Management of Brain Metastases in Metastatic Renal Cell Carcinoma

Elshad Hasanov, MD, PhD[a],*, Eric Jonasch, MD[b],*

KEYWORDS

- Renal cell carcinoma • Brain metastasis • Stereotactic radiosurgery • Craniotomy
- Immune checkpoint inhibitors

KEY POINTS

- The authors recommend early brain MRI screening at the time of localized disease diagnosis in patients with neurologic symptoms and metastatic disease diagnosis even in the absence of neurologic symptoms.
- Multidisciplinary management must be the foundation of care for patients with renal cell carcinoma (RCC) brain metastases at every major decision-making point, including the decision to initiate systemic therapy alone with close monitoring, central nervous system (CNS) radiation, or surgery.
- The algorithms described in this article for how to approach single or multiple RCC brain metastases are based on international consensus and are recommended for use in guiding individualized patient care.
- The inclusion of patients with untreated RCC brain metastases and no CNS symptoms in clinical trials testing novel RCC agents will aid in the identification of effective agents at an earlier stage of drug development.

INTRODUCTION

The presence of brain metastases is a poor prognostic feature in metastatic renal cell carcinoma (mRCC) even in the era of immunotherapy.[1–3] In older studies of mRCC, brain metastases were reported to have an incidence of 8% to 15%[1] (**Table 1**). However, two more recent studies conducted in the era of immuno-oncology (IO) therapy reported an incidence of brain metastases approaching 30%.[4,5] One of these studies involved routine MRI assessments before first-line treatment,[5] whereas the other prospectively followed patients who had undergone nivolumab plus ipilimumab therapy in

a Division of Cancer Medicine, The University of Texas MD Anderson Cancer Center, 1400 Holcombe Boulevard FC11.3055, Houston, TX 77030, USA; b Department of Genitourinary Medical Oncology, Division of Cancer Medicine, The University of Texas MD Anderson Cancer Center, 1515 Holcombe Boulevard Unit 1374, Houston, TX 77030, USA
* Corresponding authors.
E-mail addresses: ehasanov@mdanderson.org (E.H.); ejonasch@mdanderson.org (E.J.)

Hematol Oncol Clin N Am 37 (2023) 1005–1014
https://doi.org/10.1016/j.hoc.2023.04.020
0889-8588/23/Published by Elsevier Inc.
hemonc.theclinics.com

Table 1
Studies evaluating tyrosine kinase inhibitors and immune checkpoint blockers in patients with metastatic renal cell carcinoma and brain metastases

Study	Types of Study	Treatment	Number of Patients	Median OS (mo)	Other Results
Tyrosine Kinase Inhibitors					
Chevreau et al,[35] 2014	Phase II	Sunitinib	16	6.3	ORR: 0%
Peverelli et al,[36] 2019	Retrospective	Cabozantinib	12	8.8	ORR: 50%
Hirsch et al,[37] 2021	Retrospective	Cabozantinib	Cohort 1: 33 Cohort 2: 55	15 16	ORR: 55% ORR: 47%
Cochran et al,[38] 2012	Retrospective	TKI, mTORi, bevacizumab plus local therapy	24[a]	16.6	Local control rate at 12 mo: 93%
Verma et al,[39] 2013	Retrospective	Sorafenib, sunitinib plus local therapy	40[a]	6.7	Local control rate at 12 mo: 69%
Seastone et al,[40] 2014	Retrospective	Sunitinib, axitinib, sorafenib plus local therapy	166[b]	NA	Local control rate at 12 mo: 75%
Bates et al,[41] 2017	Retrospective	Sorafenib, sunitinib, pazopanib, temsirolimus plus local therapy	25[a]	6.7	Local control rate: 76%
Johnson et al,[42] 2015	Retrospective	TKI, mTORi, bevacizumab plus local therapy	24[a]	21	NA
Juloori et al,[43] 2019	Retrospective	TKI, mTORi, cytokine plus local therapy	376[b]	9.7	Incidence of local failure: 15%
Klausner et al,[44] 2019	Retrospective	TKI, mTORi, immunotherapy, chemotherapy plus local therapy	120[b]	13.5	Local control rate at 12 mo: 92%

ICB-based treatments

Flippot et al,[45] 2019	GETUG-AFU 26 NIVOREN Multicenter Phase II Study[16]	Nivolumab (cohort A) Nivolumab + SRS (cohort B)	cohort A: 39; cohort B: 34	12-mo OS in cohort A: 67%; in cohort B: 59%	• Intracranial response in cohort A: 12% (4/34) • Median intracranial PFS in cohort A: 2.7 mo; cohort B: 4.8 mo
Emamekhoo et al,[46] 2021	CheckMate 920, phase IV study	Nivolumab plus ipilimumab × 4 cycles, followed by nivolumab	28	Median OS not reached with minimum follow up of 6.5 mo	• ORR: 32% • Median PFS: 9.0 mo
Desai et al,[47] 2021	Retrospective	Nivolumab plus ipilimumab × 4 cycles, followed by nivolumab	17	Median OS was 25.6 mo	• ORR: 42% • Median PFS: 6.1 mo
Jonasch et al,[2] 2020	Post hoc analysis of phase 3 study	Avelumab + axitinib	23	12-mo OS: 83%	• ORR: 30.4% • Median PFS: 4.9 mo

Abbreviations: ICB, immune checkpoint blocker; mTORi, mTOR inhibitor; NA, not applicable; ORR, overall response rate; OS, overall survival; PFS, progression-free survival; SRS, stereotactic radiosurgery; TKI, tyrosine kinase inhibitor

Adapted from "Hasanov E, Yeboa DN, Tucker MD, et al. An interdisciplinary consensus on the management of brain metastases in patients with renal cell carcinoma. CA Cancer J Clin. Sep 2022;72(5):454-489." with permission.

the CheckMate 214 phase 3 study, revealing that 28% of patients who developed progressive disease had distant metastases in the brain.[4] Currently, there is a limited understanding of the specific biology of mRCC brain metastases, and there are insufficient data on the effectiveness of systemic agents alone. Patients with active brain metastases were excluded from recent trials and there are a lack of specific data regarding the efficacy of systemic therapy in brain metastases.[6–11] Therefore, the standard of care treatment of patients with brain metastases remains central nervous system (CNS)-targeted radiation treatment, including stereotactic radiosurgery (SRS), fractionated stereotactic radiotherapy (FSRT), or whole-brain radiation therapy (WBRT), and surgical resection.[1] Although these treatments have been effective in achieving local disease control, they are not sufficient to prevent new brain metastases from forming. In this section, the authors summarize current practices and ongoing studies for mRCC brain metastases. For more detailed information, please refer to the recently published international consensus statement.[1]

Local Therapy

Multidisciplinary management must underpin the care of patients with RCC brain metastases at every major decision-making point, including the choice to proceed with systemic therapy alone with close monitoring, CNS radiation, or surgery.[1] The approach for patients with a single brain metastasis largely depends on the size and location of the lesion, the presence of neurologic symptoms, and the patients' eligibility for surgery (**Fig. 1**). Single-fraction SRS is the standard of care for asymptomatic small brain metastasis in RCC patients; it is effective at controlling the local disease in patients with lesions ≤3 cm in size.[1] Prospective data are needed to demonstrate how to integrate systemic therapy into the management of the patients with brain metastases before SRS. Surgical resection (often followed by adjuvant SRS) is preferred for larger, symptomatic lesions with edema and mass effect.[12–15] However, with the development of FSRT, larger lesions can also be treated effectively. With this development, the role of surgery versus FSRT in larger lesions needs to be further investigated in patients who are considered eligible for surgical intervention.[16,17] Patients are considered good surgical candidates with a Karnofsky performance score greater than 70, surgically accessible brain metastasis, limited systemic disease, absence of organ-threatening disease causing a high-risk perioperative course, greater than 6 months of life expectancy, and without surgery-limiting comorbidities.[18–20]

Approximately 30% to 45% of patients with mRCC and brain metastasis have multiple lesions, which require a multidisciplinary approach to determine the best treatment course: SRS, FSRT, WBRT, surgical resection, or multimodality treatment[1,21–23] (**Fig. 2**). Although the best available data support the use of SRS for up to five lesions, the neurotoxicity and poor outcomes associated with WBRT along with technologic advances in stereotactic treatment planning and delivery systems led to increased interest in using SRS for more than 10 lesions.[24,25] In those patients who will be treated with WBRT, hippocampal avoidance is recommended for patients with good performance status and/or life expectancy, lesions at least 5 mm away from the hippocampi, the absence of leptomeningeal disease, and the ability to start hippocampal-avoiding-WBRT in a timely manner.[26,27] In terms of surgical intervention, the current practice suggests that resecting larger, dominant, and symptomatic lesions followed by adjuvant SRS to the surgical area and smaller remaining lesions is more effective than WBRT.[28,29]

Systemic Therapy

Although CNS-targeted therapy is the standard approach for mRCC brain metastases, systemic therapy remains a crucial part of treatment to prevent the formation

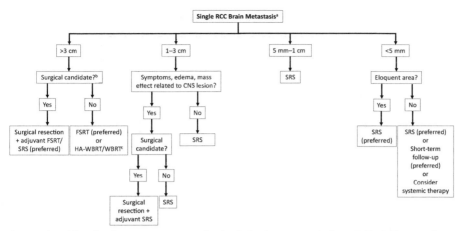

Fig. 1. Algorithm for the management of a single brain metastasis from RCC. CNS, central nervous system; FSRT, fractionated stereotactic radiotherapy; RCC, renal cell carcinoma; SRS, stereotactic radiosurgery; WBRT, whole-brain radiotherapy. [a]This flowchart is intended to provide a general overview of treatment options for patients with a single brain metastasis from RCC based on important clinical characteristics. The optimal management of each patient should be approached in a multidisciplinary fashion with input from medical oncology, radiation oncology, and neurosurgery. [b]Surgical candidates are considered as patients with Karnofsky performance score greater than 70, limited systemic disease (absence of organ-threatening disease causing a high-risk perioperative course; >6 months of life expectancy), without surgery-limiting comorbidities, and with a surgically accessible lesion. [c]Consider HA-WBRT or WBRT on the diagnosis of multiple metastases, with potential SRS as salvage therapy should disease progression occur. The factors that influence the decision to offer HA-WBRT over standard WBRT include patient performance status, life expectancy, lesion greater than 5 mm from the hippocampi, no evidence of leptomeningeal disease and timing in ability to start IMRT or HA-WBRT fast enough. (*From* "Hasanov E, Yeboa DN, Tucker MD, et al. An interdisciplinary consensus on the management of brain metastases in patients with renal cell carcinoma. CA Cancer J Clin. Sep 2022;72(5):454-489." with permission.)

of new intracranial disease and achieve extracranial disease control. Therefore, a personalized patient strategy is necessary for the optimization of systemic therapy based on prior lines of therapy, the ability of the locoregional CNS-targeted therapy to control all active brain metastases, and presence or absence of concurrent extracranial disease progression. Although there is no specific recommendation for the choice of systemic therapy, data from retrospective and prospective studies in **Table 1** can be used as a guide for decision-making. Moreover, according to recent multi-institutional real-world data from the International mRCC Database Consortium (IMDC) presented at the 2023 American Society of Clinical Oncology Genitourinary Symposium, IO-based combination regimens are associated with improved survival.[30] Specifically, combinations that include the multi-kinase inhibitors cabozantinib (NCT03967522, NCT05048212) or lenvatinib (NCT05064280, NCT04955743) could be considered and are currently being tested in clinical trials.

CURRENT STUDIES

Understanding the biology of the disease is crucial for the development of effective treatment strategies, and the significant efforts have been made in this area. The key findings include alterations in cyclin-dependent kinase inhibitor 2A (CDKN2A) and

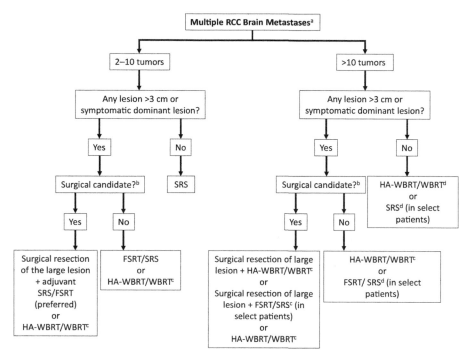

Fig. 2. Algorithm for the management of multiple brain metastases from RCC. FSRT, fractionated stereotactic radiotherapy; HA-WBRT, hippocampal-avoiding whole-brain radiotherapy; RCC, renal cell carcinoma; SRS, stereotactic radiosurgery; WBRT, whole-brain radiotherapy. [a]This flowchart is intended to provide a general overview of treatment options for patients with brain metastases from RCC based on important clinical characteristics. The optimal management of each patient should be approached in a multidisciplinary fashion with input from medical oncology, radiation oncology, and neurosurgery. [b]Surgical candidates are considered as patients with Karnofsky performance score greater than 70, limited systemic disease (absence of organ-threatening disease causing a high-risk perioperative course; more than 6 months of life expectancy) without surgery-limiting comorbidities and with surgically accessible lesions. [c]Consider HA-WBRT or WBRT on the diagnosis of multiple metastases with potential SRS as salvage therapy should disease progression occur. The factors that influence the decision to offer HA-WBRT over standard WBRT include patient performance status, life expectancy, lesion greater than 5 mm from the hippocampi, no evidence of leptomeningeal disease and timing in ability to start IMRT or HA-WBRT fast enough. [d]SRS/FSRT could be considered in select patients who have greater than 10 low-volume brain metastases with good performance status, limited extracranial disease and more than 6 to 12 months of life expectancy. (*From* "Hasanov E, Yeboa DN, Tucker MD, et al. An interdisciplinary consensus on the management of brain metastases in patients with renal cell carcinoma. CA Cancer J Clin. Sep 2022;72(5):454-489." with permission.)

phosphoinositide 3-kinase (PI3K)/AKT/the mammalian target of rapamycin (mTOR) pathway genes, activation of the PI3K/AKT/mTOR, oxidative phosphorylation (OXPHOS), and c-Met pathways, and the development of an immunosuppressive brain tumor immune microenvironment.[1,31–34] Based on these studies, the role of PI3K inhibitor paxalisib (NCT03994796), the CDK4/6 inhibitor abemaciclib (NCT03994796), cabozantinib as a single agent (NCT03967522), and combinations of nivolumab + ipilimumab + cabozantinib (NCT05048212) and pembrolizumab + lenvatinib (NCT05064280, NCT04955743) are currently being tested in clinical trials.

SUMMARY

Despite improvements in the overall survival of patients with mRCC in the immuno-therapy era, the development of brain metastasis in mRCC remains a poor prognostic feature of the disease. Therefore, it is necessary to monitor mRCC patients with brain MRIs before starting and during systemic therapy to diagnose the brain metastasis at an asymptomatic stage. The current standard of care involves treating active brain metastasis with CNS-targeted therapy. For a single brain metastasis, the choice be-tween surgery and SRS depends on the size and location of the lesion, the presence of neurologic symptoms, and the patients' eligibility for surgery. For multiple brain me-tastases, SRS is increasingly used compared with WBRT. Systemic therapy is used after treating brain metastases with CNS-targeted radiation or surgery. Numerous studies are ongoing to understand the disease biology and find more effective sys-temic treatments and multimodality approaches that can prevent intracranial disease progression while also more effectively treating extracranial disease.

CLINICS CARE POINTS

- The authors recommend early brain MRI screening at the time of localized disease diagnosis in patients with neurologic symptoms and at the time of metastatic disease diagnosis even in the absence of neurologic symptoms.

- Multidisciplinary management must be the foundation of care for patients with renal cell carcinoma (RCC) brain metastases at every major decision-making point, including the decision to initiate systemic therapy alone with close monitoring, central nervous system (CNS) radiation, or surgery.

- The algorithms described in this article for how to approach single or multiple RCC brain metastases are based on international consensus and are recommended for use in guiding Individualized patient care.

- The inclusion of patients with untreated RCC brain metastases and no CNS symptoms in clinical trials testing novel RCC agents will aid in the identification of effective agents at an earlier stage of drug development.

DISCLOSURE

E. Hasanov reports research funding to his affiliated institution from the Conquer Cancer Foundation, United States, the Kidney Cancer Association, United States, the International Kidney Cancer Coalition, and the Society for Immunotherapy of Cancer, United States, honoraria from Targeted Oncology, and advisory role from Telix Pharma-ceuticals outside the submitted work. E. Jonasch reports consulting or advisory role from Aravive, Aveo, Calithera Biosciences, Eisai, Exelixis, Merck, United States, NiKang Therapeutics, Novartis, Switzerland, Pfizer, Takeda; research funding from Arrowhead Pharmaceuticals (Inst), United States, Merck, NiKang Therapeutics, Novartis; and travel, accommodations, expenses from Pfizer.

REFERENCES

1. Hasanov E, Yeboa DN, Tucker MD, et al. An interdisciplinary consensus on the management of brain metastases in patients with renal cell carcinoma. CA Can-cer J Clin 2022;72(5):454–89.
2. Jonasch E, Hasanov E, Motzer RJ, et al. Evaluation of brain metastasis in JAVELIN Renal 101: Efficacy of avelumab + axitinib (A+Ax) versus sunitinib (S). J Clin Oncol 2020;38(6_suppl):687.

3. Achrol AS, Rennert RC, Anders C, et al. Brain metastases. Nat Rev Dis Prim 2019;5(1).

4. Tannir NM, Motzer RJ, Albiges L, et al. Patterns of progression in patients treated with nivolumab plus ipilimumab (NIVO+ IPI) versus sunitinib (SUN) for first-line treatment of advanced renal cell carcinoma (aRCC) in CheckMate 214. J Clin Oncol 2021;39(suppl 6) (abstr 313).

5. Bowman IA, Bent A, Le T, et al. Improved Survival Outcomes for Kidney Cancer Patients With Brain Metastases. Clin Genitourin Cancer 2019;17(2):e263–72.

6. Motzer RJ, Tannir NM, McDermott DF, et al. Nivolumab plus Ipilimumab versus Sunitinib in Advanced Renal-Cell Carcinoma. N Engl J Med 2018;378(14):1277–90.

7. Motzer RJ, Penkov K, Haanen J, et al. Avelumab plus Axitinib versus Sunitinib for Advanced Renal-Cell Carcinoma. N Engl J Med 2019;380(12):1103–15.

8. Motzer R, Alekseev B, Rha SY, et al. Lenvatinib plus Pembrolizumab or Everolimus for Advanced Renal Cell Carcinoma. N Engl J Med 2021;384(14):1289–300.

9. Rini BI, Plimack ER, Stus V, et al. Pembrolizumab plus Axitinib versus Sunitinib for Advanced Renal-Cell Carcinoma. N Engl J Med 2019;380(12):1116–27.

10. Choueiri TK, Powles T, Burotto M, et al. Nivolumab plus Cabozantinib versus Sunitinib for Advanced Renal-Cell Carcinoma. N Engl J Med 2021;384(9):829–41.

11. Hasanov E, Gao J, Tannir NM. The Immunotherapy Revolution in Kidney Cancer Treatment: Scientific Rationale and First-Generation Results. Cancer J 2020; 26(5):419–31.

12. Mahajan A, Ahmed S, McAleer MF, et al. Post-operative stereotactic radiosurgery versus observation for completely resected brain metastases: a single-centre, randomised, controlled, phase 3 trial. Lancet Oncol 2017;18(8):1040–8.

13. Brown PD, Ballman KV, Cerhan JH, et al. Postoperative stereotactic radiosurgery compared with whole brain radiotherapy for resected metastatic brain disease (NCCTG N107C/CEC·3): a multicentre, randomised, controlled, phase 3 trial. Lancet Oncol 2017;18(8):1049–60.

14. Al-Shamy G, Sawaya R. Management of brain metastases: the indispensable role of surgery. J Neuro Oncol 2009;92(3):275–82.

15. Akanda ZZ, Hong W, Nahavandi S, et al. Post-operative stereotactic radiosurgery following excision of brain metastases: A systematic review and meta-analysis. Radiother Oncol 2020;142:27–35.

16. Bindal AK, Bindal RK, Hess KR, et al. Surgery versus radiosurgery in the treatment of brain metastasis. J Neurosurg 1996;84(5):748–54.

17. Auchter RM, Lamond JP, Alexander E, et al. A multiinstitutional outcome and prognostic factor analysis of radiosurgery for resectable single brain metastasis. Int J Radiat Oncol Biol Phys 1996;35(1):27–35.

18. Lang FF, Wildrick DM, Sawaya R. Management of Cerebral Metastases: The Role of Surgery. Cancer Control 1998;5(2):124–9.

19. Yaeger KA, Nair MN. Surgery for brain metastases. Surg Neurol Int 2013;4(Suppl 4):S203–8.

20. Sawaya R. Surgical treatment of brain metastases. Clin Neurosurg 1999;45:41–7.

21. El Ali Z, Rottey S, Barthelemy P, et al. Brain Metastasis and Renal Cell Carcinoma: Prognostic Scores Assessment in the Era of Targeted Therapies. Anticancer Res 2019;39(6):2993–3002.

22. Shuch B, La Rochelle JC, Klatte T, et al. Brain metastasis from renal cell carcinoma: presentation, recurrence, and survival. Cancer 2008;113(7):1641–8.

23. Suarez-Sarmiento A Jr, Nguyen KA, Syed JS, et al. Brain Metastasis From Renal-Cell Carcinoma: An Institutional Study. Clin Genitourin Cancer 2019;17(6): e1163–70.

24. Yamamoto M, Serizawa T, Shuto T, et al. Stereotactic radiosurgery for patients with multiple brain metastases (JLGK0901): a multi-institutional prospective observational study. Lancet Oncol 2014;15(4):387–95.

25. Wardak Z, Christie A, Bowman A, et al. Stereotactic Radiosurgery for Multiple Brain Metastases From Renal-Cell Carcinoma. Clin Genitourin Cancer 2019; 17(2):e273–80.

26. Brown PD, Gondi V, Pugh S, et al. Hippocampal Avoidance During Whole-Brain Radiotherapy Plus Memantine for Patients With Brain Metastases: Phase III Trial NRG Oncology CC001. J Clin Oncol 2020;38(10):1019–29.

27. NCCN. National Comprehensive cancer network clinical practice guidelines in oncology: central nervous system cancers 2020 Version 3.2020. Available at: https://www.nccn.org/professionals/physician_gls/pdf/cns.pdf. Accessed January 10, 2021.

28. Pollock BE, Brown PD, Foote RL, et al. Properly selected patients with multiple brain metastases may benefit from aggressive treatment of their intracranial disease. J Neuro Oncol 2003;61(1):73–80.

29. Kayama T, Sato S, Sakurada K, et al. Effects of Surgery With Salvage Stereotactic Radiosurgery Versus Surgery With Whole-Brain Radiation Therapy in Patients With One to Four Brain Metastases (JCOG0504): A Phase III, Noninferiority, Randomized Controlled Trial. J Clin Oncol 2018;36:3282–9.

30. Takemura K, Lemelin A, Ernst MS, et al. Outcomes of patients with brain metastases from renal cell carcinoma treated with first-line therapies: results from the International Metastatic Renal Cell Carcinoma Database Consortium (IMDC), J Clin Oncol, 41 (6_suppl), 2023, 600.

31. Brastianos PK, Carter SL, Santagata S, et al. Genomic Characterization of Brain Metastases Reveals Branched Evolution and Potential Therapeutic Targets. Cancer Discov 2015;5(11):1164–77.

32. Fukumura K, Malgulwar PB, Fischer GM, et al. Multi-omic molecular profiling reveals potentially targetable abnormalities shared across multiple histologies of brain metastasis. Acta Neuropathol 2021;141(2):303–21.

33. Salmaggi A, Maderna E, Calatozzolo C, et al. CXCL12, CXCR4 and CXCR7 expression in brain metastases. Cancer Biol Ther 2009;8(17):1608–14.

34. Silva Paiva R, Gomes I, Casimiro S, et al. c-Met expression in renal cell carcinoma with bone metastases. J Bone Oncol 2020;25:100315.

35. Chevreau C, Ravaud A, Escudier B, et al. A phase II trial of sunitinib in patients with renal cell cancer and untreated brain metastases. Clin Genitourin Cancer 2014;12(1):50–4.

36. Peverelli G, Raimondi A, Ratta R, et al. Cabozantinib in Renal Cell Carcinoma With Brain Metastases: Safety and Efficacy in a Real-World Population. Clin Genitourin Cancer 2019;17(4):291–8.

37. Hirsch L, Chanza NM, Farah S, et al. Clinical Activity and Safety of Cabozantinib for Brain Metastases in Patients With Renal Cell Carcinoma. JAMA Oncol 2021; 7(12):1815–23.

38. Cochran DC, Chan MD, Aklilu M, et al. The effect of targeted agents on outcomes in patients with brain metastases from renal cell carcinoma treated with Gamma Knife surgery. J Neurosurg 2012;116(5):978–83.

39. Verma J, Jonasch E, Allen PK, et al. The impact of tyrosine kinase inhibitors on the multimodality treatment of brain metastases from renal cell carcinoma. Am J Clin Oncol 2013;36(6):620–4.

40. Seastone DJ, Elson P, Garcia JA, et al. Clinical outcome of stereotactic radiosurgery for central nervous system metastases from renal cell carcinoma. Clin Genitourin Cancer 2014;12(2):111–6.
41. Bates JE, Youn P, Peterson CR 3rd, et al. Radiotherapy for Brain Metastases From Renal Cell Carcinoma in the Targeted Therapy Era: The University of Rochester Experience. Am J Clin Oncol 2017;40(5):439–43.
42. Johnson AG, Ruiz J, Hughes R, et al. Impact of systemic targeted agents on the clinical outcomes of patients with brain metastases. Oncotarget 2015;6(22):18945–55.
43. Juloori A, Miller JA, Parsai S, et al. Overall survival and response to radiation and targeted therapies among patients with renal cell carcinoma brain metastases. J Neurosurg 2019;1–9.
44. Klausner G, Troussier I, Biau J, et al. Stereotactic Radiation Therapy for Renal Cell Carcinoma Brain Metastases in the Tyrosine Kinase Inhibitors Era: Outcomes of 120 Patients. Clin Genitourin Cancer 2019;17(3):191–200.
45. Flippot R, Dalban C, Laguerre B, et al. Safety and Efficacy of Nivolumab in Brain Metastases From Renal Cell Carcinoma: Results of the GETUG-AFU 26 NIVOREN Multicenter Phase II Study. J Clin Oncol 2019;37(23):2008–16.
46. Emamekhoo H, Olsen MR, Carthon BC, et al. Safety and efficacy of nivolumab plus ipilimumab in patients with advanced renal cell carcinoma with brain metastases: CheckMate 920. Cancer 2021.
47. Desai K, Brown L, Wei W, et al. A Multi-institutional, Retrospective Analysis of Patients with Metastatic Renal Cell Carcinoma to Bone Treated with Combination Ipilimumab and Nivolumab. Target Oncol 2021;16(5):633–42.

Novel Targeted Therapies for Renal Cell Carcinoma
Building on the Successes of Vascular Endothelial Growth Factor and mTOR Inhibition

Renée Maria Saliby, MD, MSc[a,b,1], Eddy Saad, MD, MSc[a,1],
Chris Labaki, MD[a,c], Wenxin Xu, MD[a,d], David A. Braun, MD, PhD[b],
Srinivas R. Viswanathan, MD, PhD[a,d,2,*],
Ziad Bakouny, MD, MSc[a,d,e,2,*]

KEYWORDS

- Renal cell carcinoma • Clear cell RCC • Variant histology RCC • HIF2α inhibitors
- Tyrosine kinase inhibitors • Glutaminase inhibitors • CDK4/6 inhibitors
- Targeted therapy

KEY POINTS

- Targeting the VEGFR and mTOR pathways has yielded very promising efficacy in patients with RCC, novel targeted therapies seek to build on these successes.
- HIF2α inhibition, either as monotherapy or in combination, is one of the most promising novel targets in the treatment of RCC.
- Other novel targeted therapies including MET inhibitors, glutaminase inhibitors, histone deacetylase (HDAC) inhibitors, CDK4/6 inhibitors, and AXL inhibitors are in various stages of development.

INTRODUCTION

The treatment of renal cell carcinoma (RCC) has undergone remarkable development over the past 20 years. Through the understanding of its underlying biology,[1,2]

[a] Department of Medical Oncology, Dana-Farber Cancer Institute, 450 Brookline Avenue, Boston, MA 02215, USA; [b] Center of Molecular and Cellular Oncology, Yale Cancer Center, Yale School of Medicine, 300 George Street, Suite 6400, New Haven, CT 06510, USA; [c] Department of Medicine, Beth Israel Deaconess Medical Center, 330 Brookline Avenue, Boston, MA 02215, USA; [d] Harvard Medical School, Boston, MA, USA; [e] Department of Medicine, Brigham and Women's Hospital, 75 Francis Street, Boston, MA 02115, USA
[1] Co-first authors.
[2] Co-senior authors.
* Corresponding authors. Brigham and Women's Hospital, 75 Francis Street, Boston, MA 02115.
E-mail addresses: srinivas.viswanathan@dfci.harvard.edu (S.R.V.); ziad_elbakouny@dfci.harvard.edu (Z.B.)

Hematol Oncol Clin N Am 37 (2023) 1015–1026
https://doi.org/10.1016/j.hoc.2023.05.022
0889-8588/23/© 2023 Elsevier Inc. All rights reserved.

therapies targeting the VEGF, mTOR, and PD-1 axes have transformed the treatment of this disease both in the locally advanced and metastatic settings.[3] Unfortunately, most of these patients still do not achieve sustained remissions and eventually experience tumor progression. While combining therapeutic agents targeting these pathways has been successful in delaying progression and improving survival, new targets are needed to overcome tumor resistance and achieve durable complete responses for more patients.[4] Moreover, the treatment of variant histology RCC (also known as "non-clear cell" or nccRCC) has lagged behind that of clear cell (ccRCC) owing to their rarity, molecular heterogeneity, and our poorer understanding of their underlying biology.

In this review, we will explore the most promising novel targets (excluding immunotherapy) in the treatment of RCC, including hypoxia-inducible factor 2α (HIF2α), cyclin-dependent kinases 4 and 6 (CDK 4/6), metabolic targets, epigenomic targets, and tumor surface markers targeted through antibody-drug conjugates (ADCs) (**Fig. 1**).

HYPOXIA-INDUCIBLE FACTOR 2α INHIBITION

The Von Hippel-Lindau (*VHL*) tumor suppressor gene regulates transcription factors hypoxia-inducible factor-1α (HIF-1A) and HIF-2A. Most ccRCC tumors exhibit inactivating mutations of *VHL* which leads to a constitutive activation of HIF-mediated pathways, even under normoxic conditions.[5] HIF2A drives the formation of renal cysts and hemangiomas in $VHL^{-/-}$ mouse kidneys and liver.[6–9] The pharmacologic inhibition of HIF2α with a small molecule causes tumor regression in mouse models of primary and metastatic *VHL*-defective clear cell RCC.[10]

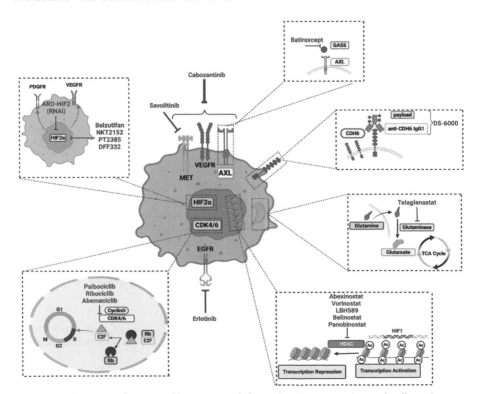

Fig. 1. Mechanisms of action of key targeted therapies in metastatic renal cell carcinoma.

Based on the results of preclinical studies, HIF2α was identified as a crucial therapeutic target, but was long viewed as "undruggable" because of the absence of a known ligand-binding site.[11] The identification of a pocket in the PAS-B domain of HIF2α that could accommodate a small molecule spurred drug discovery efforts for small molecules that disrupt HIF2α heterodimerization with HIF1β (ARNT), preventing the binding of the complex to DNA and inhibiting the transcriptional activation of downstream genes.[10,12,13] These efforts produced the specific, potent, orally bioavailable HIF2α inhibitor PT2385,[14] which was further optimized to yield belzutifan (also called PT2977 or MK-6482), a molecule with improved pharmacokinetics, bioavailability, and HIF2α affinity.[15]

PT2385 was the first HIF2α inhibitor tested in humans, in a phase I dose escalation trial in pre-treated patients with advanced ccRCC. PT2385 exhibited a favorable safety profile and promising efficacy with a disease control rate (DCR) of 66% and overall response rate (ORR) of 14%, confirming its high selectivity for HIF2α/ARNT and validating its further development in ccRCC. In a phase I trial expansion cohort, an ORR of 22% and median progression-free survival (PFS) of 7.3 months were observed in heavily pretreated patients with advanced ccRCC treated with the combination of PT2385 and nivolumab, showing that HIF2α inhibitors could be safely combined with other systemic therapies for ccRCC (**Table 1**).[16] The combination of belzutifan plus cabozantinib yielded an ORR of 57% in the first-line setting[17] and of 31% for pre-treated patients[18] in the phase II LITESPARK-003 study (NCT03634540).[19,20] The ongoing phase III LITESPARK-011 trial (NCT04586231) compares belzutifan plus lenvatinib to cabozantinib in patients with previously treated advanced ccRCC. Furthermore, another phase III trial is currently testing single-agent belzutifan versus everolimus in 736 patients with metastatic ccRCC who had previously progressed on an ICI and a VEGF-targeted agent, with PFS and OS as co-primary endpoints (NCT04195750). Other belzutifan combinations for metastatic ccRCC are being investigated in phase III studies.[20,21] Specifically, a phase III trial is currently recruiting patients and randomizing them to either belzutifan + lenvatinib + pembrolizumab, MK-1308A (quavonlimab, a CTLA-4 inhibitor, coformulated with pembrolizumab) + lenvatinib, or pembrolizumab + lenvatinib; NCT04736706.[21] Finally, belzutifan is also being studied in the adjuvant setting in combination with pembrolizumab in phase III LITESPARK-022 trial (NCT05239728).[22]

Other molecules against HIF2α are in development. NKT2152, an oral small molecule, is currently being studied in a phase I/II dose-escalation and expansion trial (NCT05119335).[23] AB521 appeared to have potent antitumor activity in animal models.[24] ARO-HIF2 is a synthetic double-stranded RNA interference trigger designed to silence HIF2A expression. Interim results from a phase Ib study in pre-treated patients with metastatic ccRCC are promising, with a good tolerance of the higher dose of 525 mg and reduced HIF2α expression on immunohistochemical analysis.[25] Across all cohorts, 7 patients (30%) achieved disease control.[25]

CYCLIN-DEPENDENT KINASE 4/6 INHIBITION

Cyclin-dependent kinase 4 and 6 (CDK4/6) are involved in the G1-to-S cell cycle checkpoint. Coactivation of the D-type cyclins and CDK4/6 holoenzyme complex phosphorylates the tumor suppressor retinoblastoma (Rb), resulting in the release of E2F proteins which finalizes the G1/S cell transition. A number of human cancers exhibit hyperactivated CDK4/6, making this pathway an attractive therapeutic target.[26] In RCC, the cyclin-dependent kinase inhibitor 2A (CDKN2A) gene encodes isoforms that negatively regulate CDK4,[27] and its deletion is a recurrent event in ccRCC[28,29]

Table 1
Published (A) and ongoing (B) trials testing the safety and efficacy of HIF-2-targeting agents

Trial ID (with Trial Name if Applicable)	Experimental HIF2 Targeted Agent	Combination Drug	Target	Line of Therapy	Phase	Primary Endpoints	Outcomes	Comments
NCT04169711[a]	ARO-HIF2			Refractory	I	AEs	DCR 30%	
NCT02974738[b] (MK-6482–001; LITESPARK-001)	Belzutifan			Previously treated with ≥1 therapy	I	AEs	ORR 25% · DCR 80%	
NCT03634540 (MK-6482–003; LITESPARK-003)[a,b]	Belzutifan	Cabozantinib	VEGFR	Cohort 1: first-line advanced ccRCC · Cohort 2: prior immunotherapy and no more than 2 prior treatments	II	ORR	ORR 57% · ORR 31%	
NCT02974738[3]	Belzutifan			Any line	I/II	MTD	ORR 24%	
NCT03401788[4]	Belzutifan			First-line	II	ORR	ORR 49%	Inclusion criteria: Patients with renal cell carcinoma associated with VHL disease
NCT02293980[5,6] (MK-3795–001)	PT2385	None (monotherapy) Nivolumab	PD-1	Refractory	I	MTD, R2PD	ORR 14% ORR 22%	

Trial ID (with trial name if applicable)	Experimental HIF2 targeted agent	Combination agent (if applicable) Drug	Target	Line of therapy	Phase	Primary endpoints		Comments
NCT04195750 (MK-6482–005; LITESPARK-005)	Belzutifan			Refractory	III	PFS, OS		Refractory

NCT number (study)	Drug	Combination	Target	Setting	Phase	Endpoints	Notes
NCT05030506 (MK-6482–010)	Belzutifan	Lenvatinib	VEGFR	Refractory	I	AEs	Patients of Chinese descent
NCT04736706 (MK-6482–012; LITESPARK-012)	Belzutifan	Lenvatinib + pembrolizumab	VEGFR + PD-1	First-line	III	PFS, OS	
NCT04846920 (MK-6482–018)	Belzutifan	Lenvatinib + pembrolizumab	VEGFR + PD-1	Refractory	II	ORR	
	Belzutifan	Pembrolizumab	PD-1	Previously treated with ≥1 therapy	I	Adverse events, DLT	
NCT05239728 (MK-6482–022; LITESPARK-022)	Belzutifan	Pembrolizumab	PD-1	Adjuvant	III	DFS	
NCT05119335	Oral NKT2152			Refractory	I/II	DLTs, RP2D, ORR	
NCT04627064	MK-6482	Abemaciclib	CDK4/6	Refractory	I	ORR, MTD	
NCT05468697 (MK-6482–024)	Belzutifan	Palbociclib	CDK4/6	Refractory	I/II	AEs, DLT, ORR	
NCT04895748	DFF332	Everolimus; Spartalizumab + Taminadenant	mTOR; PD-1 + A2A	Refractory	I	AEs, Dose intensity, DLT	In ccRCC and other malignancies
NCT04626479 (MK-3475–03A)	MK-7902	Lenvatinib + pembrolizumab; Vibostolimab + pembrolizumab	VEGFR + PD-1; TIGIT + PD-1	First-line	I/II	AEs, DLT, ORR	
NCT04626518 (MK-3475–03B)	MK-7902	Pembrolizumab; Lenvatinib	PD-1; VEGFR	Refractory	I/II	AEs, DLT, ORR	

Abbreviations: AEs, adverse events; ccRCC, clear cell renal cell carcinoma; DCR, disease control rate; DLT, dose-limiting toxicity; MTD, maximal tolerated dose; ORR, overall response rate; OS, overall survival; PFS, progression-free survival; RCC, renal cell carcinoma; RP2D, recommended phase 2 dose.

[a] Choueiri TK, McDermott DF, Merchan J, et al. Belzutifan plus cabozantinib for patients with advanced clear cell renal cell carcinoma previously treated with immunotherapy: an open-label, single-arm, phase 2 study. Lancet Oncol. 2023;0(0). https://doi.org/10.1016/S1470-2045(23)00097-9).

[b] Choueiri TK, Bauer T, Merchan J, et al. 1447O Phase II study of belzutifan plus cabozantinib as first-line treatment of advanced renal cell carcinoma (RCC): Cohort 1 of LITESPARK-003. Ann Oncol. 2022;33:S1204.doi:10.1016/j.annonc.2022.07.1550.

as well as RCC of variant histologies such as sarcomatoid, translocation, and "type 2" papillary RCC.[29–31] These mutations have been associated with worse survival, and targeting them might improve outcomes in patients with RCC.[28] The inactivation of *VHL* and loss of CDK4/6 activity are synthetically lethal in *Drosophila* and human species, as well as in in ccRCC cell lines and xenografts.[30] Building on this, inhibiting CDK4/6 pharmacologically in *VHL*−/− ccRCC pre-clinical models was synergistic with HIF2α inhibitors in HIF2α-dependent cells, and not antagonistic in those that are HIF2α-independent.[30] A phase I/II study is currently testing the combination of the CDK4/6 inhibitor palbociclib and belzutifan (NCT05468697, Supplementary Table 1). The addition of another CDK4/6 inhibitor, abemaciclib, to sunitinib resulted in increased apoptosis of 786O cells and substantial tumor regression in mice.[31] With more than 90% of ccRCC being pVHL-negative, CDK4/6 inhibition may be a promising option in this setting. A single-arm phase Ib study[32] is currently evaluating the addition of abemaciclib to sunitinib in metastatic RCC (NCT03905889). With the evolution of the standard of care in RCC, palbociclib is also now being tested in combination with axitinib and avelumab (NCT05176288).

TARGETING METABOLIC DYSREGULATION

In RCC, metabolic reprogramming results in increased consumption of glucose and glutamine, promoted by HIF1α and HIF2α.[33] The first step of glutaminolysis is the transformation of glutamine into glutamate by glutaminase, an enzyme that is often upregulated in ccRCC.[34] Glutaminase inhibition suppresses oncogenic transformation and tumor growth in preclinical models[35–37] and has been studied in RCC. Contrary to non-selective glutamine metabolism inhibitors, the oral glutaminase inhibitor telaglenastat was the first small molecule glutaminase inhibitor to show a favorable safety profile.[34] Based on preclinical data,[38] and that everolimus also inhibits key glycolytic enzymes, ENTRATA was a randomized, placebo-controlled phase II study comparing everolimus with or without telaglenastat. There was a trend toward improved PFS after the addition of telaglenastat to everolimus in patients with refractory metastatic RCC, though the clinical benefit was minimal (NCT03163667, Supplementary Table 2).[39] Telaglenastat was also combined with cabozantinib in the CANTATA trial (NCT03428217),[40] but did not meet its primary outcome of improvement in PFS.[40] Recent preclinical studies suggest that these disappointing clinical results may be due to alternative pathways leading to persistent glutamine catabolism in telaglenastat-treated tumors,[41] and the drug is no longer in development.

NOVEL RECEPTOR TYROSINE KINASE (RTK) INHIBITORS

AXL is an RTK expressed in both tumor cells and in the tumor microenvironment.[42] With its ligand GAS6, it drives metastasis and acquired resistance to treatment in various types of cancer.[42] Increased AXL expression has been shown to be associated with resistance to immune checkpoint inhibitors (ICI) and to anti-angiogenic therapies, providing rationale for the inhibition of AXL.[43,44] While some antiangiogenic treatments in RCC are tyrosine kinase inhibitors (TKIs) that also suppress the AXL pathway, the level of inhibition varies. Batiraxcept is a recombinant fusion protein containing an extracellular region of human AXL combined with the human immunoglobulin G1 heavy chain (Fc) that binds to GAS6 and inhibits the AXL/GAS6 pathway with high potency and specificity.[45] A phase Ib/II study of batiraxcept in combination with cabozantinib in previously treated patients with metastatic ccRCC showed that the combination was well tolerated and demonstrated early efficacy signals (NCT04300140),[46] with 56% ORR and all patients responded for at least 3 months.

The phase II portion of the trial evaluating batiraxcept with cabozantinib versus cabozantinib and nivolumab or batiraxcept monotherapy is ongoing (NCT04300140).[47]

XL092 is a multi-RTK inhibitor that suppresses the activity of oncogenic targets MET, VEGFR2, and TAM kinases.[48–51] Compared to cabozantinib, it has a shorter half-life at ~20 hours and has been shown to cause significant tumor shrinkage in murine models, and immunomodulatory activity both alone and in combination with ICI. The STELLAR-001[52] (NCT03845166) and STELLAR-002 (NCT05176483) trials are currently evaluating XL092 in solid tumors. A phase III trial is testing the efficacy of XL092 plus nivolumab versus sunitinib in subjects with advanced nccRCC (NCT05678673).

HISTONE DEACETYLASE PATHWAY INHIBITION

Histone deacetylases (HDACs) are epigenetic regulators that suppress gene transcription.[53] Dysregulation of this mechanism has been linked to various pathologies including cancer. HDACs are crucial for HIF-1 transcription and signaling: increased expression of HDAC in hypoxic conditions mediate the reduction of VHL expression.[54] Vorinostat is a small molecule inhibitor of HDAC that yielded promising results when combined with bevacizumab in patients with metastatic RCC, with an ORR of 18%, PFS of 48% at 6 months, and relatively good tolerability.[55] In addition, the combination of the HDAC inhibitor abexinostat with pazopanib exhibited promising durable responses, including in patients who were refractory to VEGF inhibitors.[56] A phase III trial, RENAVIV, is comparing pazopanib plus abexinostat to pazopanib plus placebo in patients with mRCC, including ICI-refractory patients (NCT03592472).[57]

ANTIBODY-DRUG CONJUGATES

Antibody-drug conjugates (ADCs) are designed to deliver high doses of a cytotoxic drug "payload" locally to a tumor via monoclonal antibodies.[58] Cadherin 6 (CDH6) is essential for the normal development of the brain and kidneys, and its expression is decreased in healthy adults but increased in RCC and ovarian cancer.[59] DS-6000a, a CDH6-targeting ADC, inhibited the growth activity of tumor cells highly expressing CDH6 in vitro. The first-in-human trial in pretreated patients with advanced ovarian cancer and RCC (NCT04707248) showed that DS-6000a was well tolerated with only one dose-limiting toxicity.[60] Among the 15 patients, 2 patients exhibited a PR (1 RCC, 1 ovarian cancer) and 9 patients had stable disease; all patients with RCC had previously received ICI. ADCs targeting ENPP3, TIM-1, and CD70 are currently being studied in RCC and are in preclinical or early clinical development.[61] While ENPP3 showed a promising signal for clinical activity in the phase I study,[62] it did not meet its primary endpoint in a phase II trial.[63] However, it is important to note that patients with various histologies of RCC (with potentially variable ENPP3 expression) were included, which may have impacted the study results. While ADCs have the advantage of being specific, thus maximizing efficacy and minimizing toxicity, payload selection should be optimized for RCC given the lack of activity for cytotoxic chemotherapy in RCC.

SUMMARY

The development of novel therapies targeting the genomic drivers of ccRCC has revolutionized the treatment of this disease over the past 2 decades and promises to continue to do so in the upcoming years. Targeting HIF2α currently stands out as the most promising novel target for patients with this disease. Other promising approaches include the targeting of epigenomic and metabolic pathways, cell cycle inhibition, and cell surface targeting using antibody-drug conjugates.

DISCLOSURE STATEMENT
Conflicts of Interest

E. Saad, R.M. Saliby., C. Labaki.: none. W. Xu reports advisory board fees from Exelixis and Jazz Pharmaceuticals, and continuing medical education honoraria from MedNet, Harborside Press, MJH Healthcare Holdings, and Academy for Continued Healthcare Learning. S.R. Viswanathan reports consulting for Jnana Therapeutics, MPM Capital, and Vida Ventures within the last 3 years and research support from Bayer, Germany. Spouse is an employee of and holds equity in Kojin Therapeutics. D.A. Braun. reports honoraria from LM Education/Exchange Services, advisory board fees from Exelixis and AVEO, personal fees from Schlesinger Associates, Cancer Expert Now, Adnovate Strategies, MDedge, CancerNetwork, Catenion, OncLive, Cello Health BioConsulting, PWW Consulting, Haymarket Medical Network, Aptitude Health, ASCO Post/Harborside, Targeted Oncology, AbbVie, and research support from Exelixis, United States and AstraZeneca, United Kingdom, outside of the submitted work. Z. Bakouny reports research support from Genentech, United States/imCORE and Bristol Myers Squibb, United States, and honoraria from UpToDate.

ACKNOWLEDGMENTS

W. Xu. acknowledges support from the Dept of Defense Early Career Investigator grant (KCRP AKCI-ECI, W81XWH-22-1-0951). S.R. Viswanathan acknowledges support from the Doris Duke Charitable Foundation, United States (Clinician-Scientist Development Award grant number 2020101), Department of Defense Kidney Cancer Research Program (W81XWH-22-1-1016), Rally Foundation for Childhood Cancer Research, United States, Kidney Cancer Association, United States, and the V Foundation, United States. D.A. Braun acknowledges support from the Dept of Defense Early Career Investigator grant (KCRP AKCI-ECI, W81XWH-20-1-0882), the Louis Goodman and Alfred Gilman Yale Scholar Fund, and the Yale Cancer Center, United States (supported by NIH, United States/NCI, United States research grant P30CA016359).

SUPPLEMENTARY DATA

Supplementary data related to this article can be found online at https://doi.org/10.1016/j.hoc.2023.05.022.

REFERENCES

1. Ricketts CJ, De Cubas AA, Fan H, et al. The cancer genome atlas comprehensive molecular characterization of renal cell carcinoma. Cell Rep 2018;23(1):313–26.e5.
2. Hsieh JJ, Le VH, Oyama T, et al. Chromosome 3p loss–orchestrated VHL, HIF, and epigenetic deregulation in clear cell renal cell carcinoma. J Clin Oncol 2018;36(36):3533–9.
3. Motzer RJ, Jonasch E, Agarwal N, et al. Kidney Cancer, Version 3.2022, NCCN clinical practice guidelines in oncology. J Natl Compr Cancer Netw 2022;20(1): 71–90.
4. Siska PJ, Beckermann KE, Rathmell WK, et al. Strategies to overcome therapeutic resistance in renal cell carcinoma. Urol Oncol 2017;35(3):102.
5. Choueiri TK, Kaelin WG Jr. Targeting the HIF2-VEGF axis in renal cell carcinoma. Nat Med 2020;26(10):1519–30.

6. Raval RR, Lau KW, Tran MGB, et al. Contrasting properties of hypoxia-inducible factor 1 (HIF-1) and HIF-2 in von hippel-lindau-associated renal cell carcinoma. Mol Cell Biol 2005;25(13):5675–86.

7. Gordan JD, Bertout JA, Hu CJ, et al. HIF-2alpha promotes hypoxic cell proliferation by enhancing c-myc transcriptional activity. Cancer Cell 2007;11(4):335–47.

8. Rankin EB, Tomaszewski JE, Haase VH. Renal cyst development in mice with conditional inactivation of the von Hippel-Lindau tumor suppressor. Cancer Res 2006;66(5):2576–83.

9. Rankin EB, Rha J, Unger TL, et al. Hypoxia-inducible factor-2 regulates vascular tumorigenesis in mice. Oncogene 2008;27(40):5354–8.

10. Cho H, Du X, Rizzi JP, et al. On-target efficacy of a HIF-2α antagonist in preclinical kidney cancer models. Nature 2016;539(7627):107–11.

11. Koehler AN. A complex task? Direct modulation of transcription factors with small molecules. Curr Opin Chem Biol 2010;14(3):331–40.

12. Benfenati F, Valtorta F, Rubenstein JL, et al. Synaptic vesicle-associated Ca2+/calmodulin-dependent protein kinase II is a binding protein for synapsin I. Nature 1992;359(6394):417–20.

13. Wallace EM, Rizzi JP, Han G, et al. A small-molecule antagonist of HIF2α is efficacious in preclinical models of renal cell carcinoma. Cancer Res 2016;76(18):5491–500.

14. Wehn PM, Rizzi JP, Dixon DD, et al. Design and activity of specific hypoxia-inducible factor-2α (HIF-2α) inhibitors for the treatment of clear cell renal cell carcinoma: discovery of clinical candidate (S)-3-((2,2-Difluoro-1-hydroxy-7-(methylsulfonyl)-2,3-dihydro-1 H-inden-4-yl)oxy)-5-fluorobenzonitrile (PT2385). J Med Chem 2018;61(21):9691–721.

15. Xu R, Wang K, Rizzi JP, et al. 3-[(1 S,2 S,3 R)-2,3-Difluoro-1-hydroxy-7-methylsulfonylindan-4-yl]oxy 5 fluorobenzonitrile (PT2977), a Hypoxia-Inducible Factor 2α (HIF-2α) Inhibitor for the Treatment of Clear Cell Renal Cell Carcinoma. J Med Chem 2019;62(15):6876–93.

16. Rini BI, Appleman LJ, Figlin RA, et al. Results from a phase I expansion cohort of the first-in-class oral HIF-2α inhibitor PT2385 in combination with nivolumab in patients with previously treated advanced RCC. J Clin Oncol 2019;37(7_suppl):558.

17. Choueiri TK, Bauer T, Merchan J, et al. 1447O Phase II study of belzutifan plus cabozantinib as first-line treatment of advanced renal cell carcinoma (RCC): Cohort 1 of LITESPARK-003. Ann Oncol 2022;33:S1204.

18. Choueiri TK, McDermott DF, Merchan J, et al. Belzutifan plus cabozantinib for patients with advanced clear cell renal cell carcinoma previously treated with immunotherapy: an open-label, single-arm, phase 2 study. Lancet Oncol 2023;0(0).

19. A Study of Belzutifan (MK-6482) in Combination With Lenvatinib Versus Cabozantinib for Treatment of Renal Cell Carcinoma (MK-6482-011) - Full Text View - ClinicalTrials.gov. Available at: https://clinicaltrials.gov/ct2/show/NCT04586231. Accessed January 19, 2023.

20. Motzer RJ, Liu Y, Perini RF, et al. Phase III study evaluating efficacy and safety of MK-6482 + lenvatinib versus cabozantinib for second- or third-line therapy in patients with advanced renal cell carcinoma (RCC) who progressed after prior anti-PD-1/L1 therapy. J Clin Oncol 2021;39(6_suppl):TPS372.

21. Choueiri TK, Plimack ER, Powles T, et al. Phase 3 study of first-line treatment with pembrolizumab + belzutifan + lenvatinib or pembrolizumab/quavonlimab + lenvatinib versus pembrolizumab + lenvatinib for advanced renal cell carcinoma (RCC). J Clin Oncol 2022;40(6_suppl):TPS399.

22. Choueiri TK, Bedke J, Karam JA, et al. LITESPARK-022: A phase 3 study of pembrolizumab + belzutifan as adjuvant treatment of clear cell renal cell carcinoma (ccRCC). J Clin Oncol 2022;40(16_suppl):TPS4602.

23. A Study of NKT2152, a HIF2α Inhibitor, in Patients With Advanced Clear Cell Renal Cell Carcinoma - Full Text View - ClinicalTrials.gov. Available at: https://clinicaltrials.gov/ct2/show/NCT05119335. Accessed January 10, 2023.

24. Lawson KV, Sivick Gauthier KE, Piovesan D, et al. 46P AB521, a clinical-stage, potent, and selective Hypoxia-Inducible Factor (HIF)-2α inhibitor, for the treatment of renal cell carcinoma. Ann Oncol 2022;33:S21.

25. Brugarolas J, Beckermann K, Rini BI, et al. Initial results from the phase 1 study of ARO-HIF2 to silence HIF2-alpha in patients with advanced ccRCC (ARO-HIF21001). J Clin Oncol 2022;40(6_suppl):339.

26. VanArsdale T, Boshoff C, Arndt KT, et al. Molecular pathways: targeting the cyclin D-CDK4/6 axis for cancer treatment. Clin Cancer Res 2015;21(13):2905–10.

27. CDKN2A cyclin dependent kinase inhibitor 2A Homo sapiens (human) - Gene - NCBI. Available at: https://www.ncbi.nlm.nih.gov/gene/1029. Accessed February 21, 2023.

28. Braun DA, Hou Y, Bakouny Z, et al. Interplay of somatic alterations and immune infiltration modulates response to PD-1 blockade in advanced clear cell renal cell carcinoma. Nat Med 2020;26(6):909–18.

29. Creighton CJ, Morgan M, Gunaratne PH, et al. Comprehensive molecular characterization of clear cell renal cell carcinoma. Nature 2013;499(7456):43–9.

30. Nicholson HE, Tariq Z, Housden BE, et al. HIF-independent synthetic lethality between CDK4/6 inhibition and VHL loss across species. Sci Signal 2019;12(601):eaay0482.

31. Small J, Washburn E, Millington K, et al. The addition of abemaciclib to sunitinib induces regression of renal cell carcinoma xenograft tumors. Oncotarget 2017;8(56):95116–34.

32. Holder SL, Warrick J, Zhu J, et al. A phase Ib study targeting PIM1 and CDK4/6 kinases in metastatic renal cell carcinoma (PICKRCC). J Clin Oncol 2020;38(6_suppl):TPS771.

33. Okazaki A, Gameiro PA, Christodoulou D, et al. Glutaminase and poly(ADP-ribose) polymerase inhibitors suppress pyrimidine synthesis and VHL-deficient renal cancers. J Clin Invest 2017;127(5):1631–45.

34. Harding JJ, Telli M, Munster P, et al. A phase I dose-escalation and expansion study of telaglenastat in patients with advanced or metastatic solid tumors. Clin Cancer Res 2021;27(18):4994–5003.

35. Gameiro PA, Yang J, Metelo AM, et al. In vivo HIF-mediated reductive carboxylation is regulated by citrate levels and sensitizes VHL-deficient cells to glutamine deprivation. Cell Metabol 2013;17(3):372–85.

36. Seltzer MJ, Bennett BD, Joshi AD, et al. Inhibition of glutaminase preferentially slows growth of glioma cells with mutant IDH1. Cancer Res 2010;70(22):8981–7.

37. Wang J Bin, Erickson JW, Fuji R, et al. Targeting mitochondrial glutaminase activity inhibits oncogenic transformation. Cancer Cell 2010;18(3):207–19.

38. Emberley E, Pan A, Chen J, et al. The glutaminase inhibitor telaglenastat enhances the antitumor activity of signal transduction inhibitors everolimus and cabozantinib in models of renal cell carcinoma. PLoS One 2021;16(11):e0259241.

39. Lee CH, Motzer R, Emamekhoo H, et al. Telaglenastat plus everolimus in advanced renal cell carcinoma: a randomized, double-blinded, placebo-controlled, phase II ENTRATA trial. Clin Cancer Res 2022;28(15):3248–55.

40. Tannir NM, Agarwal N, Porta C, et al. Efficacy and safety of telaglenastat plus cabozantinib vs placebo plus cabozantinib in patients with advanced renal cell carcinoma: the CANTATA randomized clinical trial. JAMA Oncol 2022;8(10):1411–8.

41. Kaushik AK, Tarangelo A, Boroughs LK, et al. In vivo characterization of glutamine metabolism identifies therapeutic targets in clear cell renal cell carcinoma. Sci Adv 2022;8(50). https://doi.org/10.1126/SCIADV.ABP8293/SUPPL_FILE/SCIADV.ABP8293_DATA_S1_AND_S2.ZIP.

42. Auyez A, Sayan AE, Kriajevska M, et al. AXL receptor in cancer metastasis and drug resistance: when normal functions go askew. Cancers 2021;13(19). https://doi.org/10.3390/CANCERS13194864.

43. Hahn AW, George DJ, Agarwal N. An evolving role for AXL in metastatic renal cell carcinoma. Clin Cancer Res 2021;27(24):6619–21.

44. Zhou L, Liu XD, Sun M, et al. Targeting MET and AXL overcomes resistance to sunitinib therapy in renal cell carcinoma. Oncogene 2016;35(21):2687.

45. Bonifacio L, Dodds M, Prohaska D, et al. Target-mediated drug disposition pharmacokinetic/pharmacodynamic model-informed dose selection for the first-in-human study of AVB-S6-500. Clin Transl Sci 2020;13(1):204–11.

46. Shah NJ, Beckermann K, Vogelzang NJ, et al. A phase 1b/2 study of batiraxcept (AVB-S6-500) in combination with cabozantinib in patients with advanced or metastatic clear cell renal cell (ccRCC) carcinoma who have received front-line treatment (NCT04300140). J Clin Oncol 2022;40(16_suppl):4511.

47. Beckermann K, Shah NJ, Vogelzang NJ, et al. A phase 1b/2 study of batiraxcept (AVB-S6-500) in combination with cabozantinib, cabozantinib and nivolumab, and as monotherapy in patients with advanced or metastatic clear cell renal cell carcinoma (NCT04300140). J Clin Oncol 2022;40(16_suppl):TPS4599.

48. Vegfr2 M, Hsu J, Chong C, et al. Title: Preclinical characterization of XL092, a novel receptor tyrosine kinase inhibitor of MET, Running title: Preclinical characterization of XL092. https://doi.org/10.1158/1535-7163.MCT-22-0262/3226158/mct-22-0262.pdf.

49. Graham DK, DeRyckere D, Davies KD, Earp HS. The TAM family: phosphatidylserine sensing receptor tyrosine kinases gone awry in cancer. Nat Rev Cancer 2014;14(12):769–85.

50. Gherardi E, Birchmeier W, Birchmeier C, Vande Woude G. Targeting MET in cancer: rationale and progress. Nat Rev Cancer 2012;12(2):89–103.

51. Amini A, Masoumi Moghaddam S, Morris DL, et al. The critical role of vascular endothelial growth factor in tumor angiogenesis. Curr Cancer Drug Targets 2012;12(1):23–43.

52. Sharma M, Subbiah V, Shapiro G, et al. A phase 1 first-in-human study of XL092 administered alone or in combination with immune checkpoint inhibitors (ICIs) in patients (pts) with inoperable locally advanced or metastatic solid tumors: description of genitourinary (GU) expansion cohorts. J Clin Oncol 2022; 40(6_suppl):TPS401.

53. Xu WS, Parmigiani RB, Marks PA. Histone deacetylase inhibitors: molecular mechanisms of action. Oncogene 2007;26(37):5541–52.

54. Ellis L, Hammers H, Pili R. Targeting tumor angiogenesis with histone deacetylase inhibitors. Cancer Lett 2009;280(2):145–53.

55. Pili R, Liu G, Chintala S, et al. Combination of the histone deacetylase inhibitor vorinostat with bevacizumab in patients with clear-cell renal cell carcinoma: a multicentre, single-arm phase I/II clinical trial. Br J Cancer 2017;116(7):874–83.

56. Aggarwal R, Thomas S, Pawlowska N, et al. Inhibiting histone deacetylase as a means to reverse resistance to angiogenesis inhibitors: phase i study of

abexinostat plus pazopanib in advanced solid tumor malignancies. J Clin Oncol 2017;35(11):1231–8.

57. Aggarwal RR, Thomas S, Hauke RJ, et al. RENAVIV: a randomized phase III, double-blind, placebo-controlled study of pazopanib with or without abexinostat in patients with locally advanced or metastatic renal cell carcinoma. J Clin Oncol 2019;37(7_suppl):TPS681.

58. Diamantis N, Banerji U. Antibody-drug conjugates–an emerging class of cancer treatment. Br J Cancer 2016;114(4):362–7.

59. Suzuki H, Nagase S, Saito C, et al. 10P DS-6000a, a novel CDH6-targeting anti-body-drug conjugate with a novel DNA topoisomerase I inhibitor DXd, demonstrates potent antitumor activity in preclinical models. Ann Oncol 2021;32: S363–4.

60. Hamilton EP, Jauhari S, Moore KN, et al. Phase I, two-part, multicenter, first-in-human (FIH) study of DS-6000a in subjects with advanced renal cell carcinoma (RCC) and ovarian tumors (OVC). J Clin Oncol 2022;40(16_suppl):3002.

61. Hayashi T, Hinata N. Current status and future prospects of antibody–drug conjugates in urological malignancies. Int J Urol 2022;29(10):1100–8.

62. Thompson JA, Motzer RJ, Molina AM, et al. Phase I trials of Anti-ENPP3 antibody-drug conjugates in advanced refractory renal cell carcinomas. Clin Cancer Res 2018;24(18):4399–406.

63. Kollmannsberger C, Choueiri TK, Heng DYC, et al. A randomized phase II study of AGS-16C3F versus axitinib in previously treated patients with metastatic renal cell carcinoma. Oncol 2021;26(3). 182-e361.

Novel Immune Therapies for Renal Cell Carcinoma

Looking Beyond the Programmed Cell Death Protein 1 and Cytotoxic T-Lymphocyte-Associated Protein 4 Axes

Eddy Saad, MD, MSc[a,1], Renée Maria Saliby, MD, MSc[a,1],
Chris Labaki, MD[a,b], Wenxin Xu, MD[a],
Srinivas R. Viswanathan, MD, PhD[a,c], David A. Braun, MD, PhD[d,2,*],
Ziad Bakouny, MD, MSc[a,c,e,2,*]

KEYWORDS

- Immune checkpoints • Myeloid cell targets • Immuno-metabolic pathways
- Cytokines • Adoptive cell therapies • Cancer vaccines • Renal cell carcinoma

KEY POINTS

- Immune checkpoint inhibitors improved outcomes in patients with renal cell carcinoma; however, primary and acquired resistance limit their efficacy.
- Novel immunotherapies include novel immune checkpoints, myeloid cell targets, immuno-metabolic pathways, cytokines, adoptive T cell therapy, and cancer vaccines.
- Despite multiple challenges, efforts are underway to leverage the antitumoral immune response against renal cell carcinoma.

INTRODUCTION

In metastatic renal cell carcinoma (RCC), some patients have deep and/or durable responses to immune checkpoint inhibitors (ICIs), while others seem to derive little

[a] Department of Medical Oncology, Dana-Farber Cancer Institute, 450 Brookline Avenue, Boston, MA 02115, USA; [b] Department of Medicine, Beth Israel Deaconess Medical Center, 330 Brookline Avenue, Boston, MA 02115, USA; [c] Harvard Medical School, 25 Shattuck Street, Boston, MA 02115, USA; [d] Center of Molecular and Cellular Oncology, Yale Cancer Center, Yale School of Medicine, 300 George Street, Suite 6400, New Haven, CT 06510, USA; [e] Department of Medicine, Brigham and Women's Hospital, 75 Francis Street, Boston, MA 02115, USA
[1] Co-first authors.
[2] Co-senior authors.
* Corresponding authors. Department of Medicine, Brigham and Women's Hospital, 75 Francis Street, Boston, MA 02115.
E-mail addresses: David.braun@yale.edu (D.A.B.); ziad_elbakouny@dfci.harvard.edu (Z.B.)

Hematol Oncol Clin N Am 37 (2023) 1027–1040
https://doi.org/10.1016/j.hoc.2023.05.023
0889-8588/23/© 2023 Elsevier Inc. All rights reserved.

clinical benefit or eventually develop resistance.[1] This underscores the need to identify novel immune targets that can help overcome resistance and improve outcomes for patients with RCC. The tumor microenvironment (TME) is implicated in the response to immunotherapy in RCC. Through complex interactions involving immune checkpoint expression, tumor-associated macrophages (TAMs) and cytokines, the TME fosters an immunosuppressive milieu that promotes tumor progression.[2] Furthermore, advanced RCC is associated with an immune dysfunction circuit characterized by terminally exhausted T cells and immunosuppressive M2-like macrophages.[3] These observations constitute the basis for novel immune targets in RCC. On one hand, there is a need to switch off the inhibitory signals that maintain immunosuppression. On the other hand, strategies to prime the immune system and restore antitumoral activity can also be implemented. In this review, we explore the latest research on various immune targets for RCC, focusing on lymphoid and myeloid immune checkpoints, cytokine therapy, immuno-metabolic pathway modulation, vaccines, and adoptive T-cell therapy (**Fig. 1**).

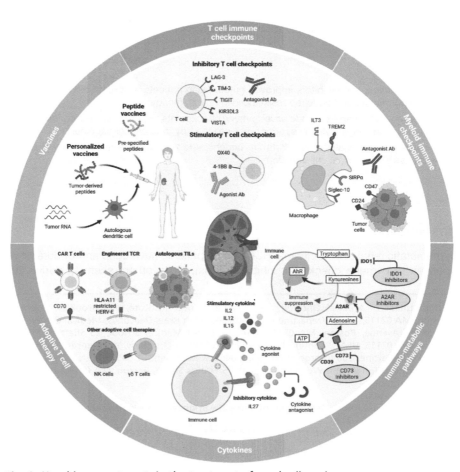

Fig. 1. Novel immune targets in the treatment of renal cell carcinoma.

IMMUNE CHECKPOINTS

Anti-tumoral T-cell activity is finely regulated by numerous inhibitory and stimulatory immune checkpoints.[4] Apart from programmed cell death protein 1/ligand 1 (PD-1/L1) and cytotoxic T-lymphocyte-associated protein 4 (CTLA-4) recent studies have uncovered several other immune checkpoints that hold promise in RCC. Several trials testing these molecules in the clinical setting have already been published, and many other trials are still ongoing (**Table 1**).

Inhibitory T-Cell Checkpoints

Lymphocyte-activation gene 3 (LAG-3) is a member of the immunoglobulin superfamily that is expressed on the surface of tumor infiltrating T cells upon stimulation.[5] It serves a double role as a negative regulator of T-cell function and an enhancer of antigen presentation by dendritic cells (DCs).[6,7] In RCC, co-expression of LAG-3 and PD-L1 is associated with a poor prognosis.[8] Dual blockade of PD-1 and LAG-3 stimulates interferon gamma (IFNγ) release *in vitro*.[9] Several LAG-3 inhibitors have been developed and tested on multiple types of tumors in the clinical setting.[10–12] Phase I/II trials assessing dual LAG-3 and PD-1 inhibition in a pan-cancer setting showed responses in patients with RCC, with some potential single agent activity also noted, and phase III data in treatment-naïve metastatic melanoma showed improved progression-free survival (PFS) with addition of relatlimab (LAG-3 inhibitor) to nivolumab (PD-1 inhibitor) versus nivolumab alone.[11,13,14] As such LAG-3 is a promising novel immune checkpoint target in RCC with multiple trials in development.

T-cell immunoglobulin and mucin-domain containing-3 (TIM-3) is a marker of exhaustion in CD8$^+$ tumor infiltrating lymphocytes (TILs) and is highly expressed by intratumoral regulatory T cells (Treg).[15] TIM-3 expression is negatively associated with survival in many solid tumors, including RCC.[16] Despite encouraging early data, in a phase I/II trial, no objective responses were observed in 87 patients treated with the TIM-3 inhibitor sabatolimab as a single agent, including 2 patients with RCC.[17]

T-cell immunoreceptor with immunoglobulin and ITIM domains (TIGIT) is a co-inhibitory receptor that is expressed by exhausted CD8$^+$ T cells in RCC, similar to LAG-3 and TIM-3.[18] In the preclinical setting, combined inhibition of TIGIT and PD-L1 led to tumor rejection.[19] While the combination of tiragolumab (anti-TIGIT antibody) and atezolizumab showed promising efficacy in the treatment of non-small cell lung cancer (NSCLC) along with a tolerable safety profile, when compared with atezolizumab alone,[20] phase III trials with the same combination did not meet the co-primary endpoint of PFS in both SCLC and NSCLC.[21,22] However, this combination continues to be assessed in a phase II trial in patients with solid tumors, including RCC.

V-domain Ig suppressor of T-cell activation (VISTA) is a member of the B7 family that acts to inhibit T-cell activation.[23] An oral inhibitor of PD-L1/2 and VISTA has been tested in a phase I clinical trial and showed an acceptable safety profile and antitumor activity; the trial included 3 patients with RCC, though none had tumor shrinkage on this therapy.[24]

Overall, despite a strong rationale and supporting preclinical findings, targeting novel negative immune checkpoints in RCC has yet to demonstrate convincing efficacy in early phase trials. Nevertheless, more trials in this space are ongoing, with LAG-3 being of greatest interest at this time.

Stimulatory T-Cell Checkpoints

OX40 (CD134) is a co-stimulatory molecule expressed on activated T cells that binds to its ligand OX40L to enhance effector T cell and NK antitumor activity.[25] Despite

Table 1
Ongoing trials testing the safety and efficacy of novel immune therapies for renal cell carcinoma

Trial ID (Trial Name)	Experimental Arm	Target	Phase
Inhibitory T-cell immune checkpoints			
NCT03744468	BGB-A425 + Tislelizumab (LBL-007)	TIM-3 + PD-1	I/II
NCT03628677	Domvanalimab (AB154) ± Zimberelimab (AB122)	TIGIT ± PD-1	I
NCT02913313	BMS-986207 ± Nivolumab	TIGIT ± PD-1	I/II
NCT03260322	ASP8374 ± Pembrolizumab	TIGIT ± PD-1	I
NCT02794571	Tiragolumab ± Atezolizumab	TIGIT ± PD-L1	I
NCT03977467	Tiragolumab + Atezolizumab	TIGIT + PD-L1	II
NCT04570839	COM701 + BMS-986207 + Nivolumab	PVRIG + TIGIT + PD-1	I/II
NCT04457778	M6223	TIGIT	I
NCT01714739	Lirilumab + Nivolumab ± Ipilimumab	KIR2DL + PD-1 ± CTLA-4	I/II
NCT04475523	CI-8993	VISTA	I
NCT04773951	JS004 + Toripalimab	B- and T-lymphocyte attenuator (BTLA) + PD-1	I
Stimulatory T-cell immune checkpoints			
NCT03071757	ABBV-368 ± ABBV-181	OX40 ± PD-1	I
NCT03893955	ABBV-927 + ABBV-368 ± ABBV-181	CD40 + OX40 ± PD-1	I
NCT04198766	INBRX-106 ± Pembrolizumab	OX40 ± PD-1	I
NCT02705482	MEDI0562 + Durvalumab	OX40 ± PD-1	I
	MEDI0562 + Tremelimumab	OX40 ± CTLA-4	
NCT02528357	GSK3174998 ± Pembrolizumab	OX40 ± PD-1	I
NCT03809624	INBRX-105	4-1BB+ PD-L1	I
NCT02253992	Urelumab + Nivolumab	4-1BB+ PD-1	I/II
Myeloid immune checkpoints			
NCT04691375	PY314 ± Pembrolizumab	TREM2 ± PD-1	I
NCT05440045	6MW3211	CD47 + PD-L1	II

NCT Number	Regimen	Target	Phase
NCT05048160	6MW3211	CD47 + PD-L1	I/II
NCT04913337	NGM707 ± Pembrolizumab	ILT2/ILT4 ± PD-1	I/II
Cytokines			
NCT03729245 (PIVOT-09)	NKTR-214 + Nivolumab	IL2 cytokine + PD-1	III
NCT04540705 (PIVOT IO 011)	NKTR-214 + Nivolumab + TKI	IL2 cytokine + PD-1 + VEGF TKI	I
NCT03501381	High dose IL2 + Entinostat	HDAC, IL2	II
NCT04235777	Bintrafusp alfa + NHS-IL12 ± SBRT	TGFβ/PD-L1 + IL12 cytokine	I
NCT02499328 (SCORES)	Durvalumab + AZD9150 / Durvalumab + AZD5069	PD-L1 + STAT3 / PD-L1 + CXCR2	I/II
Immuno-metabolic pathways			
NCT03192943	Linrodostat + Nivolumab	IDO1 + PD-1	I
NCT05501054	Ciforadenant + Nivolumab + Ipilimumab	A2AR + PD-1 + CTLA-4	I/II
NCT03454451	CPI-006 ± Ciforadenant ± Pembrolizumab	CD73 ± A2AR ± PD-1	I
NCT02754141	BMS-986179 ± Nivolumab	CD73 ± PD-1	I/II
Adoptive T cell therapy			
NCT02830724	Anti-CD70 CAR T cell	Anti-CD70 CAR T	I/II
NCT04696731 (TRAVERSE)	ALLO-316 + ALLO-647	Anti-CD70 CAR T + anti-CD52 mAb	I
NCT04969354	Anti-CAIX CAR T cell	Anti-CAIX CAR T	I
NCT03354390	HERV-E TCR Transduced Autologous T Cells	HERV-E TCR	I
Vaccines			
NCT02950766	NEOVAX + local Ipilimumab	Neoantigen peptides vaccine + CTLA-4	I
NCT03289962	RO7198457 ± Atezolizumab	Neoantigen RNA ± PDL-1	I
NCT03294083	PEXA-VEC + Cemiplimab	Oncolytic vaccine virus + PD-1	I/II
NCT04203901	CMN-001 + Ipilimumab + Nivolumab or Everolimus + Lenvatinib	Dendritic cell vaccine (amplified tumor RNA + CD40L RNA) + CTLA-4 + PD-1 or mTOR + TK	II
NCT05127824	Autologous alpha-DC1/TBVA vaccine + Cabozantinib	Autologous DC vaccine + VEGFR, c-Met, AXL	II

preclinical data, results from clinical trials assessing the effect of drugs targeting this pathway in solid tumors failed to show clear antitumor efficacy.[26] Nevertheless, in a phase I trial testing MOXR0916 (OX40 agonist) in 174 patients with advanced solid tumors, the only 2 partial responses (PR) recorded (1 confirmed by investigator) were seen in patients with RCC.[27] Furthermore, INBRX-106, a novel hexavalent OX40 agonist, seems to outperform bivalent antibodies in antitumor models and is currently being evaluated as a single agent or with pembrolizumab in patients with solid tumors, including RCC.[28]

4-1BB is an inducible T-cell co-stimulatory molecule that binds 4-1BBL on the surface of antigen presenting cells. Utomilumab, a 4-1BB agonist, combined with pembrolizumab demonstrated safety and efficacy in the treatment of advanced solid tumors, including 5 patients with RCC included in the study, one of whom achieved a complete response (CR) while another had PR as best response.[29] Moreover, a combination of anti-4-1BB antibodies and an immunostimulatory factor isolated from *Aggregatibacter actinomycetemcomitans* showed an enhanced antitumor effect in murine RCC models compared to either agent alone.[30]

Targeting other immune checkpoints such as CD40, CD27, and STING has proven to be beneficial in the preclinical setting, and ongoing trials are testing agents that target these pathways in RCC (see **Table 1**).[31–33]

MYELOID RECEPTORS

Myeloid cells in the TME play a complex role in maintaining immunosuppression.[34] TAMs in particular have been involved in ICI resistance.[35] Although targeting myeloid regulatory cells seems like a promising approach, few agents have demonstrated significant clinical activity and safety.[34]

CD47 is a marker that is overexpressed on malignant cells and inhibits phagocytosis by interacting with SIRPα on the surface of macrophages and DCs, acting like a myeloid immune checkpoint.[36] CD47 blockade showed promising results when combined with other agents *in vitro* and *in vivo*.[36] A clinical trial is set to evaluate the efficacy of 6MW3211, a bispecific antibody against CD47 and PD-L1, in patients with RCC. Another innate immune checkpoint involves interaction between tumorally expressed CD24 and sialic acid-binding Ig-like lectin 10 (Siglec-10), an inhibitory receptor on TAMs. Targeting this pathway increases tumor phagocytosis in preclinical models and offers another potential target.[37]

Therapies targeting other myeloid immune checkpoints have also shown favorable preclinical results and are being tested in RCC (see **Table 1**). NGM707, an antibody with dual Ig-like transcript 2/4 (ILT2/ILT4) specificity, has been shown to reprogram myeloid regulatory cells and enhance NK and T-cell cytotoxic activity.[38] MK-0482 is an anti-ILT3 antibody that has shown a good safety profile and modest antitumor activity in a phase I trial of heavily pretreated advanced solid tumors.[39] Anti-TREM2 antibodies, such as PY314, enhance anti-PD-1 response in ICI-resistant tumor models.[40] Finally, inhibition of colony-stimulating factor 1 can repolarize the TME and might improve response to PD-(L)1 blockade.[41,42]

CYTOKINE THERAPY

Interleukin 2 (IL-2) has historically been used in the treatment of metastatic RCC. While it was able to induce sustained CRs in a small subset of patients, it was also associated with significant high-grade toxicities.[43]

In a phase II trial of patients with metastatic clear cell RCC, the combination of high-dose IL-2 and pembrolizumab led to an objective response rates (ORR) of 70% (19 of

27 patients) and sustained treatment-free intervals.[44] Similarly, bempegaldesleukin (NTKR-214), a pegylated IL-2 construct, was tested in combination with PD-1 inhibition but development was discontinued after phase III trials in patients with metastatic melanoma (NCT03635983) and RCC (NCT03729245) showed no significant clinical benefit over ICI monotherapy. Other engineered IL-2 analogs are currently in development, with multiple strategies to uncouple clinical efficacy and toxicity.[45,46]

There are several published and ongoing trials (see **Table 1**) investigating the role of other cytokine therapies in the treatment of cancer, and specifically RCC. Recent developments include modified immunostimulatory cytokines such as NHS-IL12 (IL-12 fused to NHS76 antibody against DNA/histone complexes that are present in necrotic tumor),[47] IL-15 superagonist,[48] and decoy resistant IL-18,[49] as well as inhibitors of immunosuppressive cytokines such as CXCR4[50] and IL-27.[51] In addition, some combinations of cytokine therapy and ICI seem to offer a synergistic antitumoral effect with a tolerable side effect profile.[51]

ROLE OF THE MICROBIOME

The gut microbiome has been shown to influence ICI response in patients with cancer. In a recent phase I trial, an oral live bacterial product (CBM588) was demonstrated to increase PFS and overall survival (OS) in a small sample (n = 30) of patients on combination nivolumab and ipilimumab (PFS: 12.7 vs 2.5 months, hazard ratio 0.15 [95% CI 0.05–0.47] p = 0.001).[52] The effects of other microbiome modifications on treatment efficacy and toxicity are being evaluated in multiple clinical trials in the setting of RCC (NCT04758507, NCT05122546).

IMMUNO-METABOLIC PATHWAYS

Despite preclinical rationale for inhibition of tryptophan metabolism through Indoleamine 2,3-dioxygenase 1, clinical results have been disappointing.[53] Adenosine is generated via the degradation of extracellular ATP by CD39 and CD73 and acts as an immunosuppressive signal via its interaction with the adenosine 2A receptor on the surface of immune cells in the TME.[54] Ciforadenant (CPI-444) acts an adenosine competitive antagonist and has shown modest antitumor activity in a phase I trial combined with atezolizumab in patients with refractory RCC (ORR 11%, 4/35) for the combination versus 3% (1 of 33) for ciforadenant alone, with other trials in development.[55] BMS-986179, an anti-CD73 antibody, was evaluated in combination with nivolumab in a phase I/IIa trial in patients with advanced solid tumors and had a good safety profile with confirmed PRs in 7 of 59 patients with solid tumors, including in patients with RCC.[56]

ADOPTIVE T-CELL THERAPY

Allogeneic T cells genetically engineered to express a chimeric antigen receptor (CAR) have yielded remarkable responses in hematological malignancies.[57,58] However, these therapies have yet to reach the clinic for solid tumors, though they continue to be developed.[59] In the setting of RCC, CAR T cells directed against carbonic anhydrase IX (CAIX) combined with sunitinib had a synergistic antitumoral effect in animal models.[60] However, CAIX-CAR T-cell monotherapy resulted in high grade hepatic adverse events and no clinical responses across 12 patients in a phase I study.[61] In the COBALT-RCC trial, CAR T-cell therapy against CD70 (CTX130) showed 1 CR in 13 patients with advanced RCC.[62] ALLO-316 is another CD70-targeting CAR T-cell therapy that demonstrated an ORR of 17% and a disease control rate of 89% in 19 patients with RCC in the TRAVERSE trial.[63] Next generation CD70-targeting CAR

T cells (CTX131) with edits to regnase-1 and TGFβR2 have shown increased potency in preclinical models.[62] Furthermore, dual targeting CAR T-cell therapy against both CAIX and CD70 are being developed and seem to outperform monovalent CAR T cells in a mouse model of RCC.[64]

It has been shown that allogeneic hematopoietic stem cell transplantation can induce a sustained graft-versus-tumor response in some patients with metastatic RCC.[65] In these patients, T cells targeting an HLA-A11-restricted human endogenous retrovirus E (HERV-E)-derived peptide have been identified.[66] HERVs are DNA sequences that have been integrated into the human genome over the course of evolution.[67,68] Although transcriptionally silent in normal cells, HERVs can be expressed in cancer cells, giving rise to ERV peptides that act as neoantigens.[69] This has prompted a phase I clinical trial to investigate whether autologous T cells transduced with a HERV-E specific TCR could be effective in treating HLA-A11+ patients with metastatic RCC.

Another approach to harness T cells in RCC is autologous TIL therapy. The injection of autologous *ex vivo* expanded TILs has been performed in patients with metastatic melanoma, yielding durable clinical responses.[74] However, expanding TILs derived from RCC have proven to be challenging.[71] Even with the use of rapid expansion protocols, autologous expanded RCC-derived TILs displayed a less developed immune response than melanoma-derived TILs.[72] In addition to traditional αβ T cells, other effector immune cells are being harvested in the setting of adoptive therapy. For instance, efforts are underway to create genetically engineered NK cells with improved antitumor efficacy. Examples include the over-expression of CXCR2, which increases homing to the tumor site,[73] or the addition of a CAR-targeting CAIX (in combination with bortezomib)[74] or EGFR (in combination with cabozantinib).[75] Furthermore, γδ T cells are also emerging as major actors in the immune response to ICI, especially in HLA-I-negative tumors, and offer an encouraging mechanism to help overcome ICI resistance.[70]

VACCINES

Multiple vaccine approaches to boost the antitumoral immune response are under development. This includes peptide vaccines, personalized vaccines, and autologous DCs. IMA901 was the first peptide vaccine developed against antigens in RCC. Despite promising phase I and II trials,[76] a phase III trial comparing the combination of IMA901 and sunitinib to sunitinib alone failed to show clinical benefit in patients with RCC.[77] Other peptide vaccines are still being investigated (see **Table 1**).

Unlike IMA901, which primes the immune system to target pre-specified antigens, personalized vaccines tailor the immune response against tumor-associated and tumor-specific antigens. One approach consists in electroporating tumor RNA and CD40L into autologous DC, inducing them to express tumor-associated antigens. This autologous DC vaccine, known as CMN-001, showed promising phase I/II data, but did not show an added benefit with sunitinib in a phase III trial.[78] A retrospective analysis suggesting that the combination of CMN-001 and everolimus might have a synergistic effect[79] has prompted the development of a phase II clinical trial testing CMN-001 in combination with either nivolumab and ipilimumab, or everolimus and lenvatinib in patients with RCC. Another approach involves targeting neoantigens derived from tumor-specific mutations. HLA-binding peptides that are predicted through tumor RNA and DNA sequencing are synthesized and administered to patients to generate a tumor-specific immune response. Neovax is a personalized neoantigen vaccine that was shown to induce a persistent T-cell response in melanoma.[80] It is being tested in combination with ipilimumab in a phase I clinical trial in patients with RCC.

SUMMARY

The emergence of novel immunotherapies in RCC holds promise for the development of more effective treatments. As reviewed herein, one approach seeks to relieve the inhibition of effector cells by targeting immune checkpoints, myeloid cells, or immuno-metabolic pathways. Another approach seeks to prime the immune response using cytokines, adoptive T-cell therapy, or vaccines. Leveraging the immune system offers encouraging prospects and aims to overcome treatment resistance and improve outcomes for patients with RCC.

CLINICS CARE POINTS

- There is insufficient evidence so far for novel immunotherapies, besides PD-(L)1 and CTLA-4 inhibitors, in the treatment of metastatic renal cell carcinoma.
- Different strategies are being developped to harness the immune system and might lead to therapeutic implications in the future.

ACKNOWLEDGMENTS

W. Xu acknowledges support from the Dept of Defense Early Career Investigator grant (KCRP AKCI-ECI, W81XWH-22-1-0951). S.R. Viswanathan acknowledges support from the Doris Duke Charitable Foundation, United States (Clinician-Scientist Development Award grant number 2020101), Department of Defense Kidney Cancer Research Program (W81XWH-22-1-1016), Rally Foundation for Childhood Cancer Research, United States, Kidney Cancer Association, United States, and the V Foundation, United States. D.A. Braun acknowledges support from the Dept of Defense Early Career Investigator grant (KCRP AKCI-ECI, W81XWH-20-1-0882), the Louis Goodman and Alfred Gilman Yale Scholar Fund, and the Yale Cancer Center, United States (supported by NIH, United States/NCI, United States research grant P30CA016359).

DISCLOSURES

Conflicts of Interest: E. Saad, R.M. Saliby, C. Labaki: none. W. Xu reports advisory board fees from Exelixis and Jazz Pharmaceuticals, and continuing medical education honoraria from MedNet, Harborside Press, MJH Healthcare Holdings, and Academy for Continued Healthcare Learning. S.R. Viswanathan reports consulting for Jnana Therapeutics, MPM Capital, and Vida Ventures within the last 3 years and research support from Bayer, Germany. Spouse is an employee of and holds equity in Kojin Therapeutics. D.A. Braun reports honoraria from LM Education/Exchange Services, advisory board fees from Exelixis and AVEO, personal fees from Schlesinger Associates, Cancer Expert Now, Adnovate Strategies, MDedge, CancerNetwork, Catenion, OncLive, Cello Health BioConsulting, PWW Consulting, Haymarket Medical Network, Aptitude Health, ASCO Post/Harborside, Targeted Oncology, AbbVie, and research support from Exelixis and AstraZeneca, outside of the submitted work. Z. Bakouny reports research support from Genentech, United States/imCORE and Bristol Myers Squibb, United States, and honoraria from UpToDate.

REFERENCES

1. Rappold PM, Silagy AW, Kotecha RR, Hakimi AA. Immune checkpoint blockade in renal cell carcinoma. J Surg Oncol 2021;123(3):739–50.

2. Díaz-Montero CM, Rini BI, Finke JH. The immunology of renal cell carcinoma. Nat Rev Nephrol 2020;16(12):721–35.

3. Braun DA, Street K, Burke KP, et al. Progressive immune dysfunction with advancing disease stage in renal cell carcinoma. Cancer Cell 2021;39(5): 632–48.e8.

4. Braun DA, Bakouny Z, Hirsch L, et al. Beyond conventional immune-checkpoint inhibition — novel immunotherapies for renal cell carcinoma. Nat Rev Clin Oncol 2021;18(4):199–214.

5. Maruhashi T, Sugiura D, Okazaki IM, Okazaki T. LAG-3: from molecular functions to clinical applications. J Immunother Cancer 2020;8(2):e001014.

6. Andreae S, Buisson S, Triebel F. MHC class II signal transduction in human dendritic cells induced by a natural ligand, the LAG-3 protein (CD223). Blood 2003; 102(6):2130–7.

7. Triebel F. LAG-3: A regulator of T-cell and DC responses and its use in therapeutic vaccination. Trends Immunol 2003;24(12):619–22.

8. Lee CH, Jung SJ, Seo WI, et al. Coexpression of lymphocyte-activation gene 3 and programmed death ligand-1 in tumor infiltrating immune cells predicts worse outcome in renal cell carcinoma. Int J Immunopathol Pharmacol 2022;36. https://doi.org/10.1177/03946320221125588.

9. Zelba H, Bedke J, Hennenlotter J, et al. PD-1 and LAG-3 dominate checkpoint receptor-mediated T-cell inhibition in renal cell carcinoma. Cancer Immunol Res 2019;7(11):1891–9.

10. Brignone C, Escudier B, Grygar C, Marcu M, Triebel F. A phase I pharmacokinetic and biological correlative study of IMP321, a novel MHC class II agonist, in patients with advanced renal cell carcinoma. Clin Cancer Res 2009;15(19):6225–31.

11. Schöffski P, Tan DSW, Martín M, et al. Phase I/II study of the LAG-3 inhibitor ieramilimab (LAG525) ± anti-PD-1 spartalizumab (PDR001) in patients with advanced malignancies. J Immunother Cancer 2022;10(2):e003776.

12. Dr. Zhang on the Combination of LAG525 and Spartalizumab in Advanced Malignancies. Available at: https://www.onclive.com/view/dr-zhang-on-the-combination-of-lag525-and-spartalizumab-in-advanced-malignancies. Accessed April 22, 2023.

13. Luke JJ, Patel MR, Hamilton EP, et al. A phase I, first-in-human, open-label, dose-escalation study of MGD013, a bispecific DART molecule binding PD-1 and LAG-3, in patients with unresectable or metastatic neoplasms. J Clin Oncol 2020; 38(15_suppl):3004.

14. Tawbi HA, Schadendorf D, Lipson EJ, et al. Relatlimab and nivolumab versus nivolumab in untreated advanced melanoma. N Engl J Med 2022;386(1):24–34.

15. Wolf Y, Anderson AC, Kuchroo VK. TIM3 comes of age as an inhibitory receptor. Nat Rev Immunol 2020;20(3):173–85.

16. Zhang Y, Cai P, Liang T, Wang L, Hu L. TIM-3 is a potential prognostic marker for patients with solid tumors: A systematic review and meta-analysis. Oncotarget 2017;8(19):31705–13.

17. Curigliano G, Gelderblom H, Mach N, et al. Phase I/Ib clinical trial of sabatolimab, an anti–TIM-3 antibody, alone and in combination with spartalizumab, an anti–PD-1 antibody, in advanced solid tumors. Clin Cancer Res 2021;27(13):3620–9.

18. Takamatsu K, Tanaka N, Hakozaki K, et al. Profiling the inhibitory receptors LAG-3, TIM-3, and TIGIT in renal cell carcinoma reveals malignancy. Nat Commun 2021;12(1). https://doi.org/10.1038/s41467-021-25865-0.

19. Johnston RJ, Comps-Agrar L, Hackney J, et al. The Immunoreceptor TIGIT Regulates Antitumor and Antiviral CD8+ T Cell Effector Function. Cancer Cell 2014; 26(6):923–37.
20. Cho BC, Abreu DR, Hussein M, et al. Tiragolumab plus atezolizumab versus placebo plus atezolizumab as a first-line treatment for PD-L1-selected non-small-cell lung cancer (CITYSCAPE): primary and follow-up analyses of a randomised, double-blind, phase 2 study. Lancet Oncol 2022;23(6):781–92.
21. Genentech: Press Releases | Tuesday, May 10, 2022. Available at: https://www.gene.com/media/press-releases/14951/2022-05-10/genentech-reports-interim-results-for-ph. Accessed April 22, 2023.
22. Rudin CM, Liu SV, Lu S, et al. SKYSCRAPER-02: primary results of a phase III, randomized, double-blind, placebo-controlled study of atezolizumab (atezo) + carboplatin + etoposide (CE) with or without tiragolumab (tira) in patients (pts) with untreated extensive-stage small cell lung cancer (ES-SCLC). J Clin Oncol 2022;40(17_suppl):LBA8507.
23. Hong S, Yuan Q, Xia H, et al. Analysis of VISTA expression and function in renal cell carcinoma highlights VISTA as a potential target for immunotherapy. Protein Cell 2019;10(11):840.
24. Bang YJ, Powderly J, Patel M, et al. Phase 1 trial of CA-170, a first-in-class, orally available, small molecule immune checkpoint inhibitor (ICI) dually targeting PD-L1 and VISTA, in patients with advanced solid tumors or lymphomas. SITC 2018.
25. Croft M. Control of Immunity by the TNFR-related molecule OX40 (CD134). Annu Rev Immunol 2010;28:57–78.
26. Sadeghi S, Parikh RA, Tsao-Wei DD, et al. Phase II randomized double blind trial of axitinib (Axi) +/- PF-04518600, an OX40 antibody (PFOX) after PD1/PDL1 antibody (IO) therapy (Tx) in metastatic renal cell carcinoma (mRCC). J Clin Oncol 2022;40(16_suppl):4529.
27. Kim TW, Burris HA, de Miguel Luken MJ, et al. First-in-human phase I study of the OX40 agonist MOXR0916 in patients with advanced solid tumors. Clin Cancer Res 2022;28(16):3452–63.
28. Rowell E, Kinkead H, Torretti E, et al. 856 INBRX-106: a novel hexavalent anti-OX40 agonist for the treatment of solid tumors. J Immunother Cancer 2021; 9(Suppl 2):A897.
29. Tolcher AW, Sznol M, Hu-Lieskovan S, et al. Phase Ib Study of Utomilumab (PF-05082566), a 4-1BB/CD137 Agonist, in Combination with Pembrolizumab (MK-3475) in Patients with Advanced Solid Tumors. Clin Cancer Res 2017;23(18): 5349–57.
30. Ju SA, Park SM, Joe Y, Chung HT, An WG, Kim BS. Anti-4-1BB antibody-based combination therapy augments antitumor immunity by enhancing CD11c+CD8+ T cells in renal cell carcinoma. Oncol Lett 2022;23(2):1–11.
31. Zhang Y, Wu X, Sharma A, et al. Anti-CD40 predominates over anti-CTLA-4 to provide enhanced antitumor response of DC-CIK cells in renal cell carcinoma. Front Immunol 2022;13:4890.
32. Wu Z, Lin Y, Liu LM, et al. Identification of Cytosolic DNA Sensor cGAS-STING as Immune-Related Risk Factor in Renal Carcinoma following Pan-Cancer Analysis. Published online 2022;7978042. https://doi.org/10.1155/2022/7978042.
33. Benhamouda N, Sam I, Epaillard N, et al. Plasma CD27, a surrogate of the intra-tumoral CD27-CD70 interaction, correlates with immunotherapy resistance in renal cell carcinoma. Clin Cancer Res 2022;28(22):4983–94.
34. Jahchan NS, Mujal AM, Pollack JL, et al. Tuning the tumor myeloid microenvironment to fight cancer. Front Immunol 2019;10:1611.

35. DeNardo DG, Ruffell B. Macrophages as regulators of tumour immunity and immunotherapy. Nat Rev Immunol 2019;19(6):369–82.

36. Logtenberg MEW, Scheeren FA, Schumacher TN. The CD47-SIRPα immune checkpoint. Immunity 2020;52(5):742–52.

37. Barkal AA, Brewer RE, Markovic M, et al. CD24 signalling through macrophage Siglec-10 is a target for cancer immunotherapy. Nature 2019;572(7769):392–6.

38. Mondal K, Song C, Tian J, et al. Abstract LB156: Preclinical evaluation of NGM707, a novel anti-ILT2/anti-ILT4 dual antagonist monoclonal antibody. Cancer Res 2021;81(13_Supplement):LB156.

39. Gutierrez M, Spreafico A, Wang D, et al. Phase 1 first-in-human study of anti–ILT3 mAb MK-0482 as monotherapy and in combination with pembrolizumab in advanced solid tumors: dose escalation results. J Clin Oncol 2022; 40(16_suppl):2505.

40. Binnewies M, Abushawish M, Lee T, et al. Abstract C104: Therapeutic targeting of TREM2+ tumor-associated macrophages as a means of overcoming checkpoint inhibitor resistance. Mol Cancer Ther 2019;18:C104.

41. Cannarile MA, Weisser M, Jacob W, Jegg AM, Ries CH, Rüttinger D. Colony-stimulating factor 1 receptor (CSF1R) inhibitors in cancer therapy. J Immunother Cancer 2017;5(1):53.

42. Lin CC. Clinical development of colony-stimulating factor 1 receptor (Csf1r) inhibitors. J Immunother Precis Oncol 2021;4(2):105–14.

43. Klapper JA, Downey SG, Smith FO, et al. High-dose interleukin-2 for the treatment of metastatic renal cell carcinoma: A retrospective analysis of response and survival in patients treated in the Surgery Branch at the National Cancer Institute between 1986 and 2006. Cancer 2008;113(2):293–301.

44. Chatzkel J, Schell MJ, Chahoud J, et al. Coordinated Pembrolizumab and High Dose IL-2 (5-in-a-Row Schedule) for Therapy of Metastatic Clear Cell Renal Cancer. Clin Genitourin Cancer 2022;20(3):252–9.

45. Calvo E, Boni V, Chaudhry A, et al. Nemvaleukin alfa in patients with advanced renal cell carcinoma: ARTISTRY-1. J Clin Oncol 2022;40(6_suppl):330.

46. Moynihan K, Pappas D, Sultan H, et al. 1092 The CD8+ T cell selectivity of AB248 is essential for optimal anti-tumor activity and safety in nonclinical models. Journal for ImmunoTherapy of Cancer 2022;10:A1133. BMJ Specialist Journals.

47. Greiner JW, Morillon YM, Schlom J. NHS-IL12, a Tumor-Targeting Immunocytokine. ImmunoTargets Ther 2021;10:155–69.

48. Desbois M, Desbois M, Desbois M, et al. IL-15 superagonist RLI has potent immunostimulatory properties on NK cells: Implications for antimetastatic treatment. J Immunother Cancer 2020;8(1):e000632.

49. Zhou T, Damsky W, Weizman O El, et al. IL-18BP is a secreted immune checkpoint and barrier to IL-18 immunotherapy. Nature 2020;583(7817):609–14.

50. McDermott DF, Vaishampayan U, Matrana M, et al. Safety and efficacy of the oral CXCR4 inhibitor X4P-001 + axitinib in advanced renal cell carcinoma patients: An analysis of subgroup responses by prior treatment. Ann Oncol 2019;30:v482–3.

51. Naing A, Mantia C, Morgensztern D, et al. First-in-human study of SRF388, a first-in-class IL-27 targeting antibody, as monotherapy and in combination with pembrolizumab in patients with advanced solid tumors. J Clin Oncol 2022; 40(16_suppl):2501.

52. Dizman N, Meza L, Bergerot P, et al. Nivolumab plus ipilimumab with or without live bacterial supplementation in metastatic renal cell carcinoma: a randomized phase 1 trial. Nat Med 2022;28(4):704–12.

53. Long GV, Dummer R, Hamid O, et al. Epacadostat plus pembrolizumab versus placebo plus pembrolizumab in patients with unresectable or metastatic melanoma (ECHO-301/KEYNOTE-252): a phase 3, randomised, double-blind study. Lancet Oncol 2019;20(8):1083–97.
54. Allard D, Turcotte M, Stagg J. Targeting A2 adenosine receptors in cancer. Immunol Cell Biol 2017;95(4):333–9.
55. Fong L, Hotson A, Powderly JD, et al. Adenosine A2A receptor blockade as an immunotherapy for treatment-refractory renal cell cancer. Cancer Discov 2020; 10(1):40.
56. Siu LL, Burris H, Le DT, et al. Abstract CT180: Preliminary phase 1 profile of BMS-986179, an anti-CD73 antibody, in combination with nivolumab in patients with advanced solid tumors. Cancer Res 2018;78(13 Supplement):CT180.
57. Schuster SJ, Svoboda J, Chong EA, et al. Chimeric antigen receptor T cells in refractory B-cell lymphomas. N Engl J Med 2017;377(26):2545–54.
58. Porter DL, Levine BL, Kalos M, Bagg A, June CH. Chimeric antigen receptor-modified T cells in chronic lymphoid leukemia. N Engl J Med 2011;365(8):725–33.
59. Louis CU, Savoldo B, Dotti G, et al. Antitumor activity and long-term fate of chimeric antigen receptor-positive T cells in patients with neuroblastoma. Blood 2011;118(23):6050–6.
60. Li H, Ding J, Lu M, et al. CAIX-specific CAR-T Cells and Sunitinib Show Synergistic Effects Against Metastatic Renal Cancer Models. J Immunother 2020;43(1): 16–28.
61. Lamers CHJ, Sleijfer S, Van Steenbergen S, et al. Treatment of metastatic renal cell carcinoma with CAIX CAR-engineered T cells: clinical evaluation and management of on-target toxicity. Mol Ther 2013;21(4):904–12.
62. Pal S, Tran B, Haanen J, et al. 558 CTX130 allogeneic CRISPR-Cas9–engineered chimeric antigen receptor (CAR) T cells in patients with advanced clear cell renal cell carcinoma: Results from the phase 1 COBALT-RCC study. J Immunother Cancer 2022;10(Suppl 2):A584.
63. Researchers report on promising novel antitumor strategies in early-phase clinical trials - AACR Annual Meeting News. Available at: https://www.aacrmeetingnews.org/news/researchers-report-on-promising-novel-antitumor-strategies-in-early-phase-clinical-trials/. Accessed April 22, 2023.
64. Wang Y, Grimaud M, Buck A, et al. Abstract 6606: Develop dual-targeted CAR-T cells to achieve RCC cures. Cancer Res 2020;80(16_Supplement):6606.
65. Childs R, Chernoff A, Contentin N, et al. Regression of metastatic renal-cell carcinoma after nonmyeloablative allogeneic peripheral-blood stem-cell transplantation. N Engl J Med 2000;343(11):750–8.
66. Takahashi Y, Harashima N, Kajigaya S, et al. Regression of human kidney cancer following allogeneic stem cell transplantation is associated with recognition of an HERV-E antigen by T cells. J Clin Invest 2008;118(3):1099.
67. Hurst TP, Emmer A, Douville RN, Grandi N, Tramontano E. Human Endogenous Retroviruses Are Ancient Acquired Elements Still Shaping Innate Immune Responses. Front Immunol 2018;9:2039.
68. Rosenberg SA, Yang JC, Sherry RM, et al. Durable complete responses in heavily pretreated patients with metastatic melanoma using T-cell transfer immunotherapy. Clin Cancer Res 2011;17(13):4550–7. https://doi.org/10.1158/1078-0432.CCR-11-0116.
69. Bonaventura P, Alcazer V, Mutez V, et al. Identification of shared tumor epitopes from endogenous retroviruses inducing high-avidity cytotoxic T cells for cancer immunotherapy. Sci Adv 2022;8(4):3671.

70. de Vries NL, van de Haar J, Veninga V, et al. γδ T cells are effectors of immunotherapy in cancers with HLA class I defects. Nature 2023;1–8. https://doi.org/10.1038/s41586-022-05593-1. Published online January 11, 2023.
71. Figlin RA, Thompson JA, Bukowski RM, et al. Multicenter, randomized, phase III trial of CD8(+) tumor-infiltrating lymphocytes in combination with recombinant interleukin-2 in metastatic renal cell carcinoma. J Clin Oncol 1999;17(8):2521–9.
72. Andersen R, Westergaard MCW, Kjeldsen JW, et al. T-cell responses in the microenvironment of primary renal cell carcinoma-implications for adoptive cell therapy. Cancer Immunol Res 2018;6(2):222–35.
73. Whilding LM, Halim L, Draper B, et al. CAR T-Cells Targeting the Integrin αvβ6 and Co-Expressing the Chemokine Receptor CXCR2 Demonstrate Enhanced Homing and Efficacy against Several Solid Malignancies. Cancers (Basel) 2019;11(5):674.
74. Zhang Q, Xu J, Ding J, et al. Bortezomib improves adoptive carbonic anhydrase IX-specific chimeric antigen receptor-modified NK92 cell therapy in mouse models of human renal cell carcinoma. Oncol Rep 2018;40(6):3714–24.
75. Zhang Q, Tian K, Xu J, et al. Synergistic Effects of Cabozantinib and EGFR-Specific CAR-NK-92 Cells in Renal Cell Carcinoma. J Immunol Res 2017;2017.
76. Kirner A, Mayer-Mokler A, Reinhardt C. IMA901: A multi-peptide cancer vaccine for treatment of renal cell cancer. Hum Vaccin Immunother 2014;10(11):3179.
77. Rini BI, Stenzl A, Zdrojowy R, et al. IMA901, a multipeptide cancer vaccine, plus sunitinib versus sunitinib alone, as first-line therapy for advanced or metastatic renal cell carcinoma (IMPRINT): a multicentre, open-label, randomised, controlled, phase 3 trial. Lancet Oncol 2016;17(11):1599–611.
78. Figlin RA, Tannir NM, Uzzo RG, et al. Results of the ADAPT Phase 3 Study of Rocapuldencel-T in Combination with Sunitinib as First-Line Therapy in Patients with Metastatic Renal Cell Carcinoma. Clin Cancer Res 2020;26(10):2327–35.
79. Master VA, Uzzo RG, Bratlavsky G, Karam JA. Autologous Dendritic Vaccine Therapy in Metastatic Kidney Cancer: The ADAPT Trial and Beyond. Published online 2022. https://doi.org/10.1016/j.euf.2022.04.003.
80. Hu Z, Leet DE, Allesøe RL, et al. Personal neoantigen vaccines induce persistent memory T cell responses and epitope spreading in patients with melanoma. Nat Med 2021;27(3):515.

Statement of Ownership, Management, and Circulation
(All Periodicals Publications Except Requester Publications)

UNITED STATES POSTAL SERVICE®

1. Publication Title	2. Publication Number	3. Filing Date
HEMATOLOGY/ONCOLOGY CLINICS OF NORTH AMERICA	002 – 473	5/18/2023

4. Issue Frequency	5. Number of Issues Published Annually	6. Annual Subscription Price
FEB, APR, JUN, AUG, OCT, DEC	6	$494.00

7. Complete Mailing Address of Known Office of Publication (Not printer) (Street, city, county, state, and ZIP+4®)
ELSEVIER INC.
230 Park Avenue, Suite 800
New York, NY 10169

Contact Person: Malathi Samayan
Telephone (Include area code): 91-44-4299-4507

8. Complete Mailing Address of Headquarters or General Business Office of Publisher (Not printer)
ELSEVIER INC.
230 Park Avenue, Suite 800
New York, NY 10169

9. Full Names and Complete Mailing Addresses of Publisher, Editor, and Managing Editor (Do not leave blank)

Publisher (Name and complete mailing address)
Dolores Meloni, ELSEVIER INC.
1600 JOHN F KENNEDY BLVD. SUITE 1600
PHILADELPHIA, PA 19103-2899

Editor (Name and complete mailing address)
STACY EASTMAN, ELSEVIER INC.
1600 JOHN F KENNEDY BLVD. SUITE 1600
PHILADELPHIA, PA 19103-2899

Managing Editor (Name and complete mailing address)
PATRICK MANLEY, ELSEVIER INC.
1600 JOHN F KENNEDY BLVD. SUITE 1600
PHILADELPHIA, PA 19103-2899

10. Owner (Do not leave blank. If the publication is owned by a corporation, give the name and address of the corporation immediately followed by the names and addresses of all stockholders owning or holding 1 percent or more of the total amount of stock. If not owned by a corporation, give the names and addresses of the individual owners. If owned by a partnership or other unincorporated firm, give its name and address as well as those of each individual owner. If the publication is published by a nonprofit organization, give its name and address.)

Full Name	Complete Mailing Address
WHOLLY OWNED SUBSIDIARY OF REED/ELSEVIER, US HOLDINGS	1600 JOHN F KENNEDY BLVD. SUITE 1600 PHILADELPHIA, PA 19103-2899

11. Known Bondholders, Mortgagees, and Other Security Holders Owning or Holding 1 Percent or More of Total Amount of Bonds, Mortgages, or Other Securities. If none, check box ▸ ☐ None

Full Name	Complete Mailing Address
N/A	

12. Tax Status (For completion by nonprofit organizations authorized to mail at nonprofit rates) (Check one)
The purpose, function, and nonprofit status of this organization and the exempt status for federal income tax purposes:
☒ Has Not Changed During Preceding 12 Months
☐ Has Changed During Preceding 12 Months (Publisher must submit explanation of change with this statement)

PS Form **3526**, July 2014 [Page 1 of 4 (see instructions page 4)] PSN: 7530-01-000-9931 PRIVACY NOTICE: See our privacy policy on www.usps.com.

---

13. Publication Title			14. Issue Date for Circulation Data Below
HEMATOLOGY/ONCOLOGY CLINICS OF NORTH AMERICA			AUGUST 2023

15. Extent and Nature of Circulation			Average No. Copies Each Issue During Preceding 12 Months	No. Copies of Single Issue Published Nearest to Filing Date
a. Total Number of Copies (Net press run)			117	117
b. Paid Circulation (By Mail and Outside the Mail)	(1)	Mailed Outside-County Paid Subscriptions Stated on PS Form 3541 (Include paid distribution above nominal rate, advertiser's proof copies, and exchange copies)	58	31
	(2)	Mailed In-County Paid Subscriptions Stated on PS Form 3541 (Include paid distribution above nominal rate, advertiser's proof copies, and exchange copies)	0	0
	(3)	Paid Distribution Outside the Mails Including Sales Through Dealers and Carriers, Street Vendors, Counter Sales, and Other Paid Distribution Outside USPS®	36	56
	(4)	Paid Distribution by Other Classes of Mail Through the USPS (e.g., First-Class Mail®)	11	18
c. Total Paid Distribution (Sum of 15b (1), (2), (3), and (4))			105	105
d. Free or Nominal Rate Distribution (By Mail and Outside the Mail)	(1)	Free or Nominal Rate Outside-County Copies Included on PS Form 3541	11	11
	(2)	Free or Nominal Rate In-County Copies Included on PS Form 3541	0	0
	(3)	Free or Nominal Rate Copies Mailed at Other Classes Through the USPS (e.g., First-Class Mail)	0	0
	(4)	Free or Nominal Rate Distribution Outside the Mail (Carriers or other means)	1	1
e. Total Free or Nominal Rate Distribution (Sum of 15d (1), (2), (3) and (4))			12	12
f. Total Distribution (Sum of 15c and 15e)			117	117
g. Copies not Distributed (See Instructions to Publishers #4 (page #3))			0	0
h. Total (Sum of 15f and g)			117	117
i. Percent Paid (15c divided by 15f times 100)			89.74%	89.74%

* If you are claiming electronic copies, go to line 16 on page 3. If you are not claiming electronic copies, skip to line 17 on page 3.

16. Electronic Copy Circulation	Average No. Copies Each Issue During Preceding 12 Months	No. Copies of Single Issue Published Nearest to Filing Date
a. Paid Electronic Copies		
b. Total Paid Print Copies (Line 15c) + Paid Electronic Copies (Line 16a)		
c. Total Print Distribution (Line 15f) + Paid Electronic Copies (Line 16a)		
d. Percent Paid (Both Print & Electronic Copies) (16b divided by 16c × 100)		

☒ I certify that 50% of all my distributed copies (electronic and print) are paid above a nominal price.

17. Publication of Statement of Ownership
☒ If the publication is a general publication, publication of this statement is required. Will be printed in the OCTOBER 2023 issue of this publication. ☐ Publication not required.

18. Signature and Title of Editor, Publisher, Business Manager, or Owner

Malathi Samayan — Distribution Controller

Malathi Samayan Date 9/18/2023

I certify that all information furnished on this form is true and complete. I understand that anyone who furnishes false or misleading information on this form or who omits material or information requested on the form may be subject to criminal sanctions (including fines and imprisonment) and/or civil sanctions (including civil penalties).

PS Form **3526**, July 2014 (Page 3 of 4) PRIVACY NOTICE: See our privacy policy on www.usps.com.

Moving?

Make sure your subscription moves with you!

To notify us of your new address, find your **Clinics Account Number** (located on your mailing label above your name), and contact customer service at:

Email: journalscustomerservice-usa@elsevier.com

800-654-2452 (subscribers in the U.S. & Canada)
314-447-8871 (subscribers outside of the U.S. & Canada)

Fax number: 314-447-8029

Elsevier Health Sciences Division
Subscription Customer Service
3251 Riverport Lane
Maryland Heights, MO 63043

*To ensure uninterrupted delivery of your subscription, please notify us at least 4 weeks in advance of move.